PROGRESS IN CLINICAL AND BIOLOGICAL RESEARCH

Series Editors   Vincent P. Eijsvoogel   Seymour S. Kety
Nathan Back   Robert Grover   Sidney Udenfriend
George J. Brewer   Kurt Hirschhorn   Jonathan W. Uhr

Vol 1: Erythrocyte Structure and Function, George J. Brewer, *Editor*

Vol 2: Preventability of Perinatal Injury, Karlis Adamsons and Howard A. Fox, *Editors*

Vol 3: Infections of the Fetus and the Newborn Infant, Saul Krugman and Anne A. Gershon, *Editors*

Vol 4: Conflicts in Childhood Cancer, Lucius F. Sinks and John O. Godden, *Editors*

Vol 5: Trace Components of Plasma: Isolation and Clinical Significance, G.A. Jamieson and T.J. Greenwalt, *Editors*

Vol 6: Prostatic Disease, H. Marberger, H. Haschek, H.K.A. Schirmer, J.A.C. Colston, and E. Witkin, *Editors*

Vol 7: Blood Pressure, Edema and Proteinuria in Pregnancy, Emanuel A. Friedman, *Editor*

Vol 8: Cell Surface Receptors, Garth L. Nicolson, Michael A. Raftery, Martin Rodbell, and C. Fred Fox, *Editors*

Vol 9: Membranes and Neoplasia: New Approaches and Strategies, Vincent T. Marchesi, *Editor*

Vol 10: Diabetes and Other Endocrine Disorders During Pregnancy and in the Newborn, Maria I. New and Robert H. Fiser, *Editors*

Vol 11: Clinical Uses of Frozen-Thawed Red Blood Cells, John A. Griep, *Editor*

Vol 12: Breast Cancer, Albert C.W. Montague, Geary L. Stonesifer, Jr., and Edward F. Lewison, *Editors*

Vol 13: The Granulocyte: Function and Clinical Utilization, Tibor J. Greenwalt and G.A. Jamieson, *Editors*

Vol 14: Zinc Metabolism: Current Aspects in Health and Disease, George J. Brewer and Ananda S. Prasad, *Editors*

Vol 15: Cellular Neurobiology, Zach Hall, Regis Kelly, and C. Fred Fox, *Editors*

Vol 16: HLA and Malignancy, Gerald P. Murphy, *Editor*

Vol 17: Cell Shape and Surface Architecture, Jean Paul Revel, Ulf Henning, and C. Fred Fox, *Editors*

Vol 18: Tay-Sachs Disease: Screening and Prevention, Michael M. Kaback, *Editor*

Vol 19: Blood Substitutes and Plasma Expanders, G.A. Jamieson and T.J. Greenwalt, *Editors*

Vol 20: Erythrocyte Membranes: Recent Clinical and Experimental Advances, Walter C. Kruckeberg, John W. Eaton, and George J. Brewer, *Editors*

Vol 21: The Red Cell, George J. Brewer, *Editor*

Vol 22: Molecular Aspects of Membrane Transport, Dale Oxender and C. Fred Fox, *Editors*

Vol 23: Cell Surface Carbohydrates and Biological Recognition, Vincent T. Marchesi, Victor Ginsburg, Phillips W. Robbins, and C. Fred Fox, *Editors*

MEMBRANES, RECEPTORS, AND THE IMMUNE RESPONSE

80 YEARS AFTER EHRLICH'S SIDE CHAIN THEORY

MEMBRANES, RECEPTORS, AND THE IMMUNE RESPONSE
80 YEARS AFTER EHRLICH'S SIDE CHAIN THEORY

A Symposium Commemorating the 80th Anniversary
of Ehrlich's Side Chain Theory Held at
La Rabida—University of Chicago Institute
Chicago, Illinois, September, 1979

Editors
Edward P. Cohen
Heinz Köhler

ALAN R. LISS, INC. • NEW YORK

Address all inquiries to the publisher:

Alan R. Liss, Inc., 150 Fifth Avenue, New York, NY 10011

Copyright © 1980 Alan R. Liss, Inc.

Printed in the United States of America

Library of Congress Cataloging in Publication Data
Main entry under title:

Membranes, receptors, and the immune response.

(Progress in clinical and biological research; v. 42)
Includes bibliographical references and index.
1. Immune response — Congresses. 2. Cell receptors — Congresses.
3. Cell membranes — Congresses. I. Cohen, Edward P. II. Köhler,
Heinz, 1939— III. Series.
QR186.M44   574.2'9   80-7811
ISBN 0-8451-0042-4

Contents

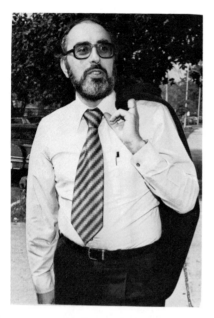

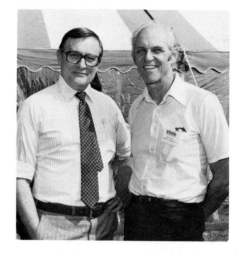

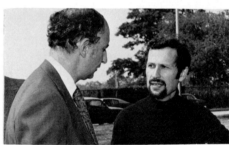

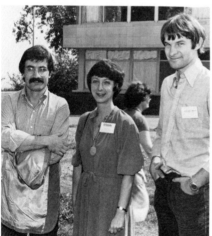

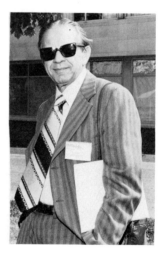

SOME PARTICIPANTS

First Row
J.D. Capra, F.J. Bollum, D.W. Talmage
Second Row
J. Quintans, B.K. Birshtein, M. Cramer,
S.C. Silverstein, H. Köhler
Third Row
A. Sehon

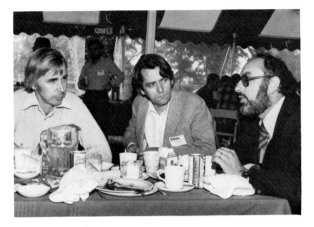
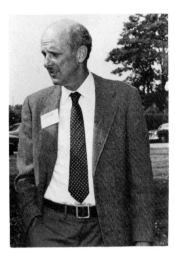
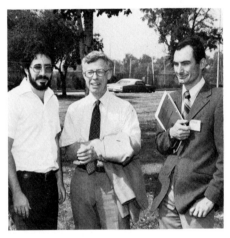
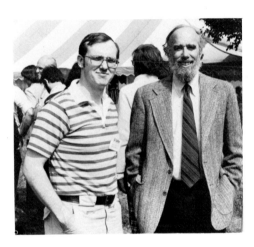
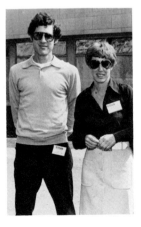

SOME PARTICIPANTS

First Row
H. Wigzell, P.A. Cazenave, J.D. Capra,
E.P. Cohen

Second Row
P.J. Leibson, D.A. Rowley, H. Schreiber,
T. McKearn, M.D. Scharff

Third Row
J.L. Claflin, K.L. Knight

Introduction

In recent years, the scope of immunology has expanded far beyond that which could have been envisioned by pioneers in the field. It is no longer sufficient to limit research in immunology to investigations relating solely to questions regarding the formation of antibodies and the appearance of cytotoxic effector cells. Studies of the most fundamental events occurring at the molecular level in the genome are being included as our understanding of the immune phenomenon broadens. Developmental and ontological aspects of cellular differentiation, membrane structure and the display of antigen receptors, control mechanisms and intercellular recognition along with the means by which foreign substances are recognized by specialized cells are studies relevant and appropriate to the study of immunity. Testimonies to the broadened scope of the phenomenon are the numbers of immunological journals, their enlarged contents and the increased numbers of investigators in the field. The frequency and duration of conferences and symposia devoted to immunology serve to emphasize the ever present need for communications between investigators involved in studies not only within the obvious scope of immunology but within a variety of related disciplines as well.

Fundamental to our thoughts on the immune phenomenon is the mechanism of antigen recognition. Approximately 80 years ago Paul Ehrlich hypothesized that immunity results through the interaction of antigen with specific, complementary, preformed receptors. The underlying concept is that specialized cells possess antigen-specific structures on their membranes before antigen exposure. Humoral immunity results, Ehrlich, theorized, as a consequence of the combination of antigen with such receptors. As Felix Horowitz so clearly pointed out in the 1967 Cold Spring Harbor Symposium, "the term receptor has survived up to the present day and has influenced the thinking of almost everyone in the society of immunologists to at least some extent." It is no less true today.

The organizers of a conference held at the LaRabida-University of Chicago Institute, September 23rd to 26th, 1979, had in mind the commemoration of Ehrlich's ingenious receptor copy theory. One of the main purposes of the meeting was to remind the members of the diverse sections

of immunological research of their common inheritance and
to provide a unifying link for their work. Membrane bio-
chemists, developmental biologists and molecular endocrino-
logists base the foundations of their research on concep-
tions analogous to Ehrlich's theory as they consider the
responsiveness of differentiated cells to varying external
ligands. Investigators in these areas were present at the
conference along with immunologists to exchange ideas,
approaches and concepts.

The somewhat remote setting of LaRabida, located on the
shores of Lake Michigan, was an ideal place to hold the
conference. A pleasant Indian summer with comfortable day
and evening temperatures was helpful for its intended purpose. It was apparent, as the meeting progressed, that
the foundations of modern immunology, with its specialized
areas and sophisticated technologies, is firmly embedded
in the classical disciplines of biochemistry and physiology. This attitude grew throughout the meeting and helped
to reinforce the unifying concept and the motivation behind
the conference itself.

The success of the meeting was possible through the
dedicated help of the LaRabida staff, especially Ms. Carole
Timkovich and Ms. Michele Townsend, as well as the work of
Ms. Rose Maloney of the University of Illinois.

The symposium was generously supported by funds re-
ceived from the Fogarty International Center, the National
Science Foundation, and by contributions received from
Miles Laboratory, Merck, Sharpe and Dohme, the Upjohn
Company, the Kroc Foundation, Ortho Pharmaceutical
Company, and Packard Instrument Corporation.

Organizers: E.P. Cohen and H. Kohler
             Chicago, Illinois, 1979

Pages 1—46, Membranes, Receptors, and the Immune Response
© 1980 Alan R. Liss, Inc., 150 Fifth Avenue, New York, NY 10011

STRUCTURAL AND GENETIC INSIGHTS INTO ANTIBODY COMPLEMENTARITY

Elvin A. Kabat

Departments of Microbiology, Human Genetics and
Development, and Neurology, and the Cancer Center/
Institute for Cancer Research, Columbia University
College of Physicians and Surgeons, New York,
N. Y. 10032; and the National Cancer Institute,
National Institutes of Health, Bethesda, Md. 20205.

The problem of antibody complementarity was very close
to the heart of Paul Ehrlich. Indeed his extension to
antigen-antibody interaction (Ehrlich, 1900 see Himmelweit
p. 179) of the lock and key mechanism which Emil Fischer
first introduced for enzyme-substrate interaction showed remarkable insight. Unlike enzyme-substrate interactions,
antigen-antibody reactions were incredibly complicated by
what we now recognize as antibody heterogeneity. They were
further complicated by the lack of purified toxins so that
one got antibodies to impurities; by the instability of diphtheria toxin and its spontaneous conversion to toxoid; by
the absence of a concept of antigenic determinants; and by
the failure to recognize that on immunization with a toxin,
one could get neutralizing antitoxin as well as non-neutral-
izing antibodies to the toxin itself. Neither Ehrlich nor
anyone else in his day could have predicted the remarkable
developments that have taken place in purification and
characterization of proteins.

Nevertheless his side-chain theory came remarkably close
to the truth. Moreover, he developed methods for the biological standardization of antitoxins that are in use today and
which are reliable despite the extraordinary heterogeneity
of antitoxins especially those produced in the horse. He
studied the toxic plant proteins ricin (Ehrlich, 1891a,b;
Himmelweit pp. 21-26) and abrin (Himmelweit pp. 27-30) now
termed lectins, which were more stable than diphtheria toxin

and was the first to show that antibodies to ricin would inhibit the toxic and the hemagglutinating properties (Himmelweit, pp. 84-85). This was an enormous simplification of the problem. Since the two properties often run parallel it permitted a more chemical approach to antigen-antibody interactions. We now know that what was called ricin was a mixture (Kabat et al. 1947) of a hemagglutinin and a toxic protein each sharing an identical α-subunit but differing in their β-subunits (Nicolson et al. 1974); the problem was further complicated by the specific receptor site of the hemagglutinin which could itself react with serum glycoproteins including normal immunoglobulins.

Ehrlich was the father of the chemical approach to the study of immune reactions and although he and Madsen invited Svante Arrhenius to collaborate so that the latter's insights into ionic interactions might be incorporated into the chemical approach, Ehrlich was adamant in refusing to accept this approach as applied to diphtheria toxin. Arrhenius (1907) attributed the difficulties to the presence of toxoid and toxin in varying proportions while Ehrlich hypothesized that there existed a complex mixture of toxins differing in their intrinsic toxicities. Although Arrhenius and Madsen were closer to the truth as concerns toxoid and toxin, Ehrlich was troubled by inconsistencies which we now know to be related to the heterogeneity of the antitoxins and to antibodies to impurities in the toxin; he thus would not abandon his biological standardization. This controversy persisted (Heidelberger, 1946; van Heyningen and Bidwell, 1948) in various forms after the quantitative flocculation curve (Pappenheimer and Robinson, 1937) was proposed as a substitute for in vivo standardization, but it has not replaced in vivo standardization as the primary method for the reasons which Ehrlich had appreciated.

Ehrlich originated selective theories of antibody formation picturing each antibody forming cell as having receptors specific for the antigenic determinant; receptors were synthesized in excess and secreted into the blood stream as antibodies. The demonstration by Landsteiner (1945) of seemingly limitless numbers of antigenic specificities led to the development of template or instructive theories which were abandoned with the emergence of our modern understanding of protein synthesis resulting from transcription and translation of a nucleotide sequence in the DNA. Selective theories as reintroduced by Jerne (1955) and modified by

Burnet (1959) into the clonal selection theory are now generally accepted. One might perhaps suspect that Ehrlich's
important work in developing histological staining reactions
for examining cells, which showed the relatively uniform
appearance of small lymphocytes constituted a difficulty in
getting others to accept the concept that each of these
smaller "look-alike" lymphocytes was programmed to react to
a different antigenic determinant and had a different
specific receptor on its surface.

The chemical approach to the understanding of antibody
structure and specificity has continued to fluorish since
Ehrlich. A sine qua non of this progress has been the development of quantitative chemical methods for the estimation
of antigens and antibodies on a weight basis by Michael
Heidelberger and his school (Heidelberger, 1939, 1956; Kabat,
1961, 1976, 1979) (See Heidelberger and Kendall, 1979 for a
background account.) now extended by radio- (Yalow and Berson,
1960) and enzyme (Engvall and Perlmann, 1971) immunoassay to
the nanogram and picogram range (see Parker, 1976; Haber and
Paulsen, 1974) which permitted antibodies to be treated as
substances rather than as properties, and led to their
purification and characterization as immunoglobulins with
defined molecular weights and electrophoretic properties
(Pedersen and Heidelberger, 1937; Kabat, 1939; Tiselius and
Kabat, 1939). Among other crucial developments were the
recognition of Bence Jones proteins as the light chains of
immunoglobulins (Edelman and Gally, 1962); the two chain
structure of immunoglobulins (Porter, 1973; Edelman, 1973)
and of fragments produced by enzymatic cleavage, and of
myeloma proteins as monoclonal products (Waldenström, 1944,
1948; Kunkel, 1965) secreted by neoplastic lymphoid cells;
the recognition of the immunoglobulin classes and subclasses in various species, the production of myeloma
proteins in BALB/c and NZB mice by injection of mineral oil
(Potter, 1972, 1977; Warner, 1975) similar to those seen in
man and many of which possessed antibody activity; the
recognition of allotypic (Oudin, 1956; Grubb, 1956) and
idiotypic (see Oudin, 1974; Kunkel, 1965) determinants on
antibodies and on immunoglobulins and the demonstration that
their inheritance was determined by classical Mendelian
genetics; the electron microscopic study of immunoglobulins
and of hapten antibody complexes (Valentine and Green, 1967;
Svehag, 1973; Parkhouse et al. 1970; Acton et al. 1971;
Beale and Feinstein, 1976); the ability to sequence myeloma
proteins and homogeneous antibodies, and the availability

of several three-dimensional structures of myeloma Fab fragments and light chain dimers from high resolution X-ray crystallography (see below for references).

The concomitant growth of molecular biology with its remarkable experimental insights (see Watson, 1976) and its development to the stage of determining the nucleotide sequence of individual genes (Sanger et al. 1977; Maxam and Gilbert, 1977) and even their synthesis (Khorana, 1968) has further expanded our horizons. The finding of intervening sequences in immunoglobulin and other eukaryotic genes has revolutionized our concept of the structure of genes and the transcription of mRNA (for references see Crick, 1979; Rabbitts, 1978, 1979). It is now possible to anticipate a reasonably early solution to the problem of the antibody complementarity and diversity and its genetic control.

Most insight into antibody combining sites has been gained with mouse and human myeloma proteins with antibody activity (see Potter, 1977; Kabat, 1978b), with homogeneous rabbit antibodies largely to type specific pneumococcal (Haber, 1970, 1971) and the group A and C specific streptococcal polysaccharides (Krause, 1970) and with various monoclonal human antibodies such as the cold agglutinins with anti-blood group I and i specificities (Feizi et al. 1971, 1978; Kabat et al. 1978). High resolution X-ray structures have given us a picture of what antibody sites look like and extensive sequencing of variable regions of light and heavy chains tabulated in Kabat et al. (1976, 1979a) has permitted important correlations between certain segments and antibody combining site structure and specificity. Nevertheless our understanding is still incomplete. We do not have a model of an antibody combining site with its site completely filled by an antigenic determinant, nor do we even have sequence data on a myeloma protein or antibody with specificity for a determinant on a naturally occurring protein of known sequence and structure. One hopes that the one myeloma protein which has an antibody site which reacts with flagellin (Smith and Potter, 1975) will ultimately be sequenced.

The hybridoma technic introduced by Köhler and Milstein (1976) has made it possible to obtain large quantities of monoclonal antibodies to any antigen and of any specificity in amounts suitable for sequencing and attempts at crystallization. Many laboratories are engaged in such studies (Melchers et al. 1978), generally not only for this purpose, but for making mouse reagents specific for single antigenic determinants of all kinds and for making anti-idiotypic sera. The technic will prove most powerful in determining the repertoires of antibody combining sites to single antigenic determinants and of anti-idiotypic sites to each of these antibody combining sites to provide estimates of the size of the network hypothesized to regulate antibody production (Jerne, 1974) and permit evaluation of such regulation at defined single nodes of the network.

ANTIBODY COMPLEMENTARITY

Our current insight into antibody complementarity and site structure is based on three general approaches. The first of these is mapping the complementarity regions of antibody combining sites by determining which of a series of low molecular weight ligands of known structure fit best into the site (Kabat, 1956, 1957, 1960, 1976; Karush, 1962). This is most often accomplished by immunochemical methods using inhibition by haptens, oligosaccharides, oligopeptides, oligonucleotides, etc. of precipitation of antibody by antigen; by direct binding of the hapten in the site, as measured by equilibrium dialysis (Marrack and Smith, 1932; Haurowitz and Breinl, 1933; Eisen and Karush, 1949; Klotz, 1953; Karush, 1956; Kabat, 1961, 1976) fluorescence quenching (Velick et al. 1960), affinity electrophoresis (Takeo and Kabat, 1978; Horejsi et al. 1977, 1979) etc. or by displacement by hapten of labeled antigen competitively from the combining site (Benjamini et al. 1972; Haber and Paulsen 1974) as in radio- or enzyme-immunoassay. The principles developed for antibody combining sites are being applied extensively to characterization of lectin combining sites (Goldstein and Hayes, 1978; Kabat, 1978a; Pereira and Kabat, 1979).

In the absence of X-ray crystallographic data (see below) and nuclear magnetic resonance data (Dwek, 1977; Dwek et al. 1977; Dower and Dwek, 1979), this is the most widely used and perhaps the only general approach to site mapping, having been applied most extensively to anti-carbohydrate sites but also to antiprotein, antipolypeptide, and antinucleotide specific sites. Among the important insights gained has been the establishment of the range of sizes of antibody combining sites. These were initially established after dextran was shown to be antigenic in

humans (Kabat and Berg, 1952; Maurer, 1953) giving rise to
precipitating antibodies. The isolation and characterization
during the same period (Jeanes et al. 1957; Turvey and Whelan,
1957) of oligosaccharides of the isomaltose (IM) series
(α1→6 linked) made it possible to use a quantitative hapten
inhibition assay and provided a molecular ruler for probing
the size of the antibody combining site (Kabat, 1954, 1956,
1957, 1960; see 1976, 1978b). Most human antidextrans, produced by injecting dextrans with very high proportions of
α1→6 linkages, were shown to be specific for α1→6 linked
chains, the upper limit being a terminal non-reducing hexa-
or hepta-saccharide of the IM series. However, the antibody
response of each individual was not homogeneous but populations
of antibody molecules were formed with combining sites which
varied in size some complementary to a tri-, others to a
tetra-, still others to a pentasaccharide etc. The combining
site sizes ranged from a lower limit of about between 1 to 2
glucoses (Arakatsu et al. 1966) to an upper limit of about
six to seven in α1→6 linkage. This size range has been found
to apply to all kinds of antigenic determinants regardless of
their nature (see Kabat, 1976, 1978b; Goodman, 1975; Atassi
and Stavitsky, 1978) and is comparable to the range of combining sites of enzymes especially at the upper end. Lysozyme
is complementary to a hexasaccharide of the bacterial cell
wall (Phillips, 1966; Rupley, 1967; Chipman et al. 1967),
enzymes such as urease may have a site smaller than the lower
limit. Most lectin sites studied tend toward the lower
limit in site size (Kabat, 1978b; Goldstein and Hayes, 1978;
Pereira and Kabat, 1979) no sites larger than a tetrasac-
charide (Bretting et al. 1976) having been reported. The
inference from studies on whole antiserum that the antibody
response to dextran was heterogeneous was verified in that
it was possible to fractionate the antidextran formed by a
given person into two populations one with sites most complementary to smaller oligosaccharides and another with sites
complementary to larger oligosaccharides (Schlossman and
Kabat, 1962; Gelzer and Kabat, 1964a,b) and similar studies
have been carried out with antibodies to synthetic polypeptides (Schechter et al. 1970). Using dextrans with higher
proportions of α1→3, α1→4, or α1→2 linkages, antisera were
obtained (Kabat, 1954; Allen and Kabat, 1956) which in
addition to α1→6 antibodies contained antibody of these other
specificities.

Although I provided seven and one-half liters of my
serum by 15 one liter plasmaphereses at weekly intervals, and

although much useful information on antibody specificity to the various antigens with which I immunized myself has been obtained, it did not prove practical to fractionate my anti-dextran into homogeneous antibody populations in quantities suitable for sequencing.

The next major advance in the study of antibody combining sites came from the recognition that myeloma proteins which were monoclonal could have antibody specificities and many of these were antidextrans (Leon et al. 1970; Lundblad et al. 1972; Cisar et al.1974, 1975) anti-levans (Cisar et al. 1974, 1975; Wu et al. 1978), anti-galactans (Jolley et al. 1974; Glaudemans, 1975) etc. Each myeloma antibody would have a specific combining site of uniform size and shape. The earliest studies on myeloma antidextrans were on antibodies of $\alpha 1 \rightarrow 3$ specificity; MOPC 104E (Leon et al. 1970) was found to be most complementary to nigerotriose $DGlc\alpha 1 \rightarrow 3DGlc\alpha 1 \rightarrow 3DGlc$ while J558 (Lundblad et al. 1972) was most specific for nigeropentaose.

Another significant development came from studying BALB/c (Cisar et al. 1974, 1975) and subsequently NZB (Wu et al. 1978) mouse myeloma antidextrans of $\alpha 1 \rightarrow 6$ specificity largely because more oligosaccharides are readily available not only to establish the upper limit of the antibody combining site but also to evaluate the effect of branching substitutions on the $\alpha 1 \rightarrow 6$ oligosaccharides (Torii et al. 1966; Cisar et al. 1974; Wu et al. 1978). One thus had a reasonable expectation of mapping the site precisely and completely.

Quantitative precipitin and precipitin inhibition assays showed two mouse IgAκ antidextran myelomas W3434 and W3129 to have sites complementary to a chain of five $\alpha 1 \rightarrow 6$ linked glucoses IM5, isomaltopentaose being the best inhibitor while another QUPC52 also an IgAκ was most complementary to a hexasaccharide of the same structure, IM6 (Cisar et al., 1974).

Measurements of association constants K^a (Cisar et al. 1975) by equilibrium dialysis and by fluorescence quenching yielded the surprising result that K^a for W3129, the protein with the smaller size site, was much higher (1×10^5 M^{-1}) than that of QUPC52 (8.4×10^3 M^{-1}). This had never been encountered in studies on antibody combining sites, antibodies with larger size sites invariably having higher K^a. To understand what was going on, we measured the relative contribution to the total binding energy of each glucose residue in the two sites. The very instructive finding was that the two glucoses at the non-reducing end, contributed 60 percent of the binding energy of the site complementary to IM5 (W3129) whereas they contributed less than five percent of the total binding energy to the site complementary to IM6 (QUPC52). Thus the smaller pentasaccharide size site was directed toward the terminal non-reducing ends of the dextran chain with the terminal one or two glucoses at the non-reducing end bound in three dimensions e.g., was a cavity type site, whereas the hexasaccharide size site was directed toward internal sequences of six αl→6 linked glucoses and thus was a groove type site resembling the lysozyme site.

Independent evidence for this conclusion was obtained using a synthetic linear dextran synthesized by Ruckel and Schuerch (1967). This dextran, which consisted of chains of about 200 αl→6 linked glucoses and had but one terminal non-reducing end, did not precipitate with W3129 since it was monovalent; however as expected it inhibited precipitation of this antidextran by a branched dextran comparably to IM5. Additional evidence for cavity type sites has been obtained by Bennett and Glaudemans (1979) using fluorescence quenching on Fab fragments, by Takeo and Kabat (1978) by affinity electrophoresis, and by Schepers et al. (1978) on MOPC104E an αl→3 antidextran.

Since the linear dextran with its 200 αl→6 linked glucoses was multivalent with respect to antibody with specificity directed toward a sequence of six internal αl→6 linkages, it would be expected to precipitate such antibodies and this was found to be the case confirming the groove-shape of the combining site.

When fractions of my antidextran obtained by isoelectric focusing were studied for precipitation by the linear dextran (Cisar et al. 1975) they were found to be mixtures of molecules with cavity and groove type sites as were rabbit antibodies (Arakatsu et al. 1966; Outschoorn et al. 1974) produced by immunization with isomaltotrionic and isomaltohexaonic acids coupled to BSA.

The existence of antibodies to other branched polysaccharides with specificity directed toward terminal non-reducing ends of chains as well as toward internal structures has demonstrated (Schalch et al. 1979) with rabbit antibodies to the group specific A variant polysaccharide of the streptococcus, composed of rhamnose with $\alpha 1 \rightarrow 2$ and $\alpha 1 \rightarrow 3$ linkages. The versatility of the antibody forming mechanism is well illustrated by the finding that the K^a of the anti-streptococcal antibodies specific for internal sequences were higher than those directed toward the terminal non-reducing ends; this was attributable to the hydrophobic interaction of the CH_3 group of carbon 6 of rhamnose.

The existence of antigenic linear polysaccharides such as certain of the pneumococcal polysaccharides S III, S VIII, S VIa (see How et al. 1964) necessitate the ability to form groove-type sites.

I have dealt elsewhere extensively with the mapping of antibody and lectin combining sites (Kabat, 1976, 1978a,b, 1979; Pereira and Kabat, 1979) and the number of such studies is too great for each to be considered. The diversity of sites may be comprehended by considering how it would increase as the complexity of the structure of the antigenic determinants increase. Antibodies with specificities for homopolymers have been shown to be different for different linkages and if several types of linkage are present in a hexasaccharide determinant the number of specificities will increase dramatically. For a chain of six glucoses, since linkages maybe $\alpha 1 \rightarrow 6$, $\alpha 1 \rightarrow 4$, $\alpha 1 \rightarrow 3$, and $\alpha 1 \rightarrow 2$, there would be 1024 different structures. If there were an antibody site specifically directed toward the hexasaccharide as well as toward smaller portions of it e.g., the di-, tri-, tetra-, and pentasaccharide units as well as groove and cavity type sites, the number of different combining site specificities would become staggering. Indeed this does not even consider the possibility that antibody combining sites could be directed toward different conformations of the hexasaccharide or smaller segments of it. Proceeding to chains involving two different sugars one might arrive at an even higher number of combining sites since it has been demonstrated for the linear type III pneumococcal polysaccharide (Mage and Kabat, 1963) that antibodies to internal segments of the chain could be of two kinds with sites specific for one or the other sugar constituent each of which could be the immunodominant group. It might be increased even further by the demonstration (Zopf et al. 1978) that antibodies to an oligosaccharide chain might be directed against two different sides of the oligosaccharide chain. If the findings of Wood et al. (1978) with lectin II of Bandeiraea simplicifolia that an internal sugar constituent may serve as a spacer, merely connecting two sugar units both of which interact with portions of the combining site, are found to hold for anti-bodies, yet another parameter of diversity of antibody com-bining sites toward a single determinant would exist.

Similar estimates may be made for antibodies to homo- and hetero-polypeptides, nucleotides, etc. With antigenic determinants of proteins, the fixed three dimensional structure of the determinants may be such as to restrict the heterogeneity of the response (Crumpton, 1975; Atassi and Stavitsky, 1978).

In considering the generation of diversity several groups have invoked unusual cross reactions (see below for references) to reduce the size of the repertoire of antibody combining sites. The extent to which this actually would effect any reduction in the number of specific combining sites is not clear. Studies on type III and type VIII rabbit anti-pneumococcal antibodies have shown very extensive differences in sequence in the complementarity determining regions (CDR) (Haber et al. 1975) indicating a substantial number of different antibody combining sites. Indeed it has not been possible to designate a single amino acid residue or segment as making contact in the site with the antigenic determinant. This emphasizes the indispensability of mapping the sites of the antibodies to be sequenced by immunochemical procedures to establish similarities and differences in site size and complementarity which might then be correlated with the sequence data.

The second major line of investigation of the structure of antibody combining sites involves the examination of sequences of the variable regions of light and heavy chains from myeloma proteins and homogeneous antibodies of various species. The magnitude of the problem may be seen in that perhaps 30 to 40 percent of the total number of amino acid residues sequenced in all proteins to date are in variable regions and several hundred investigators have devoted years to obtaining such sequence data. The variable region data have been tabulated with references, antibody specificities etc. (Kabat et al. 1976, 1979a; see also Dayhoff, 1972 including supplements 1, 1973; 2, 1976; and 3, 1978). Major early contributions were the recognition of variable (V) and constant regions (C) (Hilschmann and Craig, 1965), the existence of subgroups in human V_κ and V_λ light chains (Hood et al. 1967; Niall and Edman, 1967; Milstein, 1967) in mouse V_K chains (Potter, 1977) and in heavy chains (V_H) (Barstad et al. 1974; Capra and Kehoe, 1975), the extra-ordinary similarity of V regions from various species and the finding that certain residues showed more variability than others (Milstein and Pink, 1970; Kabat, 1970).

As sequence data on myeloma proteins from humans and from mice accumulated, it became possible to apply statistical methods to attempt to locate those amino acid residues or those segments which might be involved in antibody complemen-tarity. From the subgroup data it had become clear that the first 23 amino acids were not part of the site since several members of a given subgroup had identical sequences (Kabat, 1968).

Further insight into the problem of complementarity was gained when Wu and Kabat (1970) introduced an equation to evaluate the extent of variability at each position in the variable region. On the assumption that the antibody com-bining site in all species, like other specific receptor sites, enzyme sites, etc., would be in the same place, the sequences of all subgroups and species available which then included human V_K, V_λ and mouse V_K chains largely as Bence Jones proteins were considered as a single population and aligned for maximum homology. The equation:

$$\text{Variability} = \frac{\text{Number of different amino acids at any position}}{\text{Frequency of the most common amino acid at that position}}$$

was applied over the 107 positions in the V-regions of the light chains. In the original study at position 7, 63 proteins had been sequenced; Ser occurred 41 times and four different amino acids were present Pro, Ser, Thr, and Asp. The frequency of the most common amino acid was 41/63 = 0.65 and the variability was 4/0.65 = 6.15. In this equation an invariant residue would have a variability of 1 and the theoretical upper limit of variability for 20 amino acids occurring with equal frequency was 400. Variability was not calculated for insertions.

The variability plot obtained (Figure 1) shows three contiguous segments termed hypervariable segments consisting of residues 24-34, 50-56, and 89-97. These were predicted to be the complementarity determining regions or segments (CDR), to form the walls of the antibody combining site and

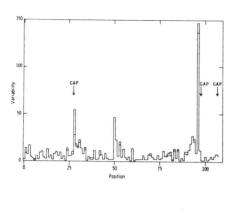

Fig. 1. Variability at different positions for the variable region of light chains. GAP indicates positions at which differences in length have been found. From Wu and Kabat (1970).

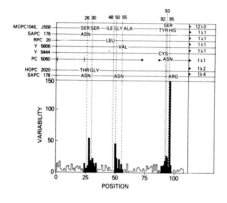

Fig. 2. Location and nature of amino acid substitutions in the mouse V_λ region superimposed on the variability plot of Fig. 1. The three CDR according to Wu and Kabat (1970) are shaded. All other residues in the sequences were identical. The number of instances of each sequence as well as the number of base changes to obtain it from λ0 are given. (From Kabat, 1978b, data from Cohn et al. 1974; Weigert and Riblet, 1976).

to contain those amino acid residues whose side chains would come into contact with the antigenic determinant and hold it in the site. These predictions were completely verified when high resolution X-ray crystallographic studies became available on Bence Jones (light chain) dimers (Schiffer et al. 1973; Edmundsen et al. 1974; Epp et al. 1974, 1975; Wang et al. 1979) and on Fab fragments (Poljak et al. 1973, 1974; Saul et al. 1978; Segal et al. 1974; Davies et al. 1975; Padlan, 1977).

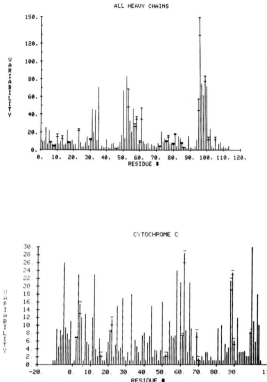

Fig. 3. Variability at different positions for the variable region of heavy chains. The plot was made by the PROPHET Computer System (Raub, 1974). From Kabat et al. (1979a).

Fig. 4. Variability plot for 67 cytochromes c. From Kabat et al. (1976).

Mouse λ chains constitute but a very small proportion of the light chain population. When mouse λ Bence Jones proteins or light chains were sequenced (Appella, 1971; Weigert et al. 1970; Weigert and Riblet, 1976) they were highly restricted in amino acid sequence over the entire V-region; indeed 12 different light chains were identical. Seven other chains showed variation in from one to three residues and, with a single exception at position 48, all were in the CDR (hypervariable regions) (Fig. 2). Position 48 was outside the CDR as originally defined from the variability plot (Fig. 1) but all mouse V$_\lambda$ chains have an insertion of three residues in the first CDR, tabulated as 27D, 27E, 27F (Kabat et al. 1976, 1979a) and it has been suggested (Kabat, 1978b) that this might move position 48 into the CDR in mouse V$_\lambda$ so that it would consist of residues 48-56. The need for a high resolution X-ray crystallographic study of a mouse Bence Jones protein or Fab fragment containing a λ chain to establish this is obvious. The delineation of CDR2 in mouse V_λ is of substantial significance in relation to nucleic acid sequences and the generation of diversity and will be discussed below.

Heavy chains were also found to show three hypervariable segments or CDRs in positions comparable to those of the light chain but displaced several residues toward the C-terminus of the chain (Fig. 3). The CDR's consisted of residues 31-35, 50-65, and 95-102; individual chains differed in length and length differences were incorporated as positions 35 A, B; 52 A, B, C; and 100 A, B, C, D, E, F, G, H. Another stretch involving length differences was at 85 A, B, C; this segment was not in the CDR.

Affinity labeling technics have shown that only residues in the CDR of the light and of the heavy chains were labeled; (for references see Givol, 1974; Kabat, 1976, 1978b) indeed when the reactive group of the label was placed at different distances from the haptenic determinant, residues in different CDRs could be labeled (Haimovitch et al. 1972).

High variability was also noted by Capra and Kehoe (1974) at positions 81, 83, 94, and 95 from plots of human heavy chains, but was less marked in plots involving all species for which sequences were available and was not seen in mouse heavy chain (Vrana et al. 1977). Residues 84 and 85 (Ansari et al. 1976; Mage, 1977) are involved in a allotypic specificity so that some variability is expected. (For other aspects of variability plots and their limitations see Kabat 1976, 1978b).

The hypervariable segments found by the variability plot are unique to light and heavy chains of immunoglobulins. Figure 4 shows a similar plot for 67 cytochromes c; there is no evidence of hypervariable segments and the site region is associated with the segment of invariant or very low variability around residues 70 to 80.

Figure 5 shows a schematic view of the immunoglobulin G molecule with the domain structure and the CDR of the light and heavy chains indicated and Figure 6 gives stereo views of the α-carbon skeleton of the V-regions of four of the five X-ray crystallographic structures. The residues of

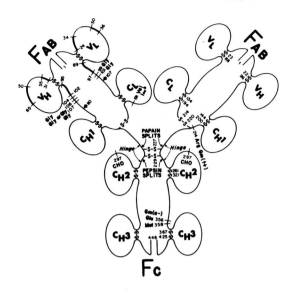

Fig. 5. Schematic view of 4-chain structure of human IgG$_K$ molecule. Numbers on right side: actual residues of protein Eu (Edelman et al. 1969; Edelman, 1970); Numbers of Fab fragments on left side aligned for maximum homology; light chains numbered as in Wu and Kabat (1970) and Kabat and Wu (1971). Heavy chains of Eu have residue 52A, 3 residues 82A, B, C and lack residues termed 100A, B, C, D, E, F, G, H and 35A, B. Thus residue 110 (end of variable region) is 114 in actual sequence. Hypervariable regions, complementarity-determining segments or regions (CDR): heavier lines. V$_L$ and V$_H$: light- and heavy-chain variable regions; C$_H$1, C$_H$2, and C$_H$3: domains of constant region of heavy chain; C$_L$: constant region of light chain. Hinge region in which 2 heavy chains are linked by disulfide bonds is indicated approximately. Attachment of carbohydrate is at residue 297. Arrows at residues 107 and 110 denote transition from variable to constant regions. Sites of action of papain and pepsin and locations of a number of genetic factors are given. From Kabat (1978b).

the CDR's are circled. All four V-regions have the same orientation of their frameworks and the differences in the CDR are clearly evident despite the absence of side chains. These sites give substantial insight into differences in site structure associated with differences in specificity.

The library of variable region sequences (Kabat et al. 1976, 1979a) has made it possible to apply statistical methods to identifying individual residues in the CDR which serve a structural role as well as those which are complementarity determining e.g., make contact with antigenic

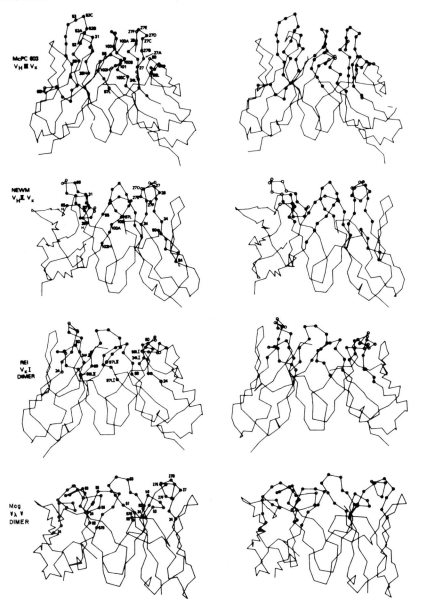

Fig. 6. Stereodrawings of the α-carbon skeletons of the V-regions of four of the five proteins studied crystallographically. Each protein is in the same orientation. With a stereo viewer it is possible to see two adjacent models at the same time, so that a comparison may be made in three dimensions. (From Kabat, 1978b).

determinants in the site or exert a conformational effect on a contacting residue. In addition it has been possible to a limited degree to identify individual residues which could be associated with specificity differences (see Kabat, 1978b). These data together with the known X-ray crystallographic structures may make it possible to fix the conformation of individual residues in the CDR in various antibodies and so define or predict the structure of individual sites more precisely.

Another important predictive approach involves the re-placement of the sequence of the CDRs in a molecule for which an X-ray crystallographic structure is available by the CDR's of a known antibody. This approach (Padlan et al. 1976; Davies and Padlan, 1977; Potter, 1977) has considerable utility since the X-ray studies available show that the non-CDR segments constitute a framework of β pleated sheet structure. Important insights into site structure are obtainable especially when other types of data are available as from nuclear magnetic resonance (Dwek, 1977, 1979). A site structure for the anti-DNP specific myeloma protein MOPC315 was proposed (Padlan et al. 1976) and was further modified (Dwek et al. 1977; Dower and Dwek, 1979). Although the two proposed structures are somewhat different, never-theless there is good definition of the DNP moiety in the site with respect to satisfying the affinity labeling and other data.

Perhaps more instructive are the findings (Davies and Padlan, 1977) on the introduction on to the framework of McPC603 of the CDR sequences of a rabbit type III anti-pneumococcal antibody; in these studies the original cavity type site of McPC603 was converted into a groove-type site; although variability plots of rabbit anti-pneumococcal (Haber et al. 1975) and anti-streptococcal antibodies showed the region of the second CDR of the light chain not to be hypervariable, nevertheless the constructed site involved the second CDR of the light chain as contacting the type III pneumococcal polysaccharide. Moreover, the size of the constructed site was complementary to a hexasaccharide in accord with earlier immunochemical studies (Mage and Kabat, 1963).

Two models of the EPC109 and ABPC47 myeloma proteins which bind β2→1 fructofuranose chains have been constructed in the same manner (Potter, 1977; Vrana et al. 1979).

From the sequence differences and idiotypic specificities of these and a third myeloma protein UPC61 binding $\beta 2\rightarrow 1$ fructofuranose chains and from H and L chain recombination data it was proposed that the hapten inhibitable cross reactive idiotypic specificity of UPC61 governed by the light chain was determined by Ser 30 and Ser 92; these two residues were about 8Å apart on the model and thus would fall well within the size of an antigenic determinant (Vrana et al. 1979). Two other non-hapten inhibitable idiotypic determinants were ascribed to framework differences. The importance of verifying inferences from hypothetical models is obvious - it will establish confidence in the predictive method and make possible the identification of complementarity determining residues and those involved in idiotypic specificity. The extensive similarities among myeloma proteins with the same or closely related specificities provides an important body of data for such studies. The most important limitation to model construction is the varying lengths of the CDR and the difficulty of orienting CDRs of different length to form a site when incorporated into the framework.

The series of eight $\beta 1\rightarrow 6$ galactan binding myeloma proteins has also been studied in an attempt to define residues involved in idiotypic specificity (Potter et al. 1979). A high resolution X-ray structure for one of these $\beta 1\rightarrow 6$ galactan binding myeloma proteins, J539, may soon be available to define the idiotypic residues more precisely and to validate predictions from models.

It is evident that much remains to be done before we have a clear understanding of the diversity in size and shape of antibody combining sites and the magnitude of the repertoire of antibody combining sites even to a single antigenic determinant.

GENETIC ASPECTS OF THE GENERATION OF DIVERSITY

Turning from structural aspects of antibody diversity to the question of what is going on in the genome, we again have an area which is exploding with new findings. Insights are coming from several approaches, especially the analysis of the extensive sequence data on immunoglobulin light and heavy chains and the use of recombinant DNA technics to obtain clones containing genes for various portions of light chains.

Both approaches have yielded important information about the genetics of V-region assembly unique and distinct from what is seen with other proteins. The finding of leader and intervening sequences in genes coding for viruses and proteins has led to the recognition of the primary transcript, an mRNA copy of the entire DNA gene including the intervening sequences from which the intervening sequences are subsequently spliced out to produce the usual mRNA copy of the coding segments (see Darnell, 1979; Crick, 1979).

Immunoglobulin light and heavy chains also have intervening sequences and their biosynthesis also involves a primary transcript and splicing (Brack and Tonegawa, 1977; Gilmore-Hebert et al. 1978; Gilmore-Hebert and Wall, 1978). Intervening sequences have been found (Tonegawa et al. 1978; Seidman et al. 1978a,b) between the precursor (Milstein et al. 1972; Swan et al. 1972; Rose et al. 1977; Burstein and Schechter, 1978; Schechter, 1979) and the V-region nucleotides and between the nucleotides coding for the C-terminal portion of the V-region and those coding for the C-region. Similarly in mouse heavy chains intervening sequences have been found by R loop mapping between V_H and C_H1 and between C_H2 and C_H3 of an α (Early et al. 1979) and a γ_1 chain (Sakano et al. 1979a). The hinge with an intervening sequence on each side separating it from the C_H1 and C_H2 domains was identified by R-loop mapping and sequencing those portions of the flanking sequences contiguous with the coding sequences (Sakano et al. 1979b). Presumably a primary transcript is made for all domains and splicing is involved in processing of the mRNA from it (Rabbits, 1978a,b; Gilmore-Hebert and Wall, 1978). These aspects appear no different from what is observed in synthesis of mRNA from other proteins.

The V-region itself however involves genetic phenomena thus far unique. In his original description of the three V_K subgroups of human light chains Milstein (1967) noted that subgroup specific residues did not extend beyond residue 94 (numbering as in Kabat et al. 1976) and that it appeared as if extensive recombination was occurring beyond residue 94. This observation was ignored or forgotten for many years perhaps because of the tendency to consider the V-domain as a separate genetic unit but appears highly significant in view of recent findings. In our original tabulation of V-region sequences (Kabat et al. 1976) sequences were listed essentially in the order in which they were reported in the literature. In preparation for the second edition and to analyze the existing data further we ordered the sequences (Kabat et al. 1978) so that all chains having a given framework segment were grouped together. For example, all chains identical in FR1 were grouped into sets. Among human V_KI chains, one set contained 18, a second set 7 and a third set 2 members; many sets had only a single member; FR2, FR3 and FR4 sets were made in a similar manner. CDR sets were not considered since very few were identical. When each V_KI chain was traced from one FR to the next, it was observed that members of the same set in FR1 could be associated with different sets in FR2, FR3, or FR4 (Fig. 7). Similar findings were obtained with BALB/c mouse V_K (Fig. 8), rabbit V_K (Fig. 9), and mouse and human V_HIII (Fig. 10) chains.

Several noteworthy findings were that:

1. FR4 sets in human V_K contained members which crossed subgroup lines; one FR4 set contained members of all four human V_K subgroups, another contained a member of V_KI and one of V_KII, and a third a member of V_KI and V_KIII (Fig. 7) (Kabat et al. 1978) confirming Milstein's (1967) original suggestion.

2. The second important finding was that one V_K FR2 set residues 35 to 49, contained one human V_KIV, 4 mouse and 8 rabbit V_K chains (Figs. 8, 9) (Kabat et al. 1978). Thus this FR2 set had been preserved unchanged for about 80 million years and might even represent the primordial sequence of the FR2 segment of the first light chain. When the sequences of NZB V_K21 myeloma proteins (Weigert et al. 1978) and additional rabbit V_K chains (Huser and Braun, 1978; Brandt and Jaton, 1978; Chersi et al. 1979) were obtained this FR2 set increased to 1 human, 20 mouse, and 13 rabbit chains (Kabat et al. 1979b).

3. The third finding was that one FR4 set of mouse V_H chains contained 2 mouse and 1 human V_HIII chains.

This apparent independent assortment of FR segments suggested that they and by inference, the CDR were the genetic units and the term minigene was introduced to describe them inasmuch as each intact V-region is generally considered to be under the control of one gene. A minigene

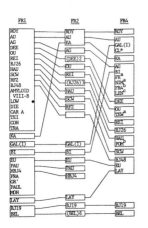

Fig. 7.   Independent assortment of framework sets in human $V_\kappa I$ chains. ●, Cold agglutinin with anti-blood group I activity; a, human κ light chain subgroup II; b, human κ light chain subgroup III; c, human κ light chain subgroup IV. From Kabat et al. 1978.

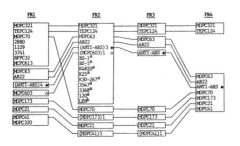

Fig. 8.   Independent assortment of framework sets in mouse V_κ chains. ●, Anti-p-azophenylarsonate; O, Anti-phosphocholine; a, rabbit κ light chain; b, human κ light chain subgroup IV.   From Kabat et al. 1978.

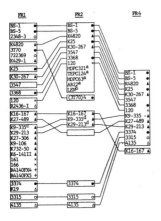

Fig. 9. Independent assortment of framework sets in rabbit V_κ chains. ●, Anti-type III pneumococcal polysaccharide; O, anti-type VIII pneumococcal polysaccharide; ▲, anti-streptococcal group A variant carbohydrate; Δ, anti-streptococcal group C carbohydrate; +, anti-p-azophenylarsonate; X, anti-Micrococcus lysodeikticus; a, mouse κ light chain; b, human κ light chain subgroup IV; c, K9-335 has the same sequence as K9-338; d, the residue at position 36 has been changed from Tyr to Phe for K29-213, K9-335, and K9-338 (Braun and Huser, 1977). From Kabat et al. 1978.

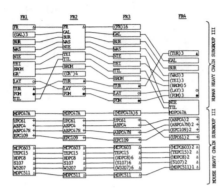

Fig. 10. Independent assortment of framework sets in
human and mouse V$_H$III chains.
●, Anti-human gamma G1 globulin; O, anti-human gamma
G1 and G3 globulin; ▲, cold
agglutinin with anti-blood
group I activity; Δ, anti-
phosphocholine; +, anti-
β2→1-fructosan. From
Kabat et al. 1978.

was defined (Kabat et al. 1979b) as a DNA segment coding
for a portion of a complete V-region and which shows evidence
of segregation as a functional unit independent of the rest
of the DNA coding for the V-region. When the CDR (hypervariable regions) were originally recognized it was proposed
(Wu and Kabat, 1970; Kabat and Wu, 1971), that the simplest
hypothesis to explain the generation of antibody diversity
would be to insert the nucleotides coding for the CDR into
those coding for the FR to assemble a complete V-region
gene. At that time the only insertional mechanism known
was episomal insertion and this was considered as a possibility. This insertion hypothesis was also advocated by
Capra and Kindt (1975; Kindt and Capra, 1978; Capra, 1976).
Such a model appeared to be consistent with the assortment
data.

While we were demonstrating assortment, Tonegawa et al.
(1978) had already sequenced nucleotides of a cloned germ
line gene from 12 day mouse embryo DNA (Igl3λ) which they
considered to be V$_λ$II finding a leader sequence coding for
the precursor, an intervening sequence and the nucleotides
coding for an amino acid sequence corresponding almost but not
exactly to residues 1-96 (numbering as in Kabat et al. 1976,
1979a) of the V-region followed by an intervening sequence
or from FR1 to within one residue from the end of CDR3.
Since residue 97 in mouse V$_λ$ chains is an invariant Val, it
was possible that CDR3 in mouse V$_λ$ extended only through
residue 96.

What we considered most interesting was that in their

comparison of the translated amino acid sequence of their clone with the established $V_\lambda I$ and $V_\lambda II$ amino acid sequences of myeloma proteins, they had two differences in FR1 and four in FR3 all corresponding to $V_\lambda II$, but the one difference in FR2 corresponded to $V_\lambda I$. It seemed to us most consistent with our assortment data and the minigene hypothesis to consider this a double recombinant rather than a somatic mutation as Tonegawa et al. (1978) had proposed. Moreover, their CDR2 corresponded to $V_\lambda I$ and their CDR3 had two residues corresponding to $V_\lambda I$, two to $V_\lambda II$ and one, residue 94, differed from both. This too would be consistent with assortment of minigenes for the CDR as well as the FR segments.

Since in the adult myeloma, the entire V-region is a contiguous sequence and since Tonegawa et al. (1977, 1978) had shown that in mouse embryo DNA the V and C regions were separated by at least 5,000 bases while in the adult V_λ myeloma immunoglobulin DNA they were separated only by 1250 nucleotides, we proposed a mechanism of somatic assembly in the genome for the joining of FR4 to the rest of the V-region sometime between the twelfth day of embryonic life and the adult. Since we had assorted only FR sequences, our findings were independent of whether one or more CDR residues assorted with FR4.

Shortly thereafter Brack et al. (1978) reported on three other DNA clones Ig99λ and Ig25λ from 12 day mouse embryo and Ig303λ from adult $V_\lambda I$ H2020. They showed by R-loop mapping and Bernard et al. (1978) showed by nucleic acid sequencing that Ig99λ coded for the precursor followed by an intervening sequence and then for nucleotides coding for the V-region from residues 1-95 that is from FR1 through to two residues from the end of CDR3. Ig25λ coded for residues 96 through 107, that is for the last 2 residues of CDR3 plus all of FR4 which they term the J segment, followed by an intervening sequence and then for the nucleotides coding for the C-region with a repetition of the codon for Gly107. The clone from adult H2020, Ig303λ, coded for the entire V-region residues 1 through 107 followed by the same intervening sequence and the nucleotides coding for the C-region with the repetition of Gly107. Thus our hypothesis of somatic assembly between the twelfth day of embryonic life and the adult myeloma was completely confirmed except that by assorting only frameworks we could not have seen that two residues of CDR3 assorted with FR4.

Accordingly the J segment conforms to our definition of a minigene.

Weigert et al. (1978) isolated and sequences a set of NZB V_K21 myeloma proteins and used the assortment principle (Kabat et al. 1978) to show that two or three residues of CDR3 plus FR4, the J segment, assorted separately from the rest of the V-region. They suggested that these CDR3 residues could contribute to the generation of diversity by recombinations involving different nucleotides of the recombining codons. Rao et al. (1979) carried out a similar assortment on the V_H region of antigalactan binding myeloma proteins and concluded that they too had a J segment composed of FR4 plus a few residues of CDR3 which could also be involved in the generation of diversity.

Subsequently Max et al. (1979) and Sakano et al. (1979b) isolated a clone coding for a series of five J segments each with intervening sequences ranging from 249 to 310 nucleotides between each J. The coding region for the five J segments translated as coding for amino acids 96-108. Sakano et al. (1979b) numbered J1 to J5 with J1 closest to the V-region whereas Max et al. (1979) numbered them with J1 closest to the C-region. Four of the J segments corresponded exactly to myeloma proteins sequenced in this region. J3 was considered to be a non-expressed J segment since it did not end with the usual GT found at the border of all coding sequences but had a CT instead; GT is generally associated with splicing out of the intervening sequences (Breathnach et al. 1978; Catterall et al. 1978; Konkel et al. 1978). Moreover J3 differed from other mouse V_K chains at positions 99, 103, and 108 and had an Asp at 104 which had never been observed. Position 99 is Gly in κ and λ chains of all species which have been studied being present in all 149 light chains (Fig. 5) (Kabat et al. 1979a). One might suspect that even if splicing could occur the chain might not be functional. The process of joining of J to the V-region by somatic recombination involving different nucleotides within a given codon has been postulated to be able to give rise to other J segments which have been recognized in mouse V_K light chains and contribute to the generation of diversity. However, each specific DNA clone results from a very low frequency event and it might be difficult to find another nucleotide stretch from the other chromosome which coded for a different set of J minigenes.

The J minigene story and its somatic assembly, it being joined to the nucleotides coding for the rest of the V-region between the twelfth day of embryonic life and the adult myeloma constitute a most exciting new development which is thus far unique to immunoglobulins.

The situation with respect to the genetics of the rest of the V-region and the generation of diversity has been much more controversial. The assortment observed by Kabat et al. (1978) for FR1, FR2, and FR3, unlike the FR4 or J assortment, appeared to be largely within individual subgroups (Figs. 7-10) and this is considered by Milstein (1979) to weaken the minigene hypothesis. Celia Milstein (1973) in analyzing sequences of human V_K subgroups did not find a significantly higher frequency of cross overs between $V_K I$ and $V_K II$ than occurred in what were considered to be two sub-subgroups of $V_K I$, termed $V_K Ia$ and $V_K Ib$ although the frequency of such cross overs was higher than expected from random point mutation. Ben-Sasson (1979) suggested as an alternative to the minigene hypothesis that massive recombination during meiosis would give the appearance of minigenes.

Seidman et al. (1978a,b) and Seidman and Leder (1978) cloned two DNA fragments of MOPC149 and these contained segments coding for the precursor sequence, an intervening sequence and what was translated as amino acids 1-97 of the myeloma protein that is exactly to the end of CDR3. They inferred from the findings that at least six EcoR1 fragments hybridized to their V-region mRNA probe of MOPC149, which encoded amino acids 44-90, that they were recognizing the genes for a V-region subgroup. Since there are 25-30 mouse subgroups (Potter, 1977), the mouse genome was estimated to contain 125-150 distinct germ line V-region genes.

Thus the recombination of J segments plus a large number of V-region genes coding for amino acids 1-95 in the genome was considered to be partly responsible for the generation of diversity plus the further assumption that diversity involved combinatorial association of V_L and V_H chains (Weigert et al. 1978). This, however, is not considered sufficient to account for the diversity and somatic mutation in the CDR is proposed as also involved. Another proposal to reduce the number of antibodies is the concept of multispecificity e.g., that antibody of a given known specificity might also react with entirely unrelated substances (Talmage, 1959; Hood and Talmage, 1970; Richards and Konigsberg, 1973; Inman, 1974, 1978; Cameron and Erlanger, 1976); however no convincing case of multispecificity has yet been found (Inman, 1978; see Kabat, 1978b).

These hypotheses fail to consider the preserved FR2 segment. Moreover, when the NZB sequences (Weigert et al. 1978) are added to those tabulated earlier (Kabat et al. 1978) a substantial improvement in the assortment is seen (Fig. 11) (Kabat et al. 1979b). If one accepts for the purpose of further analysis that there is truly a string of several hundred V_K sequences in the mouse genome each coding for positions 1 through 95, it becomes possible to count the numbers of copies of the preserved sequence by listing the differences in CDR1 and CDR2 on each side of it. When this is done it is seen that, in the BALB/c mouse of the six sequences available 5 copies and in the NZB mouse with 14 sequences, 10 copies of the preserved FR2 would be needed. Since only relatively few sequences are available these findings would imply that there might be hundreds of copies of this preserved sequence in the genome. The question immediately arises as to what would be preserving this sequence in the genome in so many copies?

This same question was originally faced when it was found that there were many V-regions all associated with a constant C-region and Dreyer and Bennett (1965) suggested that the V- and C-regions were coded by separate genes and that the C-region gene existed in but one or at most a few copies and this has proven to be the case.

The situation with respect to the preserved FR2 is even more startling (Kabat et al. 1979b). One might argue that this segment is preserved because its primary sequence is so essential to proper three-dimensional folding that any change in sequence would not give a functional chain. This is clearly not the case since there exist 12 other mouse and 8 other rabbit FR2 sets; these differ from the preserved segment in 13 of the 15 positions only Trp 35 and Gln 39 being invariant. The number of amino acid substitutions by which they differ from the preserved FR2 set vary from one to five. The other sets have been found to occur in but a single copy in 9 mouse and 8 rabbit sequences; in one instance involving a Phe at position 36 instead of a Tyr, there were six mouse and four rabbit sequences and in

FR1
1 Asp   5 Thr
12 Ala

| MOPC321 |
| TEPC124 |
| 3741 |
| 7043 |
| 7183 |
| 6308 |
| 7210 |
| TEPC111 |
| 4039 |
| 6684 |
| 7175 |
| 7940 |
| 2485 |
| 7461 |
| 2960 |
| MOPC70 |
| 2880 |
| 1229 |
| 7132 |
| B32 |
| 4999 |
| 2413 |
| C101 |
| 7769 |

1 Asn

| MOPC63 |
| AB22 |
| 7063 |
| 9245 |
| 4050 |

7 differences

| MCPC603 |

5 Ala   12 Thr

| 2154 |

FR2
36 Tyr   39 Lys
43 Pro   46 Leu

| MOPC321 |
| TEPC124 |
| 3741 |
| 7043 |
| 7183 |
| 6308 |
| 7210 |
| TEPC111 |
| 4039 |
| 6684 |
| 7175 |
| 7940 |
| 2485 |
| 7461 |
| 2960 |
| MOPC63 |
| AB22 |
| 9245 |
| 4050 |
| (Anti-Ars)3 |
| MCPC603 |
| 2154 |

36 Phe

| MOPC70 |
| 2880 |
| 1229 |
| 7132 |
| B32 |
| 4999 |
| 2413 |

39 Asn   43 Ser

| C101 |

46 Val

| 7769 |

Fig. 11. Independent assortment of FR1 and FR2 in mouse V_κ light chains. Each set of identical sequences is enclosed in a box. The positions and the amino acid residues by which it differs from the other sets, are listed above the FR1 andFR2 set with the largest number of chains. Only the positions at which differences are found are given above the other sets. From Kabat et al. 1979 b.

another there were four mouse sequences differing in five amino acids one involving a two base change ́from the pre-served FR2 set. Moreover, when one locates the position of this segment in the high resolution X-ray crystallographic structure, one sees that it is in an open portion of the molecule (Fig. 6) capable of accepting the many substitutions found.

We must therefore conclude that there is no reason to expect that the preserved sequence would remain unchanged if it occurred in so many copies in the genome nor would one expect to find the heirarchy in frequency of occurrence of the alternate FR2 segments (Kabat et al. 1979b).

If one accepts the minigene hypothesis this difficulty is clearly resolved. The preserved FR2 segment would exist in a single copy in the genome and would be expanded during differentiation as needed to generate the various different sequences which would be assembled somatically. The alternate sequences would also exist in single copies formed by the generally accepted principle of gene duplication and mutation but the primordial sequence would be used much more frequently in the assembly of the intact chains. The numbers of copies of FR1 sets required would also be extremely high based on the number associated with distinct CDR1 and a similar hierarchy of alternate FR1 sets was observed (Kabat et al. 1979b).

It should be pointed out that a human $V_\lambda II$ (Vil) and a $V_\lambda V$ (Mcg) (Wu et al. 1975) with 21 amino acid differences in the V-region had an identical first CDR of 14 residues and that a $V_\kappa I$ (Lay) and a $V_\kappa III$ (Pom) (Klapper and Capra, 1976) had an identical third CDR of 9 residues despite 30 amino acid differences throughout the V region. Capra et al. (1977) found that the three CDR of the light chains of mouse anti-p-azophenylarsonate were identical despite 16 substitutions in the framework. Braun and Huser (1977) sequenced two anti-streptococcal A variant antibodies (K9-335 and K9-335I) produced simultaneously in one rabbit differing at seven positions in FR1 and at four framework positions subsequent to CDR1; nevertheless they were identical in their CDR1 of 14 residues. These findings also are most readily explained by a minigene or insertional hypothesis. One of these two antibodies K9-335 was identical in its entire light chain sequence with another litter mate K9-338; the light chains functioned equally effectively in recombination with either heavy chain. In terms of the minigene hypothesis both rabbits would have assembled the same light chains from their repertoire of FR and CDR segments.

Although these data are completely accounted for by the minigene hypothesis and although no attempts have been made to account for them assuming that nucleotides coding for residues 1-95 of a large number of chains occur in the genome, this of course does not necessarily establish the hypothesis as correct.

Additional evidence bearing upon this issue have recently been obtained (Wu et al. 1979). The nucleotide sequences of the coding regions of three V_λ (Tonegawa et al.

From Wu et al.
1979.

Table 1. Similar short nucleotide segment pairs among the eight mouse lambda and kappa light chain DNA sequences. Identical bases are underlined.

Pair no.	Lambda DNA sequences	Amino acid positions	Kappa DNA sequences	Amino acid positions	Matches between λ and κ sequences	Number of similar sequences found elsewhere (see text)	Other nucleotide arrangements which could give same amino acid sequences λ	κ
#1	TGACTCAG	4-6	TGACTCAG C	4-6	7/8 or 8/8	2	8	2
#2	TCACTTGTCG	21-24	TCACATGTCG T	21-24	9/10 or 10/10	0	8	6
#3	TGGTCTA	45-47	TGGTCTA A	47-49	6/7 or 7/7	4 or 8	96	16
#4	GGTGTTCC	57-59	GGTGTGCC C	57-59	7/8	1	4	4
#5	TATTTCTGT	86-88	TATTACTGT	86-88	8/9	0	8	8
#6*	CCACAATGA	96-99	CCACAGTGA +	96-99	8/9	0	?	?
#7*	ATGACAT	98-100	ATGACAT A	102-104	6/7 or 7/7	3 or 10	?	?

* These sequences were found either at the junction of CDR3 and the intervening DNA sequences or in the intervening DNA sequences beyond CDR3.

+ Seidman et al 1979 have noted that a portion of this sequence CACAGTG can form an inverted repeat.

1978; Bernard et al. 1978) and five V_K cloned genes from 12 day old mouse embryo DNA (Seidman et al. 1978, 1979) were aligned and stretches of six or more nucleotides identical in all of the V_λ and the V_K clones were tabulated, allowing for one possible mismatch. Seven such sequences were found, two of which matched 6/7, two 7/8, two 8/9 and one 9/10 bases (Table 1). This finding was especially exciting because the V_K and V_λ genes are unlinked and may even be on different chromosomes (Valbuena et al. 1978). Moreover, the V_λ chains have one less amino acid residue corresponding to aligned position 10 and have an insertion of three amino acid residues following position 27 and tabulated as 27 D, E, F, and their amino acid sequences differ substantially. The nucleotide segments which matched in V_λ and V_K were located at homologous amino acid positions or off by four amino acids or less. Five of the seven sequences Nos. 2, 3, 4, 5, and 6 were positioned so that they could serve as recognition sequences for the joining by recombination or insertion of CDR and FR nucleotide segments as required by the minigene hypothesis. Of especial interest is the finding that in mouse V_λ, nucleotide segment 3 occurred in residues 45-47 whereas in mouse V_K it was found in residues 47-49. The definition of CDR2 (Wu and Kabat, 1970) based on human V_K, human V_λ, and mouse V_K delineated CDR2 as being residues 50-56 and this has generally been in accord with subsequent data. However in mouse V_λ CDR2 could consist of residues 48-56 as discussed earlier. This is in complete agreement with the finding of identical nucleotide sequence 3 at positions 45-47 in mouse V_λ and 47-49 in mouse V_κ. More remarkable is the observation that nucleotide sequence 4 is back in register matching in V_κ and V_λ at positions 57-59. Thus there is a nucleotide sequence in V_κ and V_λ located at the junction of FR1 and CDR1, of FR2 and CDR2 despite their being out of register, of CDR2 and FR3, of FR3 and CDR3 and of CDR3 and J. The question then arises why was there no such matching nucleotide sequence at the junction of FR1 and CDR2. The answer is that there is; in all light chains of all species sequenced thus far, the first residue of FR2 is Trp, for which only one codon exists and we must conclude that the DNA of mouse V_λ and V_κ chains contain nucleotide recognition signals which could be involved in the assembly of minigene segments coding for the FR, the CDR and the J.

It should be noted that four of the matching nucleotide segments are generally not in register with the nucleotides coding for their respective amino acid segments but begin at the second or third nucleotide of an amino acid codon. This may reflect the need for additional instructions, recognition signals, or points of enzyme attachment, in the genome necessary for synthesis or assembly of a functional protein. It strongly suggests that the code is not degenerate, the multiple choices of a given amino acid such as the six codons for Ser etc. being determined by the kinds of instructions etc. required in the genome for proper function while permitting the final synthesized protein to fold into the proper three dimensional structure.

To obtain further evidence for the significance of these matching mouse V_κ and V_λ nucleotide sequences, we have converted all of the alternative amino acid sequences tabulated in Kabat et al. (1976, 1979a) at these positions to see whether there were any amino acid sequences whose nucleotide sequences were unable to satisfy these matching nucleotides. Those amino acid sequences which occurred repeatedly in many light chains all gave choices satisfying the matching sequences. In some instances in which an amino acid sequence occurred only once, and since the matching nucleotides are not in the CDR so the possibility of an error in sequencing cannot be excluded, there was a reduction in the match by one nucleotide (Wu et al. 1979). This of course does not mean that when nucleotide sequences are available the matching will be maintained since there are many non-matching choices which would give the same amino acid sequence, but merely indicates that there is no disproof of these findings in the data bank of sequences.

We have also looked for these matching sequences in the nucleotides coding for φX174 (Sanger et al. 1978), SV40 (Reddy et al. 1978; Fiers et al. 1978) and G4 (Godson et al. 1978); three of the sequences Nos. 3, 5, and 6 were unique and were not found, - sequence 1 occurred twice, sequence 3 and 7 which were the shortest were found 4 or 8, or 3 or 10 times respectively depending upon whether the third nucleotide is required to be a purine (Wu et al. 1979).

The isolation of each cloned DNA segment (Tonegawa et al. 1978; Seidman et al. 1978a,b) coding for an immunoglobulin chain is a very low frequency event, every clone arising from a DNA segment coming from a single cell. A twelve day old mouse embryo is essentially a small mouse. There is no reason to believe that the small number of clones thus far isolated are giving a complete picture of the situation in the undifferentiated genome. We have suggested (Kabat et al. 1978) that sperm DNA carefully fractionated to remove somatic cells (see Schiurba and Nandi, 1979) might provide true un-differentiated genome DNA and that, with the proper probes and nucleotide sequencing, one might get evidence for the existence of small segments of DNA - our hypothesized mini-genes. Whether or not this proves eventually to be so, it is clear that a satisfying explanation of the generation of diversity must explain satisfactorily all the evidence upon which we have proposed the minigene hypothesis.

For additional insights about Paul Ehrlich see the "Paul Ehrlich Centennial," edited by R. W. Miner in the Annals of the New York Academy of Sciences, Vol. 59, pages 141-276, 1954.

ACKNOWLEDGMENTS

Work in the laboratories is supported by National Science Foundation Grant PCM 76-81029; by the Cancer Center Support grant (CA 13696) to the Institute of Cancer Research, Columbia University. The data base of variable region sequences is maintained in the PROPHET computer system (Raub, 1974) and is sponsored by the National Cancer Institute,

National Institute of Allergy and Infectious Diseases, National Institute of Arthritis, Metabolism and Digestive Diseases, and the National Institute of General Medical Sciences, Division of Research Resources (Contract no. NO1-RR-4-2117 and NO1-RR-8-2158), of the National Institutes of Health.

REFERENCES

Acton RT, Weinheimer PF, Hall SJ, Niedermeyer W, Shelton E, Bennett JC (1971). Tetrameric immune macroglobulins in three orders of bony fishes. Proc Natl Acad Sci USA 68:67.

Allen PZ, Kabat EA (1956). Immunochemical studies on dextrans. J Am Chem Soc 78:1890.

Ansari AA, Carta-Sorcini M, Mage RG, Appella E (1976). Studies on the structural localization of rabbit H chain allotypic determinants controlled by the a locus. J Biol Chem 251:6798.

Appella E (1971). Amino acid sequences of two mouse immunoglobulin lambda chains. Proc Natl Acad Sci USA 68:590.

Arakatsu Y, Ashwell G, Kabat EA (1966). Immunochemical studies on dextrans. V. Specificity and cross-reactivity with dextrans of the antibodies formed in rabbits to isomaltonic and isomaltotrionic acids coupled to bovine serum albumin. J Immunol 97:858.

Arrhenius S (1907). "Immunochemistry," New York:MacMillan.

Atassi MZ, Stavitsky AB (Ed.) (1978). "Immunology of Proteins and Peptides," New York: Plenum Press.

Barstad E, Farnsworth V, Weigert M, Cohn M, Hood L (1974). Mouse immunoglobulin heavy chains are coded by multiple germ line variable region genes. Proc Natl Acad Sci USA 71:4096.

Beale D, Feinstein A (1976). Structure and function of the constant regions of immunoglobulins. Quart Rev Biophysics 9:135.

Benjamini E, Micheli D, Young JD (1972). Antigenic determinants of proteins of defined sequences. Current Topics in Microbiol and Immunol 58:85.

Bennett LG, Glaudemans CPJ (1979). The affinity of a linear, α-D-(1→6)-linked D-glucopyranan (dextran) for homogeneous immunoglobulin A W3129. Carbohydr Res 72:315.

Ben-Sasson SA (1979). Immunoglobulin differentiation is dictated by repeated recombination sequences within the V-region prototype gene: a hypothesis. Proc Natl Acad Sci USA 76:4598.

Bernard O, Hozumi N, Tonegawa S (1978). Sequences of mouse immunoglobulin light chain genes before and after somatic changes. Cell 14:1133.

Brack C, Hirama M, Lenhard-Schuller R, Tonegawa S (1978). A complete immunoglobulin gene is created by somatic recombination. Cell 15:1.

Brack C, Tonegawa S (1977). Variable and constant parts of the immunoglobulin light chain genes of a mouse myeloma cell are 1250 nontranslated bases apart. Proc Natl Acad Sci USA 74:5652.

Brandt DCh, Jaton J-C (1978). Identical V_L region sequences of two antibodies from two outbred rabbits exhibiting complete idiotypic cross-reactivity and probably the same antigen-binding site fine structure. J Immunol 121:1194.

Braun DG, Huser H (1977). Rabbit anti-polysaccharide antibodies: structure and genetics. Prog Immunol Proc 3rd Int Cong Immunol p. 254.

Breathnach R, Benoist C, O'Hare K, Gannon F, Chambon P (1978). Ovalbumin gene: Evidence for a leader sequence in mRNA and DNA sequences at the exon- intron boundary. Proc Natl Acad Sci USA 75:4853.

Breinl F, Haurowitz F (1930). Chemische Untersuchung des Präzipitates aus Hämoglobin und Anti-Hämoglobin-Serum und Bemerkungen über die Natur der Antikörper. Z Physiol Chem 192:45.

Bretting H, Kabat EA, Liao J, Pereira MEA (1976). Purification and characterization of the agglutinins from the sponge Aaptos papillata and a study of their combining sites. Biochemistry 15:5029.

Burnet FM (1979). "The Clonal Selection Theory of Antibody Formation," Tennessee: Vanderbilt Univ Press.

Burstein Y, Schechter I (1978). Primary structures of N-terminal extra peptide segments linked to the variable and constant regions of immunoglobulin light chain precursors: implications on the organization and controlled expression of immunoglobulin genes. Biochemistry 17:2392.

Cameron D, Erlanger BF (1976). Nucleic acid reactive antibodies of restricted heterogeneity. Immunochemistry 13:263.

Capra JD (1976). The implications of phylogenetically associated residues and idiotypes on theories of antibody diversity. In Cunningham AJ (ed): "Antibody Diversity," New York: Academic Press, p 65.

Capra JD, Kehoe JM (1974). Variable region sequences of five human immunoglobulin heavy chains in the $V_H III$

subgroup: definitive identification of four heavy chain
hypervariable regions. Proc Natl Acad Sci USA 71:845.
Capra JD, Kehoe JM (1975). Hypervariable regions, idiotypy,
and the antibody-combining site. Adv Immunol 20:1.
Capra JD, Kindt TJ (1975). Antibody diversity: Can more
than one gene encode each variable region. Immunogenetics
1:417.
Capra JD, Tung AS, Nisonoff A (1977). Structural studies on
induced antibodies with defined idiotypic specificities.
V. The complete amino acid sequence of the light chain
variable regions of anti-p-azophenylarsonate antibodies
from A/J mice bearing a cross-reactive idiotype. J Immunol
119:993.
Catterall JF, O'Malley B, Robertson MA, Staden R, Tanaka Y,
Brownlee GC (1978). Nucleotide sequence homologies
at 12 intron-exon junctions in the chick ovalbumin gene.
Nature (London) 275:510.
Chersi A, Appella F, Carta S, Mage R (1979). The amino acid
sequence of a variable region of rabbit b4 light chain from
an anti-SIII antibody; comparison with light chain of the
same subgroup from anti-A variant carbohydrate antibodies
Mol Immunol 16:589.
Chipman DC, Grisaro V, Sharon N (1967). The binding of
oligosaccharide containing N-acetylglucosamine and N-acetyl-
muramic acid to lysozyme. J Biol Chem 242:4388.
Cisar J, Kabat EA, Dorner M, Liao J (1975). Binding properties of immunoglobulin combining sites specific for terminal
or non-terminal antigenic determinants in dextran. J Exp
Med 142:435.
Cisar J, Kabat EA, Liao J, Potter M (1974). Immunochemical
studies on mouse myeloma proteins reactive with dextrans
or with fructosans and on human antilevans. J Exp Med
139:159.
Crick F (1979). Split genes and RNA splicing. Science
204:264.
Crumpton MJ (1975). Protein antigens: The molecular basis
of antigenicity and immunogenicity. In Sela M (ed): "The
Antigens," New York: Academic Press, Vol II, p 1.
Darnell JE (1978). Implications of RNA·RNA splicing in
evolution of eukaryotic cells. Science 202:1257.
Davies DR, Padlan EA (1977). Correlations between antigen-
binding specificity and the three-dimensional structure of
the antibody combining sites. In Haber E, Krause RM (eds):
"Antibodies in Human Diagnosis and Therapy," New York:
Raven Press, p 119.

Davies DR, Padlan EA, Segal D (1975). Immunoglobulin
structures at high resolution. In Inman FP, Mandy WJ
(eds): "Contemporary Topics in Molecular Immunology,"
New York: Plenum Press 4:127.
Dayhoff MO (1972). "Atlas of Protein Sequence and Structure"
Washington, D.C.: National Biomedical Research Foundation
and supplements (1973) 1; (1976) 2; (1978) 3.
Dower SK, Dwek RA (1979). Phosphorus 31 nuclear magnetic
resonance probes for the combining site of the myeloma
protein 315. Biochemistry 18:3668.
Dreyer WJ, Bennett JC (1965). The molecular basis of anti-
body formation. A paradox. Proc Natl Acad Sci USA
54:865.
Dwek RA (1977). Structural studies in solution on the
combining site of the myeloma protein MOPC 315. In
Porter RR, Ada GL (eds): "Contemporary Topics in Molecular
Immunology," New York: Plenum Press, Vol 6, p 1.
Dwek RA, Wain-Hobson S, Dower S, Gettins P, Sutton B,
Perkins SJ, Givol D (1977). Structure of an antibody
combining site by magnetic resonance. Nature (London)
266:31.
Early PW, Davis MM, Kaback DB, Davidson N, Hood L (1979).
Immunoglobulin heavy chain gene organization in mice:
Analysis of a myeloma genomic clone containing variable
and α constant regions. Proc Natl Acad Sci USA 76:857.
Edelman GM (1970). The covalent structure of a human γG-
immunoglobulin. XI. Functional implications. Biochemistry
9:3197.
Edelman GM (1973). Antibody structure and molecular immunology. Science 180:830.
Edelman GM, Cunningham BA, Gall WE, Gottlieb PD, Rutishauser
U, Waxdal MJ (1969). The covalent structure of an entire
γG immunoglobulin molecule. Proc Natl Acad Sci USA
69:78.
Edelman GM, Gally JA (1962). The nature of Bence Jones
proteins. J Exp Med 116:207.
Edmundson AB, Ely KR, Girling RL, Abola EE, Schiffer M,
Westholm FA, Fausch MD, Deutsch HF (1974). Binding of
2,4-dinitrophenyl compounds and other small molecules to
a crystalline λ-type Bence Jones dimer. Biochemistry
13:3816.
Ehrlich P (1891a). Experimentelle Untersuchungen über
Immunität. I Uber Ricin. Deutsche Med Wochenschr p 976.
Ehrlich P (1891b). Experimentelle Untersuchungen über
Immunität II Über Abrin. Deutsche Med Wochenschr p 1218.

Ehrlich P (1900). On immunity with special reference to cell life. Croonian Lecture. Proc Roy Soc London Ser B 66:424.

Eisen HN, Karush F (1949). The interaction of purified antibody with homologous hapten. Antibody valence and binding constant. J Amer Chem Soc 71:363.

Engvall E, Perlmann P (1971). Enzyme linked immunosorbent assay (ELISA). Quantitative assay of immunoglobulin G. Immunochemistry 8:871.

Epp O, Colman P, Fehlhammer H, Bode W, Schiffer M, Huber R, Palm W (1974). Crystal and molecular structure of a dimer composed of the variable portions of the Bence Jones protein REI. Eur J Biochem 45:513.

Epp O, Lattman EE, Schiffer M, Huber R, Palm W (1975). The molecular structure of a dimer composed of the variable portions of the Bence-Jones protein REI refined at 2 Å resolution. Biochemistry 14:4943.

Feizi T, Kabat EA, Vicari G, Anderson B, Marsh WL (1971). Immunochemical studies on blood groups. XLIX. The I antigen complex: specificity differences among anti-I sera revealed by quantitative precipitin studies; partial structure of the I determinant specific for one anti-I serum. J Immunol 106:1578.

Feizi T, Wood E, Augé C, David S, Veyrières A (1978). Blood group I activities of synthetic oligosaccharides assessed by radioimmunoassay. Immunochemistry 15:733.

Fiers W, Contieras R, Haegeman G, Rogiers R, Vande Voorde A, Van Heuverswyn H, Van Herreweghe J, Volckaert G, Ysebaert M (1978). Complete nucleotide sequence of SV40 DNA. Nature (London) 273:113.

Gelzer J, Kabat EA (1964a). Specific fractionation of human antidextran antibodies. II. Assay of human anti-dextran sera and specifically fractionated purified antibodies by microcomplement fixation and complement fixation inhibition techniques. J Exp Med 119:983.

Gelzer J, Kabat EA (1964b). Specific fractionation of human antidextran antibodies. III. Fractionation of anti-dextran by sequential extraction with oligosaccharides of increasing chain length and attempts at subfractionation. Immunochemistry 1:303.

Gilmore-Hebert M, Hercules K, Komaromy M, Wall R (1978). Variable and constant regions are separated in the 10-kbase transcription unit coding for immunoglobulin κ light chains. Proc Natl Acad Sci USA 75:6044.

Gilmore-Hebert M, Wall R (1978). Immunoglobulin light chain mRNA is processed from large nuclear RNA. Proc Natl Acad Sci USA 75:342.

Givol D (1974). Affinity labeling and topology of the antibody combining site. Essays in Biochemistry 10:73.
Glaudemans CPJ (1975). The interaction of homogeneous im-
munoglobulins with polysaccharide antigens. Adv Carbohydr
Chem 31:313.
Godson GN, Barrell BG, Staden R, Fiddes JC (1978). Nucleotide sequence of bacteriophage G4 DNA. Nature (London)
276:236.
Goldstein IJ, Hayes CE (1978). The lectins: carbohydrate
binding proteins of plants and animals. Adv Carbohydr
Chem Biochem 35:128.
Goodman JW (1975). Antigenic determinants and antibody
combining sites. In Sela M (ed): "The Antigens," New
York: Academic Press, Vol III, p 127.
Grubb R (1956). Agglutination of erythrocytes coated with
"incomplete" anti-Rh by certain rheumatoid arthritic
sera and some other sera. The existence of human serum
groups. Acta Path Microbiol Scand 39:195.
Haber E (1970). Antibodies of restricted heterogeneity for
structural study. Fed Proc Fed Am Soc Exp Biol 29:66.
Haber E (1971). Homogeneous eluted antibodies. Induction,
characterization, isolation and structure. Ann N Y Acad
Sci 190:285.
Haber E, Margolies M, Cannon LE, Rosemblatt MS (1975).
Restricted clonal responses: A tool in understanding
antibody specificity. Miami Winter Symposium 9:303.
Haber E, Paulsen K (1974). The application of antibody to
the measurement of substances of physiological and phar-
macological interest. In Sela M (ed): "The Antigens,"
New York: Academic Press, Vol II, p 250.
Haimovich J, Eisen HN, Hurwitz E, Givol D (1972). Local-
ization of affinity-labeled residues on the heavy and
light chain of two myeloma proteins with anti-hapten
activity. Biochemistry 11:2389.
Haurowitz F, Breinl F (1933). Chemische Untersuchung der
Spezifischen Bindung von Arsanil-Eiweiss und Arsanil-
säure an Immunserum. Z physiol Chem 214:111.
Heidelberger M (1939). Quantitative absolute methods in
the study of antigen-antibody reactions. Bact Rev 3:49.
Heidelberger M (1946). Immunochemistry. In Green DE (ed):
"Currents in Biochemical Research," New York: Interscience
Publishers, Inc. p 453.
Heidelberger M (1956). "Lectures in Immunochemistry,"
New York: Academic Press.
Heidelberger M, Kendall FE (1979). The beginnings of quan-
titative immunochemistry. TIBS 4:168.

Hilschmann N, Craig LC (1965). Amino acid sequence studies with Bence Jones proteins. Proc Natl Acad Sci USA 53:1403.

Himmelweit F (Editor and Compiler) (1957). "The Collected Papers of Paul Ehrlich. Vol. II Immunology and Cancer Research." New York: Pergamon Press.

Hood L, Gray WR, Sanders BG, Dreyer WJ (1967). Light chain evolution. Cold Spring Harbor Symp Quant Biol 32:133.

Hood LW, Talmage DW (1970). Mechanism of antibody diversity: germ line basis for variability. Science 168:325.

Horejši V, Tichá M, Kocourek J (1977). Studies on lectins. XXI. Determination of dissociation constants of lectin-sugar complexes by means of affinity electrophoresis. Biochim Biophys Acta 499:290.

Horejši V, Tichá M, Kocourek J (1979). Affinity electrophoresis. TIBS 4:6.

How MJ, Brimacombe JS, Stacey M (1964). The pneumococcal polysaccharides. Adv Carb Chem 19:303.

Huser H, Braun DG (1978). Rabbit variable κ light chain regions: subgroups contain polypeptides encoded by multiple genes. Hoppe-Seyler's Z Physiol Chem 359:1473.

Inman JK (1974). Multispecificity of the antibody combining region and antibody diversity. In Sercarz EE, Williamson AR, Fox CF (eds): "The Immune System: Genes, Receptors, Signals," New York: Academic Press, p 37.

Inman JK (1978). The antibody combining region: speculations on the hypothesis of general multispecificity. In Bell GI, Perelson AS, Pimbley GH Jr., (eds): "Theoretical Immunology," New York: Marcel Dekker, Inc., p 243.

Jeanes A, Wilham CA, Jones .W, Tsuchiya HM, Rist CE (1953). Isomaltose and isomaltotriose from enzymatic hydrolysates of dextran. J Am Chem Soc 75:5911.

Jerne NK (1955). The natural-selection theory of antibody formation. Proc Natl Acad Sci USA 41:849.

Jerne NK (1974). Towards a network theory of the immune system. Ann Immunol (Inst Pasteur) 125C:373.

Jolley ME, Glaudemans CPJ, Rudikoff S, Potter M (1974). Structural requirements for the binding of derivatives of D-galactose to two homogeneous murine immunoglobulins. Biochemistry 13:3179.

Kabat EA (1939). The molecular weight of antibodies. J Exp Med 69:103.

Kabat EA (1954). Some configurational requirements and dimensions of the combining site of an antibody to a naturally occurring antigen. J Am Chem Soc 76:3709.

Kabat EA (1956). Heterogeneity in extent of the combining regions of human antidextran. J Immunol 77:377.

Kabat EA (1957). Size and heterogeneity of the combining sites of an antibody molecule. J Cell Comp Physiol 50:79 (Supplement 1).

Kabat EA (1960). The upper limit for the size of the human antidextran combining site. J Immunol 84:82.

Kabat EA (1961). "Kabat and Mayer's Experimental Immunochemistry" Second Ed. Illinois: Chas. C. Thomas.

Kabat EA (1968). Unique features of the variable regions of Bence Jones proteins and their possible relation to antibody complementarity. Proc Natl Acad Sci USA 59:613.

Kabat EA (1970). Heterogeneity and structure of antibody combining sites. Landsteiner Centennial Dec. 1968. Ann N Y Acad Sci 169:43.

Kabat EA (1976). "Structural Concepts in Immunology and Immunochemistry" Second Ed. New York: Holt, Rinehart and Winston.

Kabat EA (1978a). Dimensions and specificities of recognition sites of lectins and antibodies. J Supramol Struct 8:79.

Kabat EA (1978b). The structural basis of antibody complementarity. Adv Prot Chem 32:1.

Kabat EA (1979). Basic principles of antigen-antibody reactions. Adv Enzymol (in press).

Kabat EA, Berg D (1953). Dextran - an antigen in man. J Immunol 70:514.

Kabat EA, Heidelberger M, Bezer AE (1947). A study of the purification and properties of ricin. J Biol Chem 168:629.

Kabat EA, Liao J, Lemieux RU (1978). Immunochemical studies on blood groups. LXVIII. The combining site of anti-I Ma (group 1). Immunochemistry 15:727.

Kabat EA, Wu TT (1971). Attempts to locate complementarity-determining residues in the variable positions of light and heavy chains of immunoglobulins. Ann N Y Acad Sci 190:382.

Kabat EA, Wu TT, Bilofsky H (1976). Variable regions of immunoglobulin chains. Medical Computer Systems, Bolt, Beranek and Newman, Cambridge, Mass.

Kabat EA, Wu TT, Bilofsky H (1978). Variable region genes for the immunoglobulin framework are assembled from small segments of DNA - A hypothesis. Proc Natl Acad Sci USA 75:2429.

Kabat EA, Wu TT, Bilofsky H (1979a). "Sequences of immunoglobulin chains. Tabulation and analysis of amino acid sequences of precursors, V-regions, C-regions, J-chain, and β_2-microglobulin. Government Printing Office Publication NIH 80-2008.

Kabat EA, Wu TT, Bilofsky H (1979b). Evidence supporting somatic assembly of the DNA segments (minigenes), coding for the framework, and complementarity determining segments of immunoglobulin variable regions. J Exp Med 149:1299.

Karush F (1956). The interaction of purified antibody with optically isomeric haptens. J Am Chem Soc 78:5519.

Karush F (1962). Immunological specificity and molecular structure. Adv Immunol 2:1.

Khorana HG (1968). Synthesis in the study of nucleic acids. Biochem J 109:709.

Kindt TJ, Capra JC (1978). Gene-insertion theories of antibody diversity: A re-evaluation. Immunogenetics 6:309.

Klapper DG, Capra JD (1976). The amino acid sequence of the variable regions of the light chains from two idiotypically cross reactive IgM anti-gammaglobulins. Ann Immunol (Inst Pasteur) 127C:233.

Klotz IM (1953). Protein interactions. In Neurath H, Bailey K (eds): "The Proteins," 1B, 727, New York: Academic Press.

Köhler G, Milstein C (1976). Derivation of specific antibody-producing tissue culture and tumor lines by cell fusion. Eur J Immunol 6:511.

Konkel D, Tilghman S, Leder P (1978). The sequence of the chromosomal mouse β-globin major gene: Homologies in capping splicing and poly (A) sites. Cell 15:1125.

Krause RM (1970). The search for antibodies with molecular uniformity. Adv Immunol 12:1.

Kunkel HG (1965). Myeloma proteins and antibodies. Harvey Lectures 59:219.

Landsteiner K (1945). The specificity of serological reactions. Revised edition. Harvard, Cambridge, Mass. (1962) Paperback reprint, New York: Dover.

Leon MA, Young NM, McIntire KH (1970). Immunochemical studies of the reaction between a mouse myeloma macroglobulin and dextrans. Biochemistry 9:1023.

Lundblad A, Steller R, Kabat EA, Hirst J, Weigert MG, Cohn M (1972). Immunochemical studies of mouse myeloma proteins with specificity for dextran or for levan. Immunochemistry 9:535.

Mage RG (1977). Structure and expression of V_H and C_H allotypic determinants. In Mandel TE, Cheers C, Hosking CS, McKenzie IFC, Nossal GJV (eds): "Progress in Immunology III," Proceedings of the Third International Congress of Immunology, Australia: Australian Academy of Science, p 289.

Mage RG, Kabat EA (1963). The combining regions of the type III pneumococcus polysaccharide and homologous antibody. Biochemistry 22:1278.

Marrack JR, Smith FC (1932). Quantitative aspects of immunity reactions. The combination of antibodies with simple haptens. Brit J Exp Pathol 13:394.

Maurer PH (1953). Dextran an antigen in man. Proc Soc Exp Biol Med 83:879.

Max EE, Seidman JG, Leder P (1979). Sequences of five potential recombination sites encoded close to an immunoglobulin κ constant region gene. Proc Natl Acad Sci USA 76:3450.

Maxam AM, Gilbert W (1977). A new method for sequencing DNA. Proc Natl Acad Sci USA 74:560.

Melchers F, Potter M, Warner NL (eds) (1978). "Lymphocyte Hybridomas, Second Workshop on Functional Properties of Tumors of T and B Lymphocytes." New York: Springer.

Milstein C (1967). Linked groups of residues in immunoglobulin chains. Nature (London) 216:330.

Milstein C (1979). Remarks at the International Union of Immunological Societies. Symposium on Genetics of the Immune Response, Sesimbra, Portugal.

Milstein C, Brownlee GG, Harrison TM, Matthews MB (1972). A possible precursor of light chains. Nature New Biol 239:117.

Milstein C, Pink JRL (1970). Structure and evolution of immunoglobulins. Prog Biophys Mol Biol 21:209.

Milstein CP (1973). Crossing over and antibody diversity: the sequence of a new human κI light chain. FEBS Lett 30:40.

Niall HD, Edman P (1967). Two structurally distinct classes of kappa chains in human immunoglobulins. Nature (London) 216:262.

Nicolson GL, Blaustein J, Etzler ME (1974). Characterization of two plant lectins from Ricinus communis and their quantitative interaction with a murine lymphoma. Biochemistry 13:196.

Oudin J (1956). L' "allotypie" de certains antigenes proteidiques du serum. Comptes Rendus Acad Sci 242:2606.

Oudin J (1974). Idiotypy of antibodies. In Sela M (ed): "The Antigens," New York: Academic Press, Vol II, p 278.

Outschoorn IM, Ashwell G, Gruezo F, Kabat EA (1974). Immunochemical studies on dextrans. VIII. Specificity and cross-reactivity with dextrans of antibodies formed in rabbits to isomaltohexaonic acid coupled to bovine serum albumin. J Immunol 113:896.

Padlan EA (1977). Structural basis for the specificity of antigen-antibody reactions and structural mechanisms for the diversification of antigen-binding specificities.

Quart Rev Biophysics 10:35.
Padlan EA, Davies DR, Pecht I, Givol D, Wright C (1976).
Model building studies of antigen-binding sites. The hapten
binding site of MOPC-315. Cold Spring Harbor Symp Quant
Biol 41:627.
Pappenheimer AM, Robinson ES (1937). A quantitative study
of the Ramon diphtheria flocculation reaction. J Immunol
32:291.
Parker CW (1976). "Radioimmunoassay of Biologically Active
Compounds." New Jersey: Prentice Hall.
Parkhouse RME, Askonas BA, Dourmashkin RR (1970). Electron
microscopic studies of mouse immunoglobulin M; Structure
and reconstitution following reduction. Immunology 18:575.
Pedersen KO, Heidelberger M (1937). The molecular weight of
antibodies. J Exp Med 65:393.
Pereira MEA, Kabat EA (1979). Immunochemical studies on
lectins and their application to the fractionation of
blood group substances and cells. Critical Revs Immunol
(in press).
Phillips DC (1966). The three-dimensional structure of an
enzyme molecule. Scientific American 215 #11:78.
Poljak RJ, Amzel LM, Avey HP, Chen BL, Phizackerley RP,
Saul F (1973). Three dimensional structure of the Fab'
fragment of a human immunoglobulin at 2 Å. Proc Natl
Acad Sci USA 70:3305.
Poljak RJ, Amzel LM, Chen BL, Phizackerley RP, Saul F (1974).
The three dimensional structure of the Fab' fragment of
a human myeloma immunoglobulin at 2 Å resolution. Proc
Natl Acad Sci USA 71:3440.
Porter RR (1973). Structural studies of immunoglobulins.
Science 180:713.
Potter M (1972). Immunoglobulin-producing tumors and
myeloma proteins of mice. Physiological Revs 52:631.
Potter M (1977). Antigen binding myeloma proteins of
mice. Adv Immunol, New York: Academic Press 25:141.
Potter M, Mushinski EB, Rudikoff S, Glaudemans CPJ, Padlan
EA, Davies DR (1979). Structural and genetic basis of
idiotypy in the galactan-binding myeloma proteins. Ann
Immunol (Inst Pasteur) 130C:263.
Rabbitts TH (1978a). Primary sequence changes in the dif-
ferentiation of immunoglobulin genes. In Williamson R,
Garland PB (eds): Biochemical Society Symposium (in press).
Rabbitts TH (1978b). Evidence for splicing of interrupted
immunoglobulin variable and constant region sequences in
nuclear RNA. Nature (London) 275:291.

Rao DN, Rudikoff S, Krutzsch H, Potter M (1979). Structural evidence for independent joining region gene in immunoglobulin heavy chains from anti-galactan myeloma proteins and its potential role in generating diversity in complementarity-determining regions. Proc Natl Acad Sci USA 76:2890.

Raub WF (1974). The PROPHET system and resource sharing. Fed Proc 33:2390.

Reddy VB, Thummapay B, Dhar R, Subramanian KN, Zain BS, Pan J, Ghosh PE, Celma ML, Weissman S (1978). The genome of Simian virus 40. Science 200:494.

Richards FF, Konigsberg W (1973). Speculations - How specific are antibodies. Immunochemistry 10:545.

Rose SM, Kuehl WM, Smith GP (1977). Cloned MPC11 myeloma cells express two kappa genes, a gene for a complete light chain and a gene for the constant region polypeptide. Cell 12:453.

Ruckel ER, Schuerch C (1967). Chemical synthesis of a dextran model poly-α-(1$\rightarrow$6)-anhydro-D-glucopyranose. Biopolymers.5:515.

Rupley JA (1967). The binding and cleavage by lysozyme of N-acetyl-glucosamine oligosaccharides. Proc Roy Soc 167B:416.

Sakano H, Rogers JH, Hüppi K, Brack C, Traunecker A, Maki R, Wall R, Tonegawa S (1979a). Domains and the hinge region of an immunoglobulin heavy chain are encoded in separate DNA segments. Nature (London) 277:627.

Sakano H, Hüppi K, Heinrich G, Tonegawa S (1979b). Sequences at the somatic recombination sites of immunoglobulin light-chain genes. Nature (London) 280:288.

Sanger F, Air GM, Barrell BG, Brown NL, Coulson AR, Fiddes JC, Hutchison III CA, Slocombe PM, Smith M (1977). Nucleotide sequence of bacteriophage ϕX174 DNA. Nature (London) 265:687.

Saul FA, Amzel LM, Poljak RJ (1978). Preliminary refinement and structural analysis of the Fab' fragment from human immunoglobulin New at 2 Å resolution. J Biol Chem 25:585.

Schalch W, Wright JK, Rodkey S, Braun DG (1979). Distinct functions of monoclonal IgG antibody depend on antigen site specificities. J Exp Med 149:923.

Schechter B, Schechter I, Sela M (1970). Antibody combining sites to a series of peptide determinants of known structure. J Biol Chem 245:1438.

Schechter I, Wolf O, Zemell R, Burstein Y (1979). Structure and function of immunoglobulin genes and precursors. Fed Proc 38:1839.

Schepers G, Blatt Y, Himmelspach K, Pecht I (1978). Binding site of a dextran-specific homogeneous IgM: Thermodynamic and spectroscopic mapping by dansylated oligosaccharides. Biochemistry 17:2239.

Schiffer M, Girling RL, Ely KR, Edmundson AB $_0$(1973). Structure of a 'λ-type Bence Jones protein at 3 Å resolution. Biochemistry 12:4620.

Schiurba R, Nandi S (1979). Isolation and characterization of germ line DNA from mouse sperm. Proc Natl Acad Sci USA 76:3947.

Schlossman SF, Kabat EA (1962). Specific fractionation of a population of antidextran molecules with combining sites of various sizes. J Exp Med 116:535.

Segal DM, Padlan EA, Cohen GH, Rudikoff S, Potter M, Davies DR (1974). The three-dimensional structure of a phosphorylcholine-binding mouse immunoglobulin Fab and the nature of the antigen binding site. Proc Natl Acad Sci USA 71:4298.

Seidman JG, Leder P (1978). The arrangement and rearrangement of antibody genes. Nature (London) 276:790.

Seidman JG, Leder A, Edgell MH, Polsky F, Tilghman SM, Tiemeier DC, Leder P (1978a). Multiple related immunoglobulin variable-region genes identified by cloning and sequence analysis. Proc Natl Acad Sci USA 75:3881.

Seidman JG, Leder A, Nau M, Norman B, Leder P (1978b). Antibody diversity. The structure of cloned immunoglobulin genes suggests a mechanism for generating new sequences. Science 202:11.

Seidman JG, Max EE, Leder P (1979). A κ-immunoglobulin gene is formed by site-specific recombination without further somatic mutation. Nature (London) 280:370.

Smith AM, Potter M (1975). A BALB/c mouse IgA myeloma protein that binds Salmonella flagellar protein. J Immunol 114:1847.

Svehag S-E (1973). Structural features of immunoglobulins and complement protein Clq determined by electron microscopy. Third Int Convocation Immunol, Buffalo, New York: S. Karger-Basel, p 80.

Swan D, Aviv H, Leder P (1972). Purification and biological properties of biologically active messenger RNA for a myeloma light chain. Proc Natl Acad Sci USA 69:1967.

Takeo K, Kabat EA (1978). Binding constants of dextrans and isomaltose oligosaccharides to dextran-specific myeloma proteins determined by affinity electrophoresis. J Immunol 121:2305.

Talmage DW (1959). Immunological Specificity. Science 129:1643.

Tiselius A, Kabat EA (1939). An electrophoretic study of immune sera and purified antibody preparations. J Exp Med 69:119.

Tonegawa S, Brack C, Hozumi N, Schuller R (1977). Sequence of a mouse germ-line gene for a variable region of an immunoglobulin light chain. Proc Natl Acad Sci USA 74:3518.

Tonegawa S, Maxam AM, Tizard R, Bernard O, Gilbert W (1978). Sequence of a mouse germ-line gene for a variable region of an immunoglobulin light chain. Proc Natl Acad Sci USA 75:1485.

Torii M, Kabat EA, Weigel H (1966). Immunochemical studies on dextrans. IV. Further characterization of the determinant groups on various dextrans involved in their reactions with the homologous human antidextrans. J Immunol 96:797.

Turvey JR, Whelan WJ (1957). Preparation and characterization of isomaltodextrans. Biochem J 67:49.

Valbuena O, Marcu KB, Weigert M, Perry RP (1978). Multiplicity of germ-line genes specifying a group of related mouse κ chains with implications for the generation of immunoglobulin diversity. Nature (London) 276:780.

Valentine RC, Green NM (1967). Electron microscopy of an antibody-hapten complex. J Mol Biol 27:615.

van Heyningen WE, Bidwell E (1948). The biochemistry of the gas gangrene toxins. 4. The reaction between the α-toxin (lecithinase) and Clostridium welchii and its antitoxin. Biochem J 42:130.

Velick SF, Parker CW, Eisen HN (1960). Excitation energy transfer and the quantitative study of the antibody hapten reaction. Proc Natl Acad Sci USA 46:1470.

Vrana M, Rudikoff S, Potter M (1977). Heavy chain variable-region sequence from an inulin-binding myeloma protein. Biochemistry 16:1170.

Vrana M, Rudikoff S, Potter M (1979). The structural basis of a hapten-inhibitable κ-chain idiotype. J Immunol 122:1905.

Waldenström J (1944). Incipient myelomatosis or "essential" hyperglobulinemia with fibrinogenopenia a new syndrome. Acta Med Scand 117:216.

Waldenström J (1948). Zwei interessante Syndrome mit Hyperglobulinämie Purpura hyperglobulinaemica und Makroglobulinämie). Schweiz Med Wochenschr 78:927.

Wang B-C, Yoo CS, Sax M₀(1979). Crystal structure of Bence Jones protein Rhe (3 Å) and its unique domain - domain association. J Mol Biol 129:657.

Warner NL (1975). Autoimmunity and the pathogenesis of plasma cell tumor induction in NZB inbred and hybrid mice. Immunogenetics 2:1.

Watson JD (1976). "Molecular Biology of the Gene." Third Ed. Menlo Park, California: W. A. Benjamin.

Weigert MG, Cesari IM, Yonkovich SJ, Cohn M (1970). Variability in the lambda light chain sequences of mouse antibody. Nature (London) 228:1045.

Weigert M, Gatmaitan L, Loh E, Schilling J, Hood L (1978). Rearrangement of genetic information may product immunoglobulin diversity. Nature (London) 276:785.

Weigert M, Riblet R (1976). Genetic control of antibody variable regions. Cold Spring Harbor Symp Quant Biol 41:837.

Wood C, Kabat EA, Ebisu S, Goldstein IJ (1978). An immunochemical study of the combining sites of the second lectin isolated from Bandeiraea simplicifolia (BS II). Ann Immunol (Inst Pasteur) 129C:143.

Wu AM, Kabat EA, Weigert MG (1978). Immunochemical studies on dextran-specific and levan-specific myeloma proteins from NZB mice. Carbohydr Res 66:113.

Wu T.T, Kabat EA (1970). An analysis of the sequences of the variable regions of Bence Jones proteins and myeloma light chains and their implications for antibody complementarity. J Exp Med 132:211.

Wu TT, Kabat EA, Bilofsky H (1975). Similarities among hypervariable segments of immunoglobulin chains. Proc Natl Acad Sci USA 72:5107.

Wu TT, Kabat EA, Bilofsky H (1979). Some sequence similarities among mouse DNA segments that code for λ and κ light chains of immunoglobulins. Proc Natl Acad Sci USA 76:4617.

Yalow RS, Berson SA (1960). Immunoassay of endogenous plasma insulin in man. J Clin Invest 39:1157.

Zopf DA, Tsai C-M, Ginsburg V (1978). Antibodies against oligosaccharides coupled to proteins: characterization of carbohydrate specificity by radioimmune assay. Arch Biochem Biophys 185:61.

Session I.
Membrane Structure and Organization

Pages 49–68, Membranes, Receptors, and the Immune Response
© 1980 Alan R. Liss, Inc., 150 Fifth Avenue, New York, NY 10011

FUNCTION OF SURFACE IMMUNOGLOBULIN ON MURINE B CELLS

Jonathan W. Uhr and Ellen S. Vitetta

Department of Microbiology, University of Texas Southwestern Medical School Dallas, Texas 75235

It was postulated by Ehrlich (Ehrlich, 1900) and has been known for decades that antigen triggers lymphocytes that have antigen specific receptors on their surface to replicate and differentiate into antibody secreting cells. During the last decade, the antigen specific receptors on bursal derived lymphocytes (B cells) were formally identi- fied as immunoglobulin of various classes (isotypes) (re- viewed in Katz, 1977). The nature of the antigen specific receptors on T lymphocytes remains unknown. It appears reasonable, therefore, to select B cells for study of the mechanisms underlying triggering by antigen.

What is the importance of understanding these mech- anisms? Two major goals are to understand the transduction of immunologically induced activation and the induction of tolerance. The discrimination between signaling for trig- gering and tolerance is of considerable practical as well as theoretical importance, particularly, if we are eventually to intervene in clinical situations where there is unwanted antibody formation such as in autoimmune disease. There is another major issue, not as well appreciated, which is to understand the mechanisms that determine which pathway of differentiation is taken by a particular B cell subset after stimulation. For example, B lymphocytes can differentiate into plasma cells or into memory cells. It is unclear whether the B cell's decision to take one pathway versus another is programmed into the cell before stimulation with antigen or whether it results from the antigenic stimu- lation. If the decision has been made before contact with antigen, is it the class and quantity of the cell surface antigen specific receptors that are responsible for the programming?

Perhaps the first issue that should be raised is whether the initial triggering or tolerizing events in B cells occur on the cell surface. Because of the macromolecular nature of immunologic ligands, it has been assumed that the initial events in triggering take place on the cell surface and that a signal is transmitted subsequently through the cytoplasm to the appropriate chromosomes. This assumption appears to be a reasonable one but it does not preclude the possibility that B cells phagocytise antigens as do macrophages and that intracellular antigen could play a biological role. For example, antigens that are not easily degraded such as polysaccharides (reviewed in Katz, 1977), or d-amino acid copolymers (Katz, 1977) could be important in induction of tolerance by intercepting Ig-antigen specific receptors within the cell and thereby prevent them from becoming expressed on the cell surface. With this caveat in mind, we will assume that the molecular interactions at the B cell surface determine whether activation results.

There are two major approaches we have used to study signaling in B lymphocytes. The first approach is to determine the function of different subsets of B lymphocytes that are distinguished by their surface immunoglobin isotypes. In essence, we search for a correlation between a phenotype and a particular immunologic function e.g., what is the function of a cell that bears only IgM? These experiments involve either positive or negative selection. It is necessary to either enrich for a particular subset or delete it. The deletion is performed by killing the cell with antibody directed against a particular isotype in the presence of complement. This approach can give major clues with regard to function. The approach usually cannot give information about the role of the particular cell surface isotype in the response because most B cells carry 2 isotypes. The second approach is to remove or "blindfold" particular isotype receptors with specific antibodies and then determine the effect of this treatment upon immune responsiveness. The assumption of these experiments is that binding of receptor with antibody does not by itself signal the cell. This approach not only can give information about the role of a particular surface isotype in giving the response in question but if antibody to the isotype blocks the response, then the results indicate that that isotype is on the responder cell.

Early studies of the ontogeny of B cells in the mouse indicate that the first isotype to appear on the surface of B cells is IgM and that soon, thereafter, the majority of IgM positive cells acquire IgD and thereby bear both isotypes (reviewed in Vitetta and Uhr, 1978). The above observation led to the hypothesis (Vitetta and Uhr, 1975) that interaction of antigen with IgM on immature B cells leads to tolerance whereas interaction of antigen with cells bearing both isotypes leads to stimulation of B cells because of a triggering role played by the IgD receptor. Two major pieces of evidence have been obtained that support this idea. The first one is the effect of "blindfolding" B cells with either anti-μ or anti-δ on an in vitro primary IgM antibody response (Ligler et al., 1978). The plan of these experiments is shown in Fig. 1 and the results are described in Fig. 2. The results indicate that either anti-μ or anti-δ in sufficient concentrations can completely abolish the primary IgM response to thymus dependent (TD) antigens, i.e. the response to TNP and to SRBC stimulated by TNP-SRBC. Thus both IgM and IgD are essential for triggering TD precursors. Of course, a T cell signal is needed as well. In contrast, with TNP Brucella (TNP-BA) a class one TI antigen (Mosier, et al., 1979), anti-μ completely blocked the response whereas anti-δ had no effect (Ligler, et al., 1978).

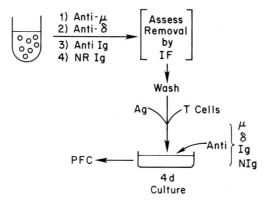

Fig. 1. Anti-Ig-Induced Blocking of the In Vitro Response

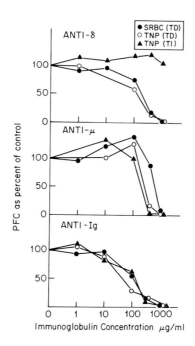

Fig. 2. Effect of antibody concentration on the
inhibition of in vitro IgM responses to TD (●,
SRBC; O, TNP) and TI (▲, TNP) antigens. Cells
were treated with the indicated antiserum and
GARIg under capping conditions and cultured with
an Ig fraction of the same antiserum used for
capping. Responses of control cultures incubated
without antibody, presented as PFC per 10^6
viable recovered cells, were as follows: anti-δ
capped, SRBC 3408, TNP(TD) 434, TNP (TI) 342;
anti-μ capped, SRBC 3905, TNP (TD) 445, TNP (TI)
215; anti-Ig capped, SRBC 2672, TNP (TD) 418,
TNP (TI) 506.

This experiment indicates, therefore, that both isotypes
are essential for stimulation of antibody formation by a TD
antigen and that the precursor bears both IgM and IgD. In
contrast, these blocking studies indicate that only the IgM
antigen-specific receptor is essential for an antibody response to the TI antigen, TNP-BA.

In adult mice, the vast majority of splenic B cells bear both IgM and IgD (Vitetta and Uhr, 1978) so it is not surprising that the TD precursor has that phenotype. In contrast, in neonates, the vast majority of B cells bear IgM only. The question arises as to whether the precursors of TD responses in neonates also bear IgD and require it for triggering? Table 1 includes the results using splenic cells from neonates. As can be seen, anti-δ completely blocked the responses to TNP and to SRBC stimulated by the TD antigen, TNP-SRBC.

Table 1. Effect of Treatment with Anti-δ on
the In Vitro TD Responses

Age of donor (B cells)	% B cells that are δ[+*]	$PFC/10^6$ viable cells			
		α-SRBC		α-TNP	
		Ig	anti-δ	Ig	anti-δ
49	83	5333	208	736	0
18	59	1476	0	284	0
7	3	302	0	29	0

* Goding et al. (1978) Transplant. Rev. 37:152.

What are the possible explanations for the observation that anti-δ does not block antibody responses to TNP-BA? One possibility is that the responder cells bear only IgM, and the second is that the responder cells bear both IgM and IgD but IgD in contrast to IgM is not essential for stimulation by TNP-BA.

To distinguish between these two interpretations, negative selection experiments were performed by Buck et al. (Buck et al., 1979). The plan of these experiments was very simple. It was to kill murine splenic populations with anti-δ and complement in order to eliminate all cells bearing IgD and to determine the effect on the resultant antibody response to TNP conjugated to TD and TI forms of immunogen.

The specificity of the hybridoma anti-δ serum (Pearson, et al., 1977) was critically examined. Thus, it was necessary to prove that the anti-δ did not react with a determinant also present on μ chain. This possibility was tested by treating lysates from radiolabeled murine splenocytes with the monoclonal anti-δ bound to sepharose and determining whether radiolabeled IgM was removed by this treatment. Fig. 3 summarizes the results of this experiment. Anti-δ removed the radioactive δ peak but not the μ peak. Anti-Ig (containing anti-κ activity) removed both the μ, δ and L chain peaks.

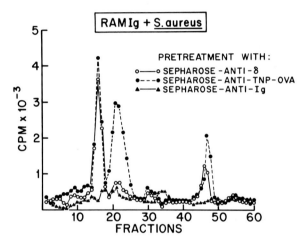

Fig. 3. Effect of treating lysates from radioiodinated C57BL/6 splenocytes with Sepharose coupled to RAMIg, RA-TNP-ovalbumin, or alloanti-δ on the subsequent recovery of IgM and IgD. Aliquots of lysate from radioiodinated cells were incubated with Sepharose-Ig, the immunoabsorbant removed by centrifugation, and the absorbed samples then treated with saturating amounts of RAMIg + S. aureus. Aliquots of each eluate were analyzed by SDS-PAGE. Pretreatment with 0, Sepharose-anti-δ; ●, Sepharose-anti-TNP; ▲, Sepharose-anti-Ig.

It was also important to prove that the anti-δ serum and C' killed all δ⁺ cells. Fig. 4 shows that anti-δ killed approximately 45% of splenic B cells [of the corresponding allotype (C57B1/6J) but not of the wrong allotype,(BALB/c)] and anti-μ approximately 60%, suggesting that all δ⁺ cells were lysed by the procedure employed.

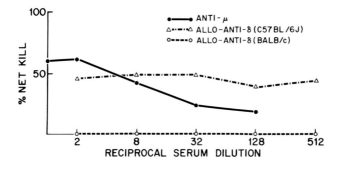

Fig. 4. Cytotoxicity of rabbit anti-μ and alloanti-δ on C57BL/6 and BALB/c splenocytes. Spleen cells were washed twice and resuspended in Eagle's minimal essential medium supplemented with 5% fetal calf serum. To 10^6 cells was added dilutions of alloanti-δ, RAμ (B6 only), normal mouse serum, normal rabbit serum, or medium, bringing the final vol to 0.05 ml per tube. After a 30-45-min incubation at 4°C, 0.05 ml of 40-50% rabbit complement (Pel-Freeze Biologicals, Inc., Rogers, Ark.) was added to each sample. Suspensions were incubated at 37°C for 30 min and then assessed for the presence of viable and dead cells by trypan blue exclusion. The results are expressed as the percent net kill where percent net kill = 100 (dead cells in experimental sample + [total cells in control sample - total cells in experimental sample])/ total cells in control sample - 100 X (dead cells in control sample/total cells in control). ●, anti-μ; Δ, allo-anti-δ(C57BL/6J); O, allo-anti-δ(BALB/c).

Using this antiserum, the results of negative selection experiments are shown in Table 2. As can be seen, approximately 3/4 of the antibody response to TNP-BA could be eliminated by prior treatment with cytotoxic anti-δ and C'. A slightly higher percentage of the response was abolished by killing with anti-μ or anti-Ig (containing anti-κ activity) and C'. The results are analogous to those obtained in the response to TNP-SRBC. Similar studies of the primary adoptive response to TNP-lipopolysaccharide (LPS) were performed. TNP-LPS is another antigen of the TI class 1 type. Again, the killing with anti-μ gave a somewhat greater

Table 2. % Inhibition of In Vitro Responses Following Depletion of B Cell Subsets

Treatment with C' + antibody against:	% Inhibition*	
	TNP-BA	TNP-SRBC
Adult** δ***	74	85
μ	85	90
μ + δ	93	97
Ig	90	85

*Calculated on the basis of the number of input cells prior to depletion

**Average of 2 experiments

***Average of 7 experiments

inhibition than that with anti-δ and, the results using TNP-LPS were strictly analogous with those using TNP-BA (Table 3).

These results indicate that the majority of precursors of the TI responders to TNP-BA or TNP-LPS bear both IgM and IgD. The difference between the extent of the inhibition of antibody responses by prior treatment with anti-μ compared to anti-δ could be significant. The difference could be due

Table 3.   Effect of C' and Anti-μ <u>vs</u> Anti-δ on the
           Primary Adoptive Response

| Antigen | Strain* | % Inhibition after treatment with C' and antiserum to | |
		δ	μ
TNP-LPS	BDF$_1$	—	96
	BDF$_1$	89	83
	C57BL/6	73	—
	C57BL/6	52	—
	AVERAGE	71	90
TNP-SRBC	BDF$_1$	96	99
	BDF$_1$	88	—
	C57BL/6	49	83
	C57BL/6	70	85
	AVERAGE	76	85

*BDF$_1$ treated with rabbit anti-δ

C57BL/6 treated with hybridoma anti-δ

to less effective killing by anti-δ compared to anti-μ, differentiation in culture of μ$^+$ cells to those bearing both
IgM and IgD or to a contribution to the TI response by cells
that bear IgM only.   If the latter explanation is correct,
then the extent of inhibition from prior killing with anti-δ
should be less in newborn mice.   The predominant B cell subset of newborn mice expresses IgM only (Vitetta and Uhr,
1978).   Buck and Vitetta (unpublished observations) demonstrated by means of the fluorescent activated cell sorter
that 3% of splenic cells from 3-5 days old mice bear small
amounts of IgD; in contrast, 25-30% bear IgM.   They, therefore, performed similar deletion experiments using neonatal
cells.

The data obtained (Table 4) were strictly analogous to
those observed using adult cells.   Thus, in the neonatal
mouse, even though the majority of cells bear only IgM, the
results indicate that the vast majority of B cells responding to TNP-BA bear IgD, <u>i.e.</u> they are derived from the
subset that accounts for 3% of splenic B cells.   In addition, the effect of anti-δ and C' pretreatment on the TNP-BA
response is not significantly different from the effect of

Table 4. Effect of C' and Anti-μ vs Anti-δ on the
Primary In Vitro Response

Age (days)	Prior treatment with C' and antiserum against	% Inhibition of Response TNP-BA	% Inhibition of Response TNP-SRBC
3		71	88
4	IgD	77	44
6		63	78
	AVERAGE	70	70
4		72	97
6	IgM	94	98
	AVERAGE	83	97

such treatment on the TNP response to the TD antigen, TNP-SRBC. No further evidence was obtained, therefore, to support the contention that cells lacking IgD contribute to the primary response against TNP-BA. The data do not exclude this possibility, but they provide no evidence to support it.

The finding that cells that bear both IgM and IgD are the major precursors for the response of at least two type 1 TI antigens even though IgD is not essential for triggering such cells is provocative. What features of TNP-BA allow it to bypass the requirement for an IgD receptor? The two most likely possibilities are its inherent mitogenicity or an increased epitope (TNP) density compared to TNP-SRBC.

There is a second finding that supports the idea that IgD plays a key role in triggering. Cambier et al. (Cambier, et al., 1976) and also Metcalf and Klinman (Metcalf and Klinman, 1976) reported independently on the susceptibility to tolerance induction of B cells from neonates compared to adults. We used an in vitro system of tolerance induction as shown in Fig. 5. The results using adult splenocytes and

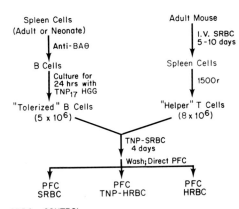

Fig. 5. Protocol for the induction and assay of tolerance in murine splenic B cells. HRBC, horse erythrocytes.

those from neonates indicate that adult B cells are highly resistant whereas neonatal B cells are highly susceptible to tolerance induction using TNP-human IgG as tolerogen and TNP-SRBC as immunogen (Fig. 6). These findings are consistent with Nossal and Pike's prediction of clonal abortion based on the differential susceptibility to tolerance of bone marrow and spleen cells (Nossal and Pike, 1978). We asked the question of whether acquisition of surface IgD on B cells contributes to this difference in tolerizability. In the following experiment, we exploited the finding that surface IgD has an unusual susceptibility to cleavage by papain, and can be cleaved in the hinge region at concentrations that do not remove IgM, H-2 or Ia molecules (Vitetta and Uhr, 1976). We treated adult B cells with papain under conditions in which IgD was cleaved but not IgM. The effect of this treatment on tolerizability was determined (Cambier, et al., 1977). As shown in Fig. 7, papain treatment rendered adult B cells more susceptible to induction of tolerance. If papain treated cells were incubated overnight, a good portion of IgD reappeared and the cells became refractory to tolerance induction. These results argue that acquisition of IgD contributes to the change in a cell from one that is easily tolerizable to one that is refractory to induction of tolerance. Similar

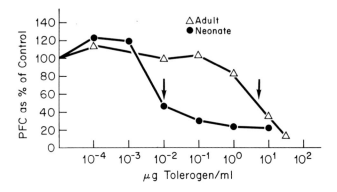

Fig. 6. Differential susceptibility of adult and neonatal TD precursors to induction of tolerance. Cells were treated with tolerogen (TNP-HGG) for 24 hours; washed and cultured with T cells and TNP-SRBC. PFC to TNP were determined after 4 days of culture. % inhibition of the responses was determined by comparing the PFC of tolerized and control cells which received no tolerogen.

results were obtained by ourselves (Vitetta, et al., 1977) and Scott et al. (Scott, et al., 1977) when treatment with anti-δ was used to remove surface IgD. Obviously, this is a more selective method for removing IgD. Treatment with anti-μ did not increase the tolerizability of the cells. This is additional evidence that IgM and IgD perform different functions in the same cell.

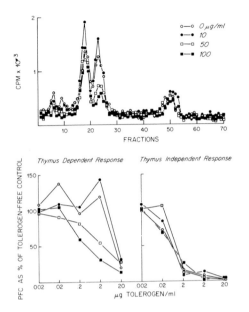

Fig. 7. SDS-polyacrylamide electropherogram (top panel) of cell membrane-associated immunoglobulins from murine splenocytes treated with varying concentrations of papain. Lower left panel:dose responses to tolerogen of papain-treated murine splenic B cells which are responsive to TD immunogen. Lower right panel: dose responses to tolerogen of papain-treated murine splenic B cells which are responsive to TI immunogen. Response to tolerogen-free controls (direct PFC/10^6 viable recovered cells) were as follows: Lower left; 0 papain 280, 10 µg papain 168, 50 µg papain 180, 100 µg papain 169. Lower right; 0 papain 695, 10 µg papain 690, 50 µg papain 557, 100 µg papain 654.

The observations on induction of tolerance together with those on triggering have led to the working hypothesis summarized in Fig. 8. Interaction of antigen with IgM on a neonatal cell results in the induction of tolerance. Interaction of antigen with IgM and IgD on an adult cell is essential for triggering with a TD antigen. A T cell signal is, of course, also needed (Katz, 1977). For certain TI

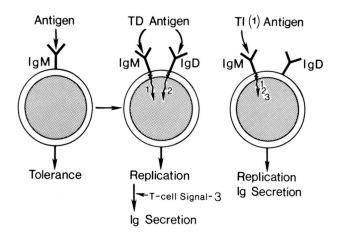

Fig. 8. Postulated role of surface immunoglobulin in delivering tolerogenic and triggering signals to B cells.

type I antigens, only interaction with surface IgM is required; some property of the antigen allows it to bypass the
requirement for both IgD and the T cell signal.

Certain points about this concept deserve further
comment. Thus, why does IgM on a neonatal cell give a
tolerizing signal after interaction with ligand and yet is
essential for triggering on an adult cell? One possibility
is that IgM may behave differently on an adult cell compared
to a neonatal cell. There is considerable evidence consistent with this possibility (Raff, et al., 1975; Sidman
and Unanue, 1979) that indicates that neonatal cells cannot
reexpress surface IgM after it has been removed by several
waves of capping whereas adult cells can. Another possibility is that IgD permits IgM to trigger; IgM cannot trigger by itself.

The role of Ig receptors in activating B cells is controversial. It is unlikely that the receptors just focus
antigen because treatment with affinity purified anti-μ can
directly activate B cells to replicate (Sieckmann, et al.,

1978; Sidman and Unanue, 1978). In particular, the findings of Parker (Parker, et al., 1979) that anti-Ig bound to acrylamide beads can stimulate B cells directly whereas phytohemagglutinin-conjugated beads also bind to B cells but do not stimulate them suggests that ligand-Ig receptor interaction is critical to the activation of B cells by specific antigen.

How is this concept reconciled with the capacity of T cell factors to stimulate B cells to differentiate into Ig secreting cells? In Parker's studies, anti-Ig bound to acrylamide beads did not lead to Ig secretion unless con-canavalin induced T cell factors were added after stimulation by Ig. One possible explanation, first advanced by Dutton (Dutton, 1975) is that antigen is needed for initial activation for replication, and that such activated cells then become capable of accepting T cell help which is required for differentiation into antibody secreting cells.

There is a provocative relationship of IgD to the reception of T cell help. As discussed above, surface IgD plays an essential role for antigens that utilize T cell help but does not appear to be required for those antigens that are not influenced by T cell help namely, some of the Type I-TI antigens. There is a second correlation between IgD and T cell help. Papain-treated cells that lack surface IgD give a plaque forming response to TNP-SRBC in which the high affinity clones are absent (Kettman, et al., 1979) (Fig. 9). If papain treated cells are incubated for 24 hours before immunogen is added, then much of surface IgD is reexpressed and high affinity clones are generated. It is possible that IgD is physically involved in some way in the reception of T cell help or alternatively, IgD and the receptor for T cell hlep may simply be coexpressed during differentiation. Clearly, the nature of this relationship warrants further investigation.

Ehrlich closed his Croonian Lecture to the Royal Society in 1900 in which he discussed his side-chain theory with a quotation from Bacon. He said...."we no longer find ourselves lost on a boundless sea but that we have already caught a distinct glimpse of the land which we hope, nay, which we expect, will yield rich treasures for biology and

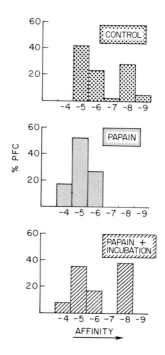

Fig. 9. Effect of papain treatment of spleen cells on the affinity of antibody made in response to TD antigen. Splenocytes from adult BDF_1 mice were treated with papain and cultured with TNP-SRBC and excess T cells. After 4 days, the affinity of the anti-TNP PFC was determined. In addition, an aliquot of papain treated cells was cultured for 24 h prior to the addition of antigen and T cells. The affinity of these anti-TNP PFC was determined as above, 4 days after the addition of antigen.

therapeutics." I must report 79 years later that we have still not landed; indeed, it is not yet clear which is the quickest way to shore. But we can expect that the distant terrain will be full of surprises and, as Ehrlich predicted, substantial rewards.

ACKNOWLEDGEMENTS

We are grateful to Drs. Cambier, Ligler, Yuan, Kettman and Buck for their invaluable collaborations, to M. Bagby, Y. Chinn, Y.M. Tseng, M. Neal and D. Richardson for technical assistance and Ms. J. Hahn for secretarial assistance. These studies were supported by NIH grants AI-12789, AI-11851 and AI-10967.

REFERENCES

Buck, LB, Yuan, D, Vitetta, ES (1979). A dichotomy between the expression of IgD on B cells and its requirement for triggering such cells with two T-independent antigens. J Exp Med 149:987.

Cambier, JC, Kettman, JR, Vitetta, ES, Uhr, JW (1976). Differential susceptibility of neonatal and adult murine spleen cells to in vitro induction of B-cell tolerance. J Exp Med 144:293.

Cambier, JC, Vitetta, ES, Kettman, JR, Wetzel, GM, Uhr, JW (1977). B cell tolerance III. Effect of papain-mediated cleavage of cell surface IgD on tolerance susceptibility of murine B cells. J Exp Med 146:107.

Dutton, RW (1975). Separate signals for the initiation of proliferation and differentiation in the B cell response to antigen. Transplant Rev 23:66.

Ehrlich, P (1900). "On Immunity with Special Reference to Life". Proc roy Soc.

Katz, D (1977). "Lymphocyte Differentiation, Recognition, and Regulation". New York: Academic Press.

Kettman, JR, Cambier, JC, Uhr, JW, Ligler, F, Vitetta, ES (1979). The role of receptor IgM and IgD in determining triggering and induction of tolerance in murine B cells. Immunol Rev 43:69.

Ligler, FS, Cambier, JC, Vitetta, ES, Kettman, JR, Uhr, JW (1978). Inactivation of antigen-responsive clones with antisera specific for IgM or IgD. J Immunol 120:1139.

Metcalf, ES, Klinman, NR (1976). In vitro induction of tolerance in neonatal murine B cells. J Exp Med 143:1327.

Mosier, DE, Goldings, EA, Bottomly, K (1979).In Cooper, M, Mosier, DE, Scher, Vitetta, ES (eds): "B Lymphocytes in the Immune Response", Elsevier North Holland, p. 91.

Nossal, GJV, Pike, BL (1978). Mechanisms of clonal abortion tolerogenesis. I. Response to immature hapten-specific B lymphocytes. J Exp Med 148:1161.

Parker, DC, Fothergill, JJ, Wadsworth, DC (1979). B lymphocyte activation by insoluble anti-immunoglobulin: induction of immunoglobulin secreton by a T cell-dependent soluble factor. J Immunol 123:931.

Pearson, T, Galfre, G, Ziegler, A, Milstein, C (1977). A myeloma hybrid producing antibody specific for an allotypic determinant on "IgD-like" molecules of the mouse. Eur J Immunol 7:684.

Raff, MC, Owen, JJT, Cooper, MD, Lawton, AR, Megson, M, Gathings, WE (1975). Differences in susceptibility of mature and immature mouse B lymphocytes to anti-immuno-globulin-induced immunoglobulin suppression in vitro. Possible implications for B-cell tolerance to self. J Exp Med 142:1052.

Scott, DW, Layton, JE, Nossal, GJV (1977). Role of IgD in the immune response and tolerance. I. Anti-δ pretreatment facilitates tolerance induction in adult B cells in vitro. J Exp Med 146:1473.

Sidman, CL, Unanue, ER (1978). Proliferative response to anti-IgM antibodies of various B lymphocyte subpopulations isolated by cell sorting. J Immunol 121:2129.

Sidman, CL, Unanue, ER (1979). Requirements for mitogenic stimulation of murine B cells by soluble anti-IgM antibodies. J Immunol 122:406.

Sieckmann, DG, Asofsky, R, Mosier, DE, Zitron, IA, Paul, WE (1978). Activation of mouse lymphocytes by anti-immunoglobulin. I. Parameters of the proliferative response. J Exp Med 147:814.

Vitetta, ES, Cambier, JC, Ligler, FS, Kettman, JR, Uhr, JW (1977). B cell tolerance. IV. Differential role of surface IgM and IgD in determining tolerance suscepti-bility of murine B cells. J Exp Med 146:1804.

Vitetta, ES, Uhr, JW (1975). Immunoglobulin-receptors re-visited. Science 189:964.

Vitetta, ES, Uhr, JW (1976). Cell surface immunoglobulin. XIX. Susceptibility of IgD and IgM on murine spleno-cytes to cleavage by papain. J Immunol 117:1579.

Vitetta, ES, Uhr, JW (1978). IgD and B cell differentiation. Immunol Rev 37:50.

UNKN: In what species was the formation of monoclonal IgD induced?

Uhr: Milstein provided us with murine monoclonal antibodies specific to the $Ig5^a$ allotype of IgD.

Gearhart: Layton and Nossal have recently published that cells that are IgD^- are as resistant to tolerance induction as cells that are IgD^+. What is the mechanism?

Uhr: These authors separated splenocytes from 19-day-old neonates into IgD^+ and IgD^- subsets by means of the fluorescence-activated cell sorter. They claim that 50% of the cells were delta-positive and 50% delta-negative. We have examined similar strains and found that 90% of B cells are IgD^+ at this time! Hence, we believe they have included in their IgD^- subset a large proportion of IgD^+ cells, thereby rendering their conclusions invalid. We believe we can explain how this situation came about. Their selection of an arbitrary cut-off point and their failure to discard fractions around the cut-off point may be responsible. A second major problem with their studies is that B cells treated with two layers of anti-body and passed through cell sorters are damaged and their subsequent functions reduced. They do not have a satisfactory quantitative method for dealing with this problem and therefore for comparing "delta-negative" subsets which were not bound by antibody with the delta-positive subset. A third problem is that anti-delta-coated cells may home differently than "delta-negative" cells in the Klinman fragment assay which they used for some of their experiments.

Hood: Only 3% of 5-day neonatal cells bear delta. Yet, anti-delta blocked their response. Are you saying that FACS is not sensitive? That the cells actually have delta?

Uhr.   No. We conclude that the precursors are from the 3%, not the 97%.

Bona: The fact that delta is not required for T independence is based on TNP Brucella experiments. What about other T-independent antigens, like TNP-Ficoll?

Uhr: The response to TNP-Ficoll, a Type 2 thymus-independent antigen, is blocked by anti-delta. Type 2 TI antigens apparently behave like TD antigens with regard to IgD. I want to emphasize that many TI-2 antigens can accept T cell help. For example, the in vitro antibody response to TNP-Ficoll can be raised ten-fold with T cell help, as shown by Jack Kethman. I find the term "thymus-independent" unsatisfactory for that reason.

Coutinho: I assume that you consider IgM and IgD to have identical specificity. How can a single cell with IgM and IgD distinguish the TNP-distinct carriers?

Uhr: They might distinguish the epitope density, or the inherent mitogenicity might be detectable by other molecules on the B cells.

Pages 70—94, Membranes, Receptors, and the Immune Response
© 1980 Alan R. Liss, Inc., 150 Fifth Avenue, New York, NY 10011

MOLECULAR IDENTIFICATION AND PROPERTIES OF TWO CELL SURFACE RECEPTORS PLAYING ROLES IN MITOGENESIS AND EPIGENESIS

C. Fred Fox, Beate Landen* and Michael Wrann*#

Molecular Biology Institute and the Department of Microbiology, University of California, Los Angeles, CA 90024, USA

SUMMARY

Studies leading to the identification of cell surface receptor macromolecules which specifically recognize a hormone, epidermal growth factor (EGF), or gp70, the coat antigen of the C-type RNA tumor viruses, have been described. EGF receptors are internalized and processed by lysosomal protease action after interaction of receptor and EGF. Other hormones, which resemble EGF in their ability to trigger mitogenesis in cultured cells, interact with the EGF receptor in a yet to be defined, but probably indirect way, decreasing the number of EGF binding sites on the cell surface. The evidence at this point indicates that these hormones interact with EGF receptors through the communal utilization of a shared cellular mechanism for internalization of their receptors and the EGF receptors.

The receptor for gp70 is not internalized in response to gp70 binding, but is instead shed into the medium by cultured cells. This receptor protein BPgp70 has now been isolated and purified to apparent homogeneity. Antibodies to BPgp70 completely block gp70 binding to cells at low concentration, indicating that BPgp70 is the physiological receptor for gp70.

* Fellows of the Max Kade Foundation
# Current Address: Sandoz Forschungsinstitut, Brunner Strasse 59, A-1235 Wien, Austria

INTRODUCTION

Both immunologists and cell biologists study regulation of cell growth and differentiation at two levels: at
the endocrine level, where ligands secreted by one population of cells influence events in another; and at the
level of direct intercellular contact. Our laboratory has
approached both these areas through the identification and
characterization of cell surface receptors.

A number of polypeptide hormones are effective induc-
ers of cell growth and share the property of stimulating
quiescent cells to synthesize DNA and multiply in number
when provided in the culture medium at less than nM concentration (Gospodarowicz and Moran, 1977; Ross and Vogel,
1978; Carpenter and Cohen, 1979). Epidermal growth factor
(EGF) is one of the best characterized of these hormones
(Carpenter and Cohen, 1979). It is also one of the most
effective hormones for binding studies with cells or isolated membranes; ninety percent or more of the EGF that
binds does so specifically to EGF receptors. Since EGF
receptors are present on the cell surface at a relatively
high density, they were ideal candidates for initial attempts at receptor affinity labeling (Das et al., 1977).
Our initial success in specifically radiolabeling the EGF
receptor has led to a better understanding of its down
regulation behavior when cells are exposed to hormone (Das
and Fox, 1978; Fox and Das, 1979; Fox et al., 1979). In
this report we describe another response of the EGF receptor, its modulation by polypeptide mitogenic hormones
other than EGF. These studies point to the existence of
"communities" of mitogenic hormone receptors that cluster
together on the cell surface.

The interactions between C-type viruses and their host
cells provide a useful prototype for the study of intercellular recognition. Both components of the interacting
system, the viral antigen and its receptors, are membrane
associated. The viral antigen, gp70, has been solubilized
and purified to apparent homogeneity (Ihle et al., 1976;
Moennig et al., 1974; Strand and August, 1973). In this
form, it retains binding activity for its specific recognition sites on cells or isolated cell surface membranes
(DeLarco and Todaro, 1976; Bishayee et al., 1978; Kalyanaraman et al., 1978; Bishayee and Strand, 1979). The major
envelope glycoproteins (gp70's) of the murine C-type viruses, comprise a large polymorphic family of antigens which
carry the type-, group- and interspecies-specific determin-

ants that provide the basis for viral classification (Strand and August, 1974). Elder, et al. (1977) have presented fingerprinting evidence that shows that structurally different species of gp70 are expressed by mouse gene-encoded proviruses as differentiation antigens. This raises the possibility that the receptors for these different gp70 species comprise a second polymorphic family of proteins that has arisen through a parallel evolutionary process. We report here the identification and preliminary characterization of a receptor protein for the gp70 of Rauscher murine leukemia virus (RMuLV).

MATERIALS AND METHODS

Growth of Cells

Murine 3T3 cell systems were used in the studies described here. Clone 42 Swiss mouse 3T3 cells (from George Todaro) were used in studies on EGF receptors. In studies on the receptors for Rauscher murine leukemia virus (RMuLV), we used a population of cells derived from clone 31 BALB/c 3T3 cells (American Type Culture Collection). Cells were grown on Dulbecco's modified Eagle's Minimal Essential Medium (DMEM) supplemented with 10% fetal calf serum. In physiological studies on EGF receptor kinetics, the cells were incubated for 24 hr prior to hormone addition in DMEM + 0.5% fetal calf serum. Cells for EGF receptor studies were grown to approximately 80% confluence; cells used for studies on gp70 receptors were grown to confluence.

Preparation and Radiolabeling of EGF and gp70

Rauscher murine leukemia virus gp70 was prepared by the method of Strand and August (1976) and contained a single gp70 band with no significant contaminating polypeptides upon characterization by sodium dodecyl sulfate polyacrylamide gel electrophoresis. Radioiodinated preparations of gp70 were prepared essentially as described by Markwell and Fox (1978), and had a specific activity of approximately 10^4-10^5 cpm/ng. Epidermal growth factor was prepared by the method of Savage and Cohen (1972) from male mouse submaxillary glands and radioiodinated by a published procedure (Das et al., 1977). The specific activity was approximately 10^5 cpm/ng.

Specific Binding of Labeled EGF and gp70

Specific binding of radioiodinated EGF was measured by previously described procedures. The Swiss 3T3 cells had a receptor density of approximately 150,000 binding sites per cell. Specific gp70 binding was determined essentially as described by Bishayee et al. (1978). All binding assays for gp70 or BPgp70 were conducted in DMEM containing 0.1 mg/ml of bovine serum albumin. The 0.3 ml binding assay system contained 100 ng of labeled gp70. Specific binding was assayed at 24° unless otherwise specified, and was the difference in binding in the absence and presence of 1 ug of unlabeled gp70. Specific binding was generally not less than 80% of total binding.

Preparation of BPgp70

BPgp70 was prepared from spent culture medium used for the growth of BALB/c 3T3 cells. This medium was concentrated by lyophilization, and the concentrated medium was dialyzed and applied to a gp70 Sepharose affinity column. The BPgp70 was eluted from the column in a solution containing high salt concentration, and this was dialyzed against dilute phosphate buffered solution. The preparations used in the experiments described here were not purified further and contained albumin as a major contaminant (approximately 50% of the total protein). The precise procedural details for BPgp70 preparation will be described elsewhere (Landen and Fox, submitted for publication). Radiolabeled BPgp70 was prepared by the chloroglycoluril method (Markwell and Fox, 1978). The specific activity of radioiodinated BPgp70 was 1×10^5 cpm/ug of protein. Specific binding of BPgp70 was the difference in binding occurring in the absence and presence of 50 ug of BPgp70, and was generally not less than 75% of total binding. The labeled albumin contaminant in the preparation did not contribute significantly to the bound radioactivity.

RESULTS AND DISCUSSION

The EGF Receptors

The decreased cellular capacity to bind a hormone after cells have been incubated with it is a commonly observed phenomenon. This "down regulation" of binding activity has been observed with EGF, insulin and human growth hormone to name but a few examples. One of the models proposed to explain this phenomenon was based on observations that degradation of bound, radiolabeled EGF accompanied the loss of cellular EGF binding activity, and that the degredation of the EGF was blocked by a drug which was a known inhibitor of lysosomal protease action in cells (Carpenter and Cohen, 1976). This model proposed that EGF receptors were internalized by cells and degraded in the lysosomes. One of the experiments which provided a direct test of this hypothesis, using the photoaffinity couplers PAPDIP & NAPEDE is described in Figure 1. High specific activity radiolabeled EGF was first bound covalently to EGF receptors on viable cells at low temperature to arrest receptor down regulation (Das and Fox, 1978). The temperature was then raised to permit down regulation of receptor to proceed. As shown in Figure 1A the labeled receptor was lost gradually during this incubation, and this loss of radioactivity in the receptor band was accompanied by a quantitative parallel loss of cellular EGF

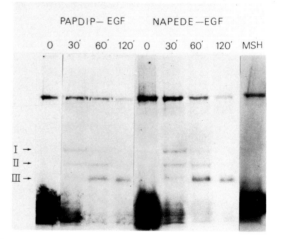

1A

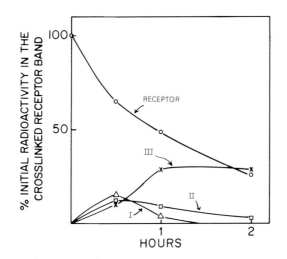

1B

Figure 1A. (OPPOSITE). Metabolic fate of affinity labeled EGF receptors on viable murine 3T3 cells. Autoradiograph of an acrylamide slab electrophoretic gel showing EGF receptors affinity labeled on viable cells at 0^0 with ^{125}I-EGF-PAPDIP, followed by incubation of the cells at 37^0. Viable Swiss 3T3 cells were incubated at 0^0 in the dark with a photoaffinity reagent of ^{125}I-EGF to achieve saturation binding with EGF receptors. The samples were then photolyzed to couple EGF and its receptors covalently. Two different photoaffinity reagents were used: PAPDIP, which couples to the amino terminus of EGF; and NAPEDE, which couples to carboxyl residues. After photolysis, some cell monolayers were incubated at 37^0 for an additional 30-120 min prior to solubilization in sodium dodecyl sulfate solution for gel electrophoresis. An additional sample (MSH) was boiled in 5% 2-mercaptoethanol prior to electrophoresis. The single band shows that the high molecular weight receptor is not a disulfide linked oligomer. From Das and Fox (1978).

Figure 1B. (ABOVE). Quantitative distribution of label in the receptor band and in the proteolytic products (bands I, II and III) that are derived from EGF receptors. The regions in the electrophoretic gel corresponding to receptor and Bands I, II and III were excised, and the radioactivity was determined. From Das and Fox (1978).

binding activity (Das and Fox, 1978). The loss of labeled receptor was also accompanied by the appearance of three receptor-derived bands of lower molecular weight. These enjoy a precursor-product relationship with receptor (Figure 1B). These bands cofractionated with the lyso-somes upon density gradient separation of the organelles produced by cellular disruption, but the receptor band separated solely with the cell surface membrane fraction (Das and Fox, 1978). The internalization and proteolytic degradation of receptor was not a response to the affinity labeling procedure. The same degradation products were revealed intralysosomally when the photolysis step was performed last so that the only EGF-receptor complexes formed would be those present during the photolysis step. Formation of the lower molecular weight receptor-derived bands has also been observed in cells where coupling of EGF to receptor occurred through the naturally occurring "direct linkage" process (Linsley et al., 1979; Baker et al., 1979).

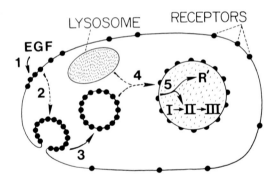

Figure 2.
Schematic representation of the fate of EGF and its recep-tors after EGF is incubated with cells. The binding of EGF to receptors 1) results in enhanced clustering of EGF re-ceptors 2) leading to their internalization in pinocytic vesicles 3). These vesicles then fuse with lysosomes 4) in which the internalized EGF receptors and the associated EGF are degraded by lysosomal protease action 5). Product R' is a polypeptide of approximately 80,000 daltons which turns over slowly once formed. From Fox and Das, (1979).

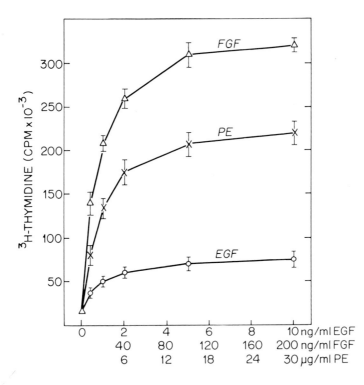

Figure 3. Stimulation of DNA synthesis in murine 3T3 cells after incubation with the mitogenic hormones EGF, FGF (fibroblast growth factor) and PDGF (platelet derived growth factor, supplied here as PE, the heated, clarified human platelet extract described by Antoniades and Scher (1975). The incorporation of ^{3}H-thymidine into DNA (Das and Fox, 1978) was determined during a one hr incubation period 24 hr after the cells had been exposed to the indicated mitogenic hormones. All cells were incubated for 24 hr in DMEM + 0.5% fetal calf serum prior to the addition of hormones at the concentrations indicated. From Fox, et al. (1979b).

The receptor-related events which transpire when EGF is added to cells are described schematically in Figure 2. EGF addition and binding to receptor leads first to receptor clustering, which has been monitored using flourescent (Haigler, et al., 1978; Maxfield et al., 1978) or ferritin labeled (Haigler et al., 1979) EGF derivatives to reveal the distribution of EGF binding sites. The observation of the eventual fate of these marker derivatives in the lysosomes supports the view that receptors and EGF are cotransported to the lysosomes and degraded there. The internalization and transport of labeled ligands to the lysosomes is not restricted to EGF. When differentially fluorescent labeled EGF, insulin and alpha $_2$-macroglobulin are added together to cells, the added species are internalized, appearing together in internalized vesicles (Maxfield, et al. 1978). This gives rise to the proposal that receptors may share common pathways for intracellular transport.

EGF is but one of a heterogeneous group of polypeptide mitogenic hormones which stimulate DNA synthesis in cultured cells. With cells of the Swiss mouse clone 42 line, EGF is less effective as a mitogen than fibroblast growth factor (FGF) or platelet derived growth factor (PDGF). The response of Swiss clone 42 3T3 cells to these three hormones is described in Figure 3. These data compare well with the results of nuclear labeling experiments performed autoradiographically (not shown). PDGF or FGF stimulate nearly 100% of the cells to enter the S phase of the cell cycle, but less than 50 of the cells to respond similarly to EGF (P. Linsley, unpublished results). The induction of DNA synthesis in Swiss 3T3 cells by these three hormones could occur through their acting on a single receptor. This led us to test for perturbations in EGF binding activity by FGF, PDGF or both. Since reliable specific binding assays have not been developed for either FGF or PDGF, reciprocal tests were not performed. Since

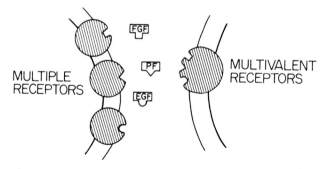

Figure 4. Scheme contrasting concepts of multiple vs. multivalent hormone receptors. See text for details.

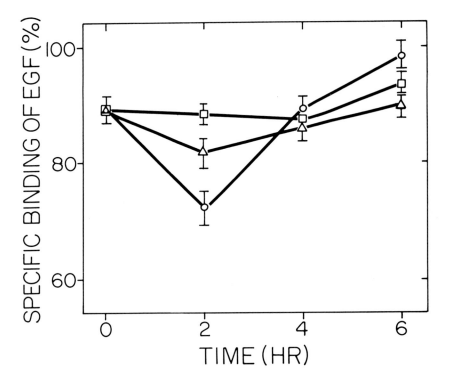

Figure 5. Transient down regulation of EGF receptors by FGF. Cells which had been incubated with 0.02 nM EGF in DMEM + 0.5% calf serum to achieve a partly (10%) down regulated steady state of EGF binding activity were treated with 0, 50 or 100 ng/ml of purified pituitary FGF, (supplied courtesy of D. Gospodarowicz, Univ. of California, Medical Center). Samples were processed for assay of EGF binding activity at the indicated times by aspirating the medium from the cells and washing the cells three times prior to addition of 10 nM radiolabeled EGF.

all three hormones induce similar effects on cells, a test for FGF- or PDGF-induced perturbation of EGF binding activity could reveal the existence of a common receptor which shares binding sites for all three, i.e., a multivalent receptor (Figure 4). Alternatively, the failure to

observe this predicted response might indicate the existence of multiple receptors which share no apparent direct
interaction of these hormones. The response of the EGF
receptors to FGF is shown in Figure 5 and reveals a phenomenon that corresponds to neither of the stated proposi-
tions. FGF does down regulate EGF receptors, but it does
so transiently. EGF receptor down regulation reached a
maximum 2 hr after FGF addition, rebounding to initial and
even greater levels, within an additional 2-4 hr. This
down regulation behavior is unlike that which occurs in
response to EGF, where down regulation of EGF receptors
occurs to a minimal level and remains there so long as the
EGF concentration is not changed (Das and Fox, 1978; Aharonov et al., 1978). Another unusual property of the transient down regulation of EGF receptors by FGF is the syn-
ergistic effect of EGF in this response. In the experiment shown, the EGF receptors were in a state of equilibrium for down regulation with a small amount of EGF. When
this experiment was done without EGF addition, no down
regulation of EGF receptors was observed at these levels
of FGF. Our observations on transient down regulation
lead to the conclusion that the EGF and FGF receptors are
localized on different polypeptide chains, but share a
common component required for their internalization (Fox
et al., 1979a).
    The response of the EGF receptors to PDGF is more pro-
nounced, with 60% of the EGF receptors participating in
transient down regulation (Wrann, Vale and Fox, manuscript
in preparation). We also recently have observed that a
substantial fraction of the EGF receptors exist in very
high molecular weight structures that are not disrupted in
nonionic detergent solution (P. Linsley, manuscript in
preparation). The formation of clustered regions of EGF
receptors has also been observed untrastructurally with
ferritin-labeled EGF on cells not exposed previously to
EGF (Haigler et al., 1979). These data indicate that
transient down regulation might occur through the enhanced
internalization of preexisting clusters of receptors in
response to any hormone that is reactive with one of the
receptor species in the clusters.
    The current status of our understanding of the kine-
tics of EGF receptor turnover are illustrated in Figure
6. EGF receptors exist in an equilibrium state which is a
balance between receptor synthesis and turnover. The addition of inhibitors of protein synthesis to cells results
in a rapid (half time = 6 hr in Swiss 3T3 cells) loss of

EGF binding activity (Aharonov et al., 1978; Fox et al., 1979b) which has an initial rate similar to that of the initial rate of restoration of EGF binding activity following maximal EGF-induced down regulation of EGF receptors (Fox et al., 1979b). This steady state level of receptor display can be modified in at least two ways: First, by EGF which gives rise to down regulation with the establishment of a new, lower steady state receptor level; Second, by hormones such as FGF or PDGF, which give rise to transient down regulation of EGF receptors. While the changes in receptor levels brought about by transient down regulation must certainly affect cell physiology, it is not possible at this point to predict the direction of the response. If the EGF receptors which are transiently down regulated by FGF or PDGF are "spare" receptors and refractory to EGF for induction of the biological response(s), transient down regulation might enhance the response of the remaining, responsive EGF receptors to EGF. On the other hand, if the receptors inactivated by FGF or PDGF are those which respond to EGF by producing the "second

Figure 6. EGF receptor turnover in the absence and presence of EGF or other mitogenic polypeptide hormones. After Fox, et al. (1979b)

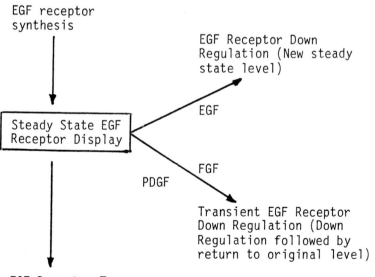

messengers" of hormone action, the effects of transient receptor down regulation by FGF or PDGF would reduce cellular responsiveness to EGF. This last proposal has obvious consequences in a system where two receptors share an internalization mechanism and are competitors for inducing alternative directions of differentiation of a single stem cell class.

The gp70 Receptors

Solubilization and purification of gp70 (Strand and August, 1973; Moennig et al., 1974; Ihle et al., 1976) the major viral antigen of Rauscher MuLV (RMuLV), has led to the demonstration of its specific binding to cells or isolated membranes by three independent groups of investigators (DeLarco and Todaro, 1976; Bishayee et al., 1978; Kalyanaraman et al., 1978; Bishayee and Strand, 1979). All have reported saturable binding with K values less than 10^{-8}M. Both binding and retention of bound gp70 by cells or membranes requires Ca++, and bound gp70 does not readily dissociate from cells when gp70 is withdrawn from the medium under otherwise optimal conditions for binding (Bishayee et al., 1978; Kalyanaraman et al., 1978).

A typical time course for gp70 binding to BALB/c 3T3 cells is shown in Figure 7. Maximal binding is achieved in approximately 2 hr at 24o. When gp70 is withdrawn at various times and the courses of dissociation of gp70 from cells followed, two kinetic components are revealed: one represents dissociable, and the second, undissociable gp70 binding. The amount of dissociable gp70 remained relatively constant throughout the experiment, but the fraction of dissociable readily was relatively constant as a function of the temperature of binding and dissociation (Figure 8). Since association experiments reveal only a single kinetic component (Bishayee et al., 1978; Kalyanaraman et al., 1978), the basis for the existence of these two classes of binding is not clear. Binding of gp70 at 37o presents an interesting curve which is reminiscent of the curves obtained when down regulation of EGF receptors occurs at 37o during incubation of cells with EGF, leading to EGF degradation (Carpenter and Cohen, 1976; Aharonov et al., 1978). However, with gp70, this behavior does not represent down regulation. At 37o, the gp70 that is lost from cells is largely intact. Bound gp70 has been reported to be not degraded extensive-

DISSOCIATION OF ^{125}I-gp70
FROM BALB/C 3T3 CELLS

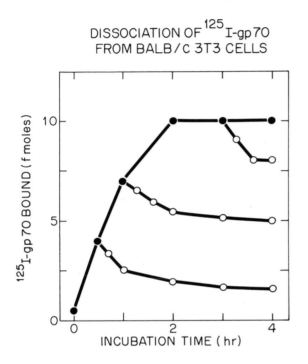

Figure 7. Kinetics of gp70 binding to cells.
Association of gp70 with cells. Specific binding of Rauscher MuLV gp70 to murine 3T3 cells and dissociation of the specifically bound ligand. BALB/c 3T3 cells (1 x 10^5/cm^2 surface area) were incubated with 100 ng of ^{125}I-gp70 in 300 ul of reaction buffer (50 mM BES, pH 7.3, 1% BSA in DMEM) at 24°C for the indicated time periods (●——●).
Dissociation of specifically bound gp70 from cells. Cells from an identical set of association assay samples were washed 3 times to remove unbound ^{125}I-gp70 at 30, 60 or 150 min; 300 ul of reaction buffer was added back to each sample and incubation at 24°C was continued as indicated (o——o). The binding plotted is specific binding, which was the difference in ^{125}I-gp70 binding in the absence and presence of 1 ug of unlabeled gp70.

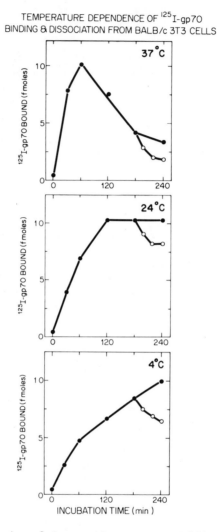

TEMPERATURE DEPENDENCE OF ^{125}I-gp70
BINDING & DISSOCIATION FROM BALB/c 3T3 CELLS

Figure 8. Effects of temperature on specific gp70 binding to cells and its subsequent dissociation. The conditions of association of ^{125}I-gp70 with BALB/c 3T3 cells were as described for Fig. 7, except that temperature was varied (●——●). After a 3 hr incubation, identical sets of samples were tested for dissociation of ^{125}I-gp70 as described for Fig. 7 (O——O); dissociation was studied at the same temperatures used for association.

EFFECT OF TRYPSIN ON THE BINDING OF ^{125}I-gp70
TO BALB/c 3T3 CELLS

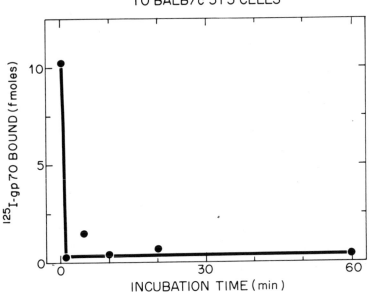

Figure 9. Sensitivity of the gp70 binding sites on BALB/c 3T3 cells to extracellular proteolysis by trypsin. BALB/c 3T3 cells were incubated with 300 ul of reaction buffer containing 10 ug/ml trypsin at 24°C for the indicated time periods. The albumin component of reaction buffer was present during the incubation with trypsin, and no morphological change occurred at the level of light microscopic observation. The cells were washed 3 times in reaction buffer and incubated with 100 ng of ^{125}I-gp70 in 300 ul reaction buffer for 60 min at 24°C.

ly (Bishayee et al., 1978; Kalyanaraman et al., 1978), and our observations are in agreement with those in the published studies.

The gp70 receptor is extremely sensitive to treatment with protease (Figure 9). Treatment with trypsin under conditions which produce no morphological change in the cells by light microscopic observation results in a rapid and complete inactivation of the cellular ability to bind

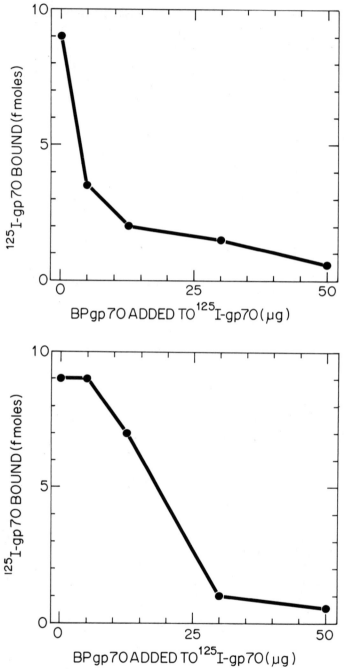

Figure 10 (OPPOSITE). Inhibition of specific gp70 binding to cells or purified cell membranes by a preparation of BPgp70, the putative cell surface receptor for gp70 on murine BALB/c 3T3 cells. Top. Samples of 100 ng of ^{125}I-gp70 were incubated with the indicated amounts of BPgp70 in a final volume of 300 ul of reaction buffer. After 60 min at 24°C, the mixture was added to 1 x 10^5 BALB/c 3T3 cells for 60 min at 24°C.

Bottom. Samples of 100 ng of ^{125}I-gp70 were incubated with the indicated amounts of BPgp70 in reaction buffer (final volume 200 ul) for 60 min at 24°C. The mixture was then added to 100 ul of reaction buffer containing 100 ug of a BALB/c 3T3 membrane preparation (Perdue, 1974) for 60 min at 24°C. The membranes were filtered over glass filters (Whatman GF/c) and the filters were counted for ^{125}I-radioactivity.

gp70. It is not clear whether this indicates receptor destruction, or release of receptor from the cell surface. The unusual gp70 dissociation properties at 37° (Figure 8) and the high sensitivity of the binding reaction to trypsin suggested to us that gp70 receptors might not be attached to the cell surface with great avidity and might therefore be shed by cultured cells into the medium. We therefore performed our initial attempts at gp70 receptor identification using spent medium from the growth of BALB/c 3T3 cells. Affinity chromatography on gp70-Sepharose yielded a high activity preparation of a gp70 binding protein which we have called BPgp70 (Binding Protein for gp70). This protein has since been purified to apparent homogeneity. The binding activity of the affinity column eluate was sufficiently high to permit an initial characterization of this putative receptor protein for gp70.

Figures 10 (Top and Bottom) describe the ability of BPgp70 to inhibit the binding of gp70 to BALB/c 3T3 cells or membranes isolated from 3T3 cells. The binding of gp70 to cells was inhibited by over 50% when as little as 1 ug of partially purified BPgp70 was incubated with gp70 prior to its addition to cells. With isolated membranes, on the other hand, nearly 20 times as much BPgp70 was required to achieve the same result. The time course for binding of gp70 to BPgp70 is described in Figure 11, and is based on the assay which measures the BPgp70-mediated inhibition of

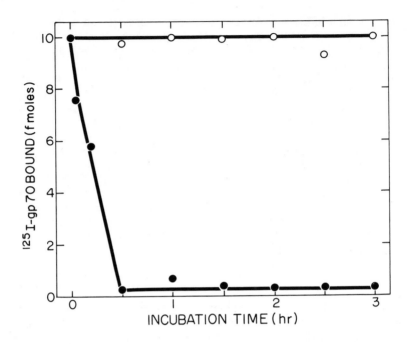

Figure 11. Rate of onset of inhibition of gp70 binding to BALB/c 3T3 cells as a function of the time of incubation of gp70 with BPgp70 prior to addition of this mixture to cells. Samples of 100 ng of ^{125}I-gp70 were incubated with 24 ug of BPgp70 in 300 ul reaction buffer for the indicated time periods at 24° and then added to 1 x 10^5 BALB/c 3T3 cells for a 60 min incubation at 24°C (●—●). As a control, a parallel set of ^{125}I-gp70 samples was incubated under the same conditions in 300 ul of reaction buffer containing no BPgp70 prior to addition to the cells (○—○).

gp70 binding to cells. The action of BPgp70 on gp70 that leads to inhibition of gp70 binding to cells is reversible, indicating that incubation of BPgp70 with gp70 does not lead to gp70 destruction. Furthermore, incubation of high quantities of BPgp70 with trace quantities of labeled gp70 did not lead to detectable gp70 degradation. These

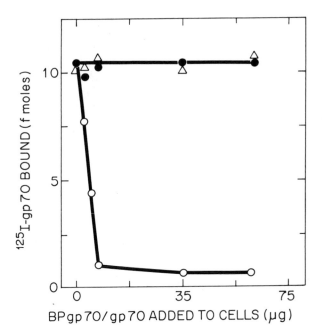

Figure 12. Competition of gp70 and BPgp70, respectively, for the specific binding of ^{125}I-gp70 to BALB/c 3T3 cells. Parallel samples of 1 x 10^5 BALB/c 3T3 cells were incubated with the indicated amounts of either BPgp70 (●—●) or unlabeled gp70 (O—O) or with none (△—△) in 300 ul of reaction buffer for 60 min at 24°C. After 3 washes in reaction buffer, the cells were exposed to 100 ng of ^{125}I-gp70 in 300 ul of reaction buffer for 60 min at 24°C.

experiments show that BPgp70 inhibits gp70 binding to cells by sequestering gp70, and not by degrading it.

The experiment in Figure 12 shows that BPgp70 does not block gp70 binding to cells by interacting with a cellular component. In this experiment either BPgp70 or gp70 was first incubated with cells; the medium was then removed and the cells were washed thoroughly to remove excess added ligand. The subsequent binding of labeled gp70 to these cells was blocked effectively, and in fact, was blocked completely by small amounts of gp70. BPgp70 had no effect whatsoever on this binding reaction when incubated with cells prior to a shift to medium containing labeled gp70 (Figure 12). It can therefore be concluded that BPgp70 blocks gp70 binding by interacting with gp70 and not with a cellular component. Figure 13 describes an experiment in which BPgp70 was radiolabeled and then added to cells. No binding of radioactive protein to cells was demonstrated unless unlabeled gp70 was incubated with them previously. Gel electrophoretic analysis of the component which bound to cells incubated with gp70 showed that the labeled material which bound had the same molecular weight as BPgp70 purified to apparent homonogeneity (Landen and Fox, submitted for publication).

When antisera were raised against BPgp70 and incubated with cells prior to addition of gp70, a complete blockade of gp70 binding was achieved. This occured with less than a 100:1 ration of crude IgG-anti BPgp70 per gp70 binding site, and 50% inhibition was achieved at a ratio of less than 30:1, providing strong support for the view that BPgp70 is the physiological receptor for the binding of RMuLV to cells.

GENERAL DISCUSSION

We have described the properties and behavior of two membrane receptors on the plasmalemma of murine 3T3 cells. One of these, the EGF receptor triggers a mitogenic response upon hormone binding. EGF may act as a mitogen in animals, though there is as yet no definitive demonstration of an EGF requirement for the growth and proliferation of any given population of cells in animals. The gp70 receptors are of obvious importance in tumor biology, and a protein that we have identified and purified to apparent homogeneity (Landen and Fox, submitted for publication) has properties expected of this receptor.

The EGF receptor is internalized in response to its specific hormone (Das and Fox, 1978; Fox and Das, 1979; Linsley et al., 1979; Baker, et al., 1979). The ability of other hormones, e.g., FGF and PDGF, to down regulate EGF receptors suggests that these hormones are members of a community of receptors which have the property of forming common clusters as an intermediate stage in their internalization and cellular processing. We have treated the biological implications of receptor internalization and processing elsewhere (Das and Fox, 1978; Fox and Das,

BINDING OF ^{125}I-BPgp70 TO BALB/c 3T3 CELLS

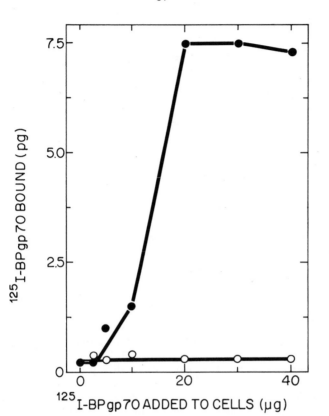

Figure 13. Binding of labeled BPgp70 to BALB/c 3T3 cells incubated previously in medium containing gp70 or no gp70. Samples of 1 x 10^5 BALB/c 3T3 cells were treated with 50 pmoles of gp70 in 300 ul of reaction buffer for 60 min at 24ºC. After 3 washes 300 ul of reaction buffer containing the indicated amounts of ^{125}I-BPgp70 were added to the cells for 60· min at 24º (●──●). An identical set of samples was incubated with 300 ul of reaction buffer containing no gp70 prior to addition of the ^{125}I-BPgp70 (O──O).

1979; Fox et al., 1979a; Fox et al., 1979b; Wrann et al., 1979), and some aspects of the possible functional conseq-uences of receptor cointernalization are treated in the EGF receptor section of RESULTS AND DISCUSSION. Though additional information is needed to permit a definitive description of the biological role(s) played by receptor internalization, our data suggest that many previously apparent "specific" responses to hormones could be mediat-ed through communal receptor modulation such as that des-cribed here.

The gp70 receptors differ from EGF receptors in their biological fate. EGF receptors, and many other mitogen receptors as well, appear to be designed for eventual in-ternalization, and while internalization of these hormones has not yet been definitively established as obligatory for their action, it must be strongly considered. It seems unlikely that cells have evolved a complex and in-teractive receptor internalization mechanism simply to dispose of circulating polypeptide hormones. The gp70 re-ceptors, on the other hand, show no propensity for inter-nalization and are instead shed in abundance. We estimate that synthesis of BPgp70, which has been shown to be of cellular origin by metabolic labeling studies (Landen and Fox, submitted for publication), may account for as much as a few tenths of a percent of the total protein synthes-ized by BALB/c 3T3 cells. Thus the normal role of BPgp70 may be that of a secreted protein which plays some yet to be defined role in intercellular recognition.

It will be interesting to test the possibility that BPgp70 species constitute a polymorphic gene family. Ex-tensive polymorphism has been observed in gp70 species (Elder et al., 1977), the other component of this recogni-tion scheme. By chance the C-type tumor viruses may have established recognition interactions between their major coat antigen and cell surface receptor(s) that play a phy-siological role other than gp70 binding. However, the other side of the coin holds the chance that the C-type viruses have established through their relationships be-tween the viral antigen and a cell surface receptor, a synergism which provides cells with a driving force for tissue evolution through enhanced rates of recombination in the receptor protein gene(s). The detailed protein chemistry of BPgp70 from BALB/c 3T3 cells and other cells lines may hold interesting prospects for the developmental geneticist.

ACKNOWLEDGEMENTS

The work on EGF receptors was supported by research grant VC-314 from the American Cancer Society and by research grants from the Muscular Dystrophy Association of America. The work on gp70 receptors was supported by contract N01 CP9 1010 and facilitated by the provision of biological material resources from the Division of Cancer, Cause and Prevention, National Cancer Institute, USPHS. We are grateful to Dr. Denis Gospodarowicz for provision of purified FGF. We thank Susan Gerber and Debra Bright for their expert technical assistance.

REFERENCES

Aharonov, A, Pruss, RM and Herschman, HR (1978) J Biol Chem 253:3970-3977

Antoniades, HN, Scher, CD (1975) Proc Natl Acad Sci, USA 74:1973-1975

Baker, JV, Simmer, R, Glenn, KC and Cunningham, DD (1979) Nature 278:743-745

Bishayee, S, Strand, M and August, JT (1978) Arch Biochem Biophys 189:161-171

Bishayee, S and Strand, M (1979) in Bitensky, M, Collier, RJ, Steiner, DF, Fox, CF (eds): "Progress in Clinical and Bioliogical Research", Vol 31, pp 721-731, Alan R Liss, Inc, NY

Carpenter, G and Cohen, S (1976) J Cell Biol 71: 159-171

Carpenter, G and Cohen, S (1979) Ann Rev Biochem 48:193-216

Das, M, Miyakawa, T, Fox, CF, Pruss, RM Aharonov, A and Herschman, HR (1977) Proc Natl Acad Sci, USA 74:2790-2794

Das, M and Fox, CF (1978) Proc Natl Acad Sci, USA 75:2644-2648

DeLarco, J and Todaro, G (1976) Cell 8:365-371

Elder, JH, Jensen, FC, Bryant, ML and Lerner, RA (1977) Nature 267:23-28

Fox, CF and Das, M (1979) J Supramol Struct 10: 199-214

Fox, CF, Vale, R, Peterson, SW and Das, M (1979a), in Sato, C, Ross, R (eds): "Hormones and Cell Culture": Cold Spring Harbor Conferences on Cell Proliferation, Vol 6 pp 143-157

Fox, CF, Wrann, M, Vale, R and Linsley, P (1979b) J Supramol Struct 12 (in press)

Gospodarowicz, D and Morna, JS (1977) Ann Rev Biochem 45: 531-538

Haigler, H, Ash, JF, Singer, SJ and Cohen, S (1978) Proc Natl Acad Sci, USA 75:3317-3321

Haigler, HR, McKanna, JA and Cohen, S (1979) J Cell Biol 81:382-395

Ihle, JN, Denny, TP and Bolognesi, DP (1976) J Virol 17: 727-736

Kalyanaraman, VS, Sarngadharan, MA and Gallo, RC (1978) J Virol 28:686-696

Linsley, P, Blifeld, C, Wrann, M and Fox, CF (1979) Nature 278:745-748

Markwell, MAK and Fox, CF (1978) Biochemistry 17:4807-4817

Maxfield, FR, Schlessinger, YJ, Shechter, Y, Pastan, I and Willingham, MC (1978) Cell 14:805-810

Moennig, V, Frank, H, Hunsmann, A, Schneider, I and Schafer, W (1974) Virology 61:100-111

Perdue, JF (1974) Methods Enzymol 31:162-168

Ross, R and Vogel, A (1978) Cell 14:203-210

Savage, CR and Cohen, S (1972) J Biol Chem 247:7609-7611

Strand, M and August, JT (1973) J Biol Chem 248:5627-5633

Strand, M and August, JT (1974) J Virol 13:171-180

Strand, M and August, JT (1976) J Biol Chem 251:559-564

Wrann, M, Linsley, PS and Fox CF (1979) FEBS Letters 104: 415-419

Pages 95–105, Membranes, Receptors, and the Immune Response
© 1980 Alan R. Liss, Inc., 150 Fifth Avenue, New York, NY 10011

THE I REGION OF THE MURINE MAJOR HISTOCOMPATIBILITY COMPLEX: GENETICS AND STRUCTURE

Richard G. Cook, Ellen S. Vitetta, Jonathan W. Uhr and J. Donald Capra[1]
Department of Microbiology, The University of Texas Southwestern Medical School, Dallas, Texas 75235

INTRODUCTION

The murine Ia alloantigens are cell surface glycoproteins encoded by the I-region of the H-2 complex (Klein, 1975; Cullen et al. 1976). Their relationship to the various immune responses controlled by the I-region has become increasingly evident through numerous studies showing inhibition of function by anti-Ia alloantisera (Schwartz et al. 1976; Frelinger et al. 1975). This suggests that the Ia antigens may function as receptor molecules which mediate interactions among cells or between cells and antigens.

Two I-subregions, A and E/C[2], encode products which can be detected by biochemical techniques. These molecules are found predominantly on B lymphocytes (Cullen et al. 1975; Vitetta and Capra, 1978) and are coexpressed on the same cell as demonstrated by both functional (Frelinger et al. 1978) and biochemical techniques (Vitetta and Cook, 1979). Both the A and E/C alloantigens consist of two subunits, α and β, with apparent MW of 31-34,000 and 26-29,000 daltons, respectively. In an effort to gain insight into the extent and nature of structural variation which exists in these putative receptor molecules, our laboratories over

[1] This work was supported in part by generous grants from the National Institutes of Health, American Cancer Society, and the National Science Foundation.

[2] Due to our present uncertainty as to whether Ia specificity 7 is encoded by the I-E or I-C subregions, the designation E/C will be utilized.

the past two years have studied the A and E/C antigens at the primary structural level. This article will describe recent structural data on these molecules and present a tentative model for the genetic organization of the genes encoding Ia antigens.

METHODS

Splenocytes from various congenic strains were either radiolabeled for 6-8 hr with ^{3}H- or ^{14}C-amino acids (Vitetta et al. 1976; Cook et al. 1978a,b; 1979a,b,c) or surface labeled with ^{125}I by the lactoperoxidase catalyzed iodination technique (Vitetta et al. 1971). Cells were lysed and chro-matographed on lentil lectin-sepharose to enrich for glycoproteins (Cook et al. 1978a). The lectin adherent glycoprotein pools were cleared of Ig and non-specific material with rabbit anti-mouse Ig and Staphylococcus aureus (S. aureus), and then the I-A and/or I-E/C alloantigens were immunopreci-pitated with appropriate alloantisera and S. aureus. The Ia α and β subunits were resolved by sodium dodecyl sulfate polyacrylamide gel electrophoresis (SDS-PAGE) (Cook et al. 1978a).

RESULTS AND DISCUSSION

Studies on the I-A Alloantigens.

Peptide maps comparing the α and β subunits of the A^k and A^b antigens are shown in Figure 1. The ^{14}C-labeled A^k α and β chains were mixed with H-labeled A^b α and β chains, digested with trypsin, and the resulting peptides separated by ion exchange chromatography. Of the 14 peptides visualized for both the k and b α chains, only nine coeluted; this represents a 63% coincidence of elution. For the k and b β chains, 18 and 22 tryptic peptides were detected, respectively, and only nine peptides (45%) coeluted. The peptide(s) which do not adhere to the resin (fall through, fractions 5-10) are considered as coincident. The final peak on each profile represents material eluted with 2 N NaOH and is not scored in these analyses.

In further experiments, the A^d and A^s subunits were also compared to those of A^k by ion exchange chromatography. The α subunits showed about 65% coelution and the β subunits

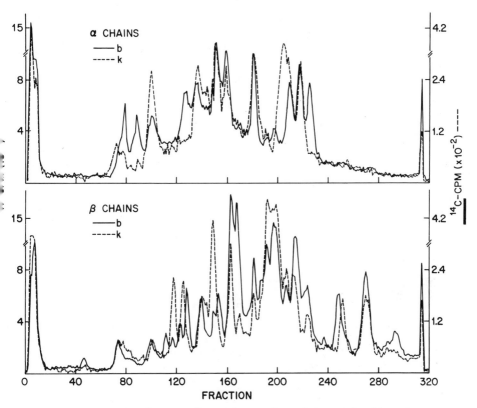

I-A α and β CHAINS

Figure 1. Ion exchange chromatography of tryptic digests of the α (upper panel) and β (lower panel) subunits of the A^k and A^b alloantigens. ^{3}H-labeled A^b α and β subunits are compared with ^{14}C-labeled A^k α and β subunits.

about 50% coelution.

We have also examined tryptic digests of the A allo-antigens by an HPLC system, which resolves peptides by differences in hydrophobicity rather than the charge diff-erences detected by ion exchange chromatography. In general, this HPLC system resolves about 75% the number of peptides detected by ion exchange chromatography. In control experi-ments, ^{3}H-labeled A^b α and β chains were compared with ^{14}C-labeled A^b α and β chains and there was coelution of all peptides. When the A^k and A^b products were compared by this technique, significant differences were seen, equivalent to those observed by ion exchange chromatography, i.e., 30-40% variation in α chains and 40-50% variation in β chains. A

comparison of the β chains from k and r haplotypes is shown
in Figure 2. Of the 15 and 17 peptides seen for the k and r
products, only 8 coelute, yielding a 50% coincident elution.

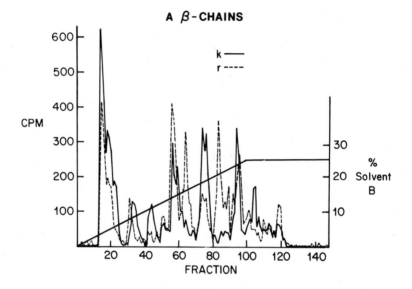

Figure 2.   HPLC of tryptic digests of the A^k and A^r β polypeptides. ^{3}H-labeled (———) A^k β is compared with [14]C-
labeled (----) A^r β. Solvent B is acetonitrile.

     Thus, both the α and β polypeptides of the A alloanti-
gens display allelic associated structural variation. This
implies that the A α and β chains are encoded within the
major histocompatibility complex (MHC) since, by definition, the B10 congenic strains utilized have the same "back-

ground genes" and differ only at their MHC.

To test whether both the A α and β chains are encoded within the A subregion, we compared the A alloantigen subunits from B10.A with those from two intra H-2 recombinants, B10.A(4R) and A.TL. All three strains are k haplotype in the A subregion; however, B10.A(4R) differs to the right of A (b haplotype in B) and A.TL differs to the left of A (s haplotype in H-2K). If both the A α and β chains are encoded within the A subregion, then the tryptic peptide profiles of the α and β subunits from the recombinants should be identical to those from B10.A. If both subunits are not encoded by A, then structural differences should be observed, since the α and β polypeptides of the b and s alleles are distinct from those of the k allele. When these studies were done, the α and β chains, respectively, from B10.A(4R) and A.TL recombinants were identical to those of B10.A. This indicates that both the α and β subunits of the A alloantigens are encoded within the A subregion.

Studies on the I-E/C Alloantigens.

The E/C alloantigens of k, r, p, and d haplotypes have been examined structurally by comparative mapping of tryptic peptides (Cook et al. 1979b). A small degree of variation (∼10%) was detected in the α chains. In contrast, the E/C β chain comparisons showed significant allelic variation — 48%, 48% and 69% coincident elution of d, p, and r tryptic peptides when compared to k. These results indicate that both chains of the E/C alloantigens are encoded within the MHC.

Using the technique of 2-dimensional (2-D) gel analysis, Jones et al. (1978) have shown that the E/C alloantigens are controlled by two different I-region loci — one in A and the other in E/C. In an effort to confirm and extend these observations to the more conventional α-β subunit nomenclature, and also to determine the possible nature of the electrophoretic variations observed by 2-D gels, we have compared the E/C α and β subunits from appropriate I-region recombinants by peptide mapping (Cook et al. 1979c). A summary of these studies is shown in Table 1; all strains were k/d haplotype in E/C, but varied in A (k, b or s). The E/C α chains from B10.A, B10.A(3R), B10.A(5R), and B10.HTT showed coelution of all tryptic peptides. However, there

TABLE I
SUMMARY OF PEPTIDE MAPPING DATA ON THE E/C ANTIGENS FROM RECOMBINANT STRAINS[a]

| Strains | H-2 Haplotypes | | | | | | | | | % of Coelution of Tryptic Peptides with B10.A E/C Subunits | |
	K	A	B	J	E	C	S	G	B	α	β
			I								
B10.A	k	k	k	k	k	d	d	d	d	100	100
B10.AQR	q	k	k	k	k	d	d	d	d	ND	100
B10.A(5R)	b	b	b	k	k	d	d	d	d	100	60
B10.A(3R)	b	b	b	b	k	d	d	d	d	100	60
B10.HTT	s	s	s	s	k	k	k	k	d	100	56

[a]The arrows indicate that the β chain must be encoded to the right or left of that locus.

were notable differences among the β subunits. The differences between 5R and B10.A indicate that the β chain is encoded to the left of I-J. In other experiments, we found that the β chains of 3R and 5R are identical (both are b in I-A,B); also the E/C β subunit from B10.HTT is distinct from the β chains of both B10.A and 3R (or 5R). Thus, the E/C β subunit is encoded in the I-A or B subregion, while the E/C α chain by definition must be encoded in the E/C subregion. This implies that allospecificities mapped to the E/C subregion are controlled by the α subunit.

Hybrid E/C alloantigens can be detected in F₁ splenocytes.

Using 2-D gel analysis of anti-E/C immunoprecipitates, Jones et al. (1978) demonstrated that in F₁ heterozygotes E/C encoded polypeptides (α chain) could associate in the cytoplasm with A encoded polypeptides (β chain) derived from both of the parental alleles. To examine this question at the primary structural level, the E/C alloantigen from (b x d) F₁ splenocytes (C57B1/6 x DBA/2J) was analyzed for the association of the E/C[d] α polypeptide with both b and $\underline{d}$ encoded β polypeptides. The $\underline{b}$ haplotype parental strain does not produce a serologically or biochemically detectable E/C antigen — SDS-PAGE analysis of anti-E/C immunoprecipitates of lysates of the $\underline{b}$ haplotype are negative. This apparently results from a failure of the $\underline{b}$ haplotype to synthesize an E/C α chain since $\underline{b}$ encoded β chains can be detected in the cytoplasm (Jones $\underline{et}$ $\underline{al}$. 1978). Also, the β polypeptides encoded by $\underline{b}$ are expressed in the 3R and 5R recombinant strains which are $\underline{k}$ in the $\underline{E/C}$ subregions. Thus the $\underline{b}$ haplotype β chain can be "rescued" if an α chain positive allele is present at $\underline{E/C}$.

In Figure 3, the β subunit derived from the $(\underline{b} \times \underline{d})$ F_1 is compared with the β subunit encoded by the $\underline{d}$ (top panel) and $\underline{b}$ (middle panel) haplotypes; $β^b$ was from the B10.A(5R) recombinant. Peptide differences between the F_1 and parental β subunits are denoted by arrows. If the parental $\underline{b}$ and $\underline{d}$ β chains were mixed 1:1 and then compared with the $\overline{F}_1$ β chains, no differences were detected (bottom panel). The α polypeptide from the $(\underline{b} \times \underline{d})$ F_1 was identical to that of the $\underline{d}$ parental strain (not shown). This demonstrates that in a $(\underline{b} \times \underline{d})$ F_1 there are two types of E/C alloantigens — one consists of $α^dβ^d$ subunits and the other $α^dβ^b$ subunits.

CONCLUSIONS

1. Allelic variation has been detected in the α and β subunits of both the A and E/C antigens. There are multiple amino acid sequence differences between allelic β chains of the A and E/C molecules; thus far no allelic variation in the α subunits has been detected by sequence analysis (Cook $\underline{et}$ $\underline{al}$. 1979a). Comparative tryptic peptide analysis has demonstrated marked allelic variation (∼40-50%) in the A α, A β, and E/C β chains and detectable (∼10%) variation in the E/C α allelic products. Since congenic mouse strains, which theoretically differ only at the MHC, have been utilized, the allelic variation observed indicates that all four subunits (A α and β, E/C α and β) are encoded within the MHC.

2. While both the α and β subunits of the A alloantigen are encoded in the $\underline{I-A}$ subregion, the E/C α and β subregions are encoded by the $\underline{E/C}$ and $\underline{A}$, $\underline{B}$ subregions, respectively. Figure 4 presents our current interpretation of the genetic organization and expression of the A and E/C

E/C β-CHAINS

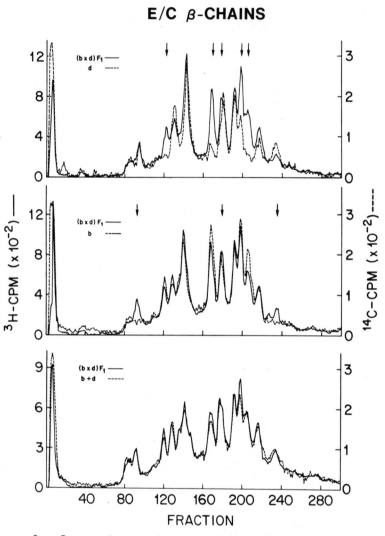

Figure 3. Ion exchange chromatography of tryptic digests of E/C β polypeptides. ³H-labeled E/C β chains from a (b x d) F₁ animal ((C57 Bl/6 x DBA/2J)F₁) are compared with ¹⁴C-labeled E/C β chains from DBA/2J (d haplotype, top panel) and B10.A(5R) (b haplotype, middle panel). In the lower panel the ³H-labeled E/C β chains from the (b x d) F₁ are compared with a 1:1 cpm mixture of the parental (b + d) ¹⁴C-labeled E/C β chains. Peptide differences are denoted by arrows.

I REGION

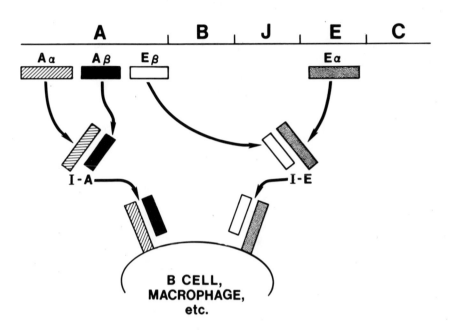

Figure 4. Interpretive model of the genetic organization and expression of the A and E/C alloantigens. The order of the A α, A β, and E β "genes" in the A subregion is not known; also, our results have not eliminated the B sub-region as the locus which encodes E β. For simplicity, E is used instead of E/C.

alloantigens.

3. Finally, although there is presently no obvious explanation for why linked genes should encode the Ia α and β subunits, the two gene (A and E/C) control of the E/C antigens does offer a possible molecular mechanism for the observed Ir gene complementation requirement for responsiveness to certain antigens.

ACKNOWLEDGMENTS

We wish to thank S. Wray and Y.-M. Tseng for excellent technical assistance during various phases of this work, and K. Able for careful and patient preparation of this manuscript. Some of the experiments were performed with the assistance of Mr. M. Siegelman.

REFERENCES

Cook RG, Vitetta ES, Capra JD, Uhr JW (1977). Structural studies on the murine Ia alloantigens. I. The partial amino acid sequence of a murine Ia molecule. Immunogen 5:437.
Cook RG, Uhr JW, Capra JD, Vitetta ES (1978a). Structural studies on the murine Ia alloantigens. II. Molecular weight characterization of the products of the I-A and I-E/C subregions. J Immunol 121:2205.
Cook RG, Vitetta ES, Uhr JW, Klein J, Wilde CE, Capra JD (1978b). Structural studies on protein products of murine chromosome 17. III. Partial amino acid sequence of an H-2K^q molecule. J Immunol 121:1015.
Cook RG, Siegelman MH, Capra JD, Uhr JW, Vitetta ES (1979a). Structural studies on the murine Ia alloantigens. IV. NH$_2$-terminal sequence analysis of allelic products of the I-A and I-E subregion. J Immunol 122:2232.
Cook RG, Uhr JW, Vitetta ES, Capra JD (1979b). Structural studies on the murine Ia alloantigens. III. Tryptic peptide comparisons of allelic products of the I-E/C subregion. Mol Immunol 16:29.
Cook RG, Vitetta ES, Uhr JW, Capra JD (1979c). Structural studies on the murine Ia alloantigens. V. Evidence that the structural gene for the E/C beta polypeptide is encoded within the I-A subregion. J Exp Med 149:981.
Cullen SE, Freed JH, Nathenson SG (1976). Structural and serological properties of murine Ia alloantigens. Transplant Rev 30:236.
Frelinger JA, Neiderhuber JE, Shreffler DC (1975). Inhibition of immune responses in vitro by specific anti-serums to Ia antigens. Science 188:258.
Frelinger JA, Hibbler FJ, Hill SW (1978). Expression of I-A and I-E/C region encoded Ia antigens on functional B cell populations. J Immunol 121:2376.
Jones PP, Murphy DB, McDevitt HO (1978). Two-gene control of the expression of a murine Ia antigen. J Exp Med 148:925.

Klein J (1975). "Biology of the Mouse Histocompatibility-2 Complex." New York: Springer-Verlag.

Vitetta ES, Baur S, Uhr JW (1971). Cell surface immunoglobulin. II. Isolation and characterization of Ig from mouse splenic lymphocytes. J Exp Med 134:242.

Vitetta ES, Capra JD, Klapper DG, Klein J, Uhr JW (1976). The partial amino acid sequence of an H-2K molecule. Proc Natl Acad Sci USA 73:905.

Vitetta ES, Capara JD (1978). The protein products of the murine 17th chromosome: Genetics and structure. Adv in Immunol 26:148.

Vitetta ES, Cook RG (1979). Surface expression and synthesis of I-A and I-E/C encoded molecules by B lymphocytes and Ig-secreting cells. J Immunol 122:2122.

Schwartz RH, David CS, Sachs DH, Paul WE (1976). T lymphocyte-enriched murine peritoneal exudate cells. III. Inhibition of antigen-induced T lymphocyte proliferation with anti-Ia antisera. J Immunol 117:531.

Session II.
Antigenic Modulation and Down-Regulation

Pages 109—126, Membranes, Receptors, and the Immune Response
© 1980 Alan R. Liss, Inc., 150 Fifth Avenue, New York, NY 10011

MODULATION OF THE INSULIN RECEPTOR BY INSULIN RECEPTOR
AUTOANTIBODIES

Len C. Harrison, Emmanuel Van Obberghen, Carl
Grunfeld, George L. King, C. Ronald Kahn
Diabetes Branch, NIAMDD, The National Institutes
of Health, 9000 Rockville Pike, 10/8S-243
Bethesda, Maryland 20205 U.S.A.

INTRODUCTION

The concept of cell surface receptors as stereospecific
molecules which recognize and bind complementary ligands,
and which effect ligand action, was clearly defined at the
beginning of this century by Paul Ehrlich (Ehrlich, 1906).
The receptor concept then evolved in a parallel but independent fashion in a number of disciplines, notably pharmacology, endocrinology, and immunology. During the past
decade, Ehrlich's receptor hypothesis has been validated and
its impact has been felt in all areas of biology. Physicochemical evidence obtained by studying the direct binding of
isotope-labeled ligands has been complemented by morphology
studies in which the binding of ligands is directly visualized using the techniques of electron microscopic autoradio-
graphy and fluorescence microscopy. In addition, antibodies
to some receptors now provide the basis for measuring these
receptors by radioimmunoassay, independently of the receptor
binding function.

The insulin receptor has served as a prototype for
studies of receptor function and a variety of physiologic
and pathologic factors are known to alter its expression and
concentration, as well as its affinity for insulin (Roth,
1973; Bar, et al., 1979). The first clear indication of the
importance of receptors in disease states came from the
studies of obesity in rodents, (Kahn, et al., 1973) and in
man (Bar, et al., 1976; Harrison, et al., 1976; Olefsky,
1976). In obesity, there is an increased prevalence of
glucose intolerance despite increased plasma insulin levels,

and a diminished response to exogenous insulin consistent with the presence of an insulin-resistant state. The insulin resistance in obesity was shown to be related to a decrease in the concentration of insulin receptors on target cells. A major factor regulating receptor concentration in obesity appeared to be insulin itself since the concentration of receptors was reciprocally related to the ambient concentration of insulin. In cultured lymphocytes insulin could induce "down-regulation" of its receptor in a specific, dose-dependent fashion; this process was shown to be energy and temperature-dependent and involved increased degradation of the receptor molecule, not simply inactivation of its binding function in situ (Gavin, et al., 1974; Blackard et al., 1978; Harrison, et al., 1979a). Other conditions associated with elevated insulin levels e.g. maturity-onset type diabetes, acromegaly, and insulinoma are also associated with decreased concentrations of insulin receptors and insulin resistance. When insulin levels return toward normal, e.g. after caloric restriction in obesity, receptor concentrations also return toward normal. Other insulin resistant states, e.g. acidosis and glucocorticoid excess, are associated with a decrease in insulin receptor affinity.

Recently, a form of diabetes caused by circulating autoantibodies to the insulin receptor has been described (Flier, et al., 1975; Kahn, et al., 1976). Autoantibodies to receptors have also been documented in three other disease states: to the TSH (thyrotropin) receptor in Graves' disease (Smith & Hall, 1974; Manley, et al., 1974), to the ACh (acetylcholine) receptor in myasthenia gravis (Appel, et al., 1975; Aharonov, et al., 1975; Lindstrom, et al., 1976), and to the β_2-adrenergic receptor in allergic rhinitis and asthma (Venter, et al., 1979, see also this volume). Clearly, receptor antibodies are part of a larger spectrum of autoimmunity, but have a special significance because the development of functional receptor assays has enabled the mechanism of action of these autoantibodies to be studied in detail. In this Chapter, we will discuss the cellular and molecular mode of action of insulin receptor autoantibodies and demonstrate their unique properties as probes of receptor structure and function.

CLINICAL SYNDROMES ASSOCIATED WITH AUTOANTIBODIES TO THE INSULIN RECEPTOR

Insulin receptor antibodies were initially discovered

in three patients with the syndrome (designated Type B) of severe insulin resistance and the skin disorder acanthosis nigricans (Flier, et al., 1975; Kahn, et al., 1976). A total of sixteen cases have now been documented, ten of these having been evaluated by us. In addition, we have also found insulin receptor antibodies in one patient who presented with hypoglycemia (L. C. Harrison, unpublished observation), in a number of other patients with the syndrome of ataxia-telangiectasia associated with insulin resistance (Bar, et al., 1978; Harrison, et al., 1979b), and in the New Zealand Obese (NZO) mouse, a model of obesity and insulin-resistant diabetes (Harrison & Itin, 1979c). The clinical details of the patients with the Type B syndrome are summarized in Table 1.

TABLE 1   CLINICAL DETAILS OF PATIENTS WITH RECEPTOR ANTIBODIES

Age at presentation:	12-62 yrs, mean 39yrs	
Sex	: 12 female, 4 male	
Race	: 10 black, 3 white, 2 Japanese, 1 Mexican-American	
Clinical features	: Symptomatic diabetes	9
	(tendency to ketosis)	(5)
	Moderate to severe glucose intolerance	14
	Marked hyperinsulinemia ($>100\mu U/ml$) and extreme resistance to exogenous insulin	16
	Acanthosis nigricans	12
	Evidence of general autoimmunity (↑globulins, ↑ESR, ↓leukocytes, ↓complement, proteinuria, antibodies to DNA, vitiligo, alopecia, enlarged submandibular glands)	16
	Lupus syndrome	2
	Sjogren's syndrome	2

INSULIN RECEPTOR STUDIES IN PATIENTS WITH RECEPTOR ANTIBODIES

The interaction of insulin with its receptor in these patients has been studied using circulating mononuclear leukocytes. Most of the binding to cells in this preparation is to the monocyte subpopulation and the binding properties of insulin receptors on monocytes are identical to those on traditional target tissues such as liver, muscle and fat

(Bar, et al., 1979). There is a marked decrease in insulin
binding to receptors from affected patients, due mainly to
a decrease in receptor affinity. Thus, the concentration of
unlabeled insulin required to displace 50% of bound tracer
[125]I-insulin in a competition assay is markedly increased
(Figure 1, left panel). Under normal circumstances the binding of insulin is a negatively cooperative process, i.e.
increasing occupancy of receptors is associated with decreasing affinity of the insulin-receptor interaction (De Meyts,
et al., 1976). This is reflected in the concave Scatchard
plot for normal binding (Figure 1, center panel). The
Scatchard plot for insulin binding to the patients' monocytes
is flat due to a loss of the high affinity component and
the absence of negative cooperativity, but there is no change
in the abscissa intercept (maximum binding capacity or
receptor concentration, R_O). The average affinity profile
shows that the receptors are "locked" in a low affinity
state (Figure 1, right panel). Kinetic experiments indicate
that this low affinity is mainly due to an increase in the
spontaneous rate of dissociation, with a inability of insulin
to further accelerate dissociation consistent with the loss
of negative cooperativity. The antibodies, therefore,
appear to act mainly like competitive antagonists. However,
some patients have had virtually no detectible binding
suggesting that the antibodies may also decrease the apparent
receptor concentration.

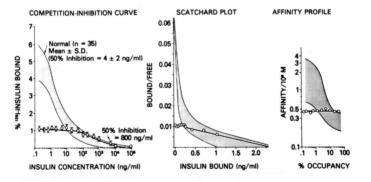

Figure 1   Insulin binding to monocytes from a patient (B-6)
with insulin receptor autoantibodies

The binding defect on the patients' cells can be partially

reversed in vivo by plasmapheresis (Muggeo, et al., 1979a) and in vitro by an acid-wash procedure designed to elute surface immunoglobulins (Muggeo, 1979b). Finally, it should be noted that in cells from two patients with ataxia-telangiectasia (Harrison, et al., 1979b), and in one patient with insulin resistance and acanthosis nigricans who developed hypoglycemia (Flier, et al., 1978) there was an increase in the number of low affinity binding sites.

EFFECTS OF RECEPTOR AUTOANTIBODIES ON INSULIN BINDING IN VITRO

The antibodies from patients with the Type B syndrome of severe insulin resistance and acanthosis nigricans are polyclonal and predominantly of the IgG class (Flier, et al., 1976). In patients with ataxia-telangiectasia and in the NZO mouse the antibodies are IgM (Harrison, et al., 1979b; Harrison and Itin, 1979c). The effects of high titer IgG antibodies on the function of the receptor in vitro have been studied in isolated adipocytes, 3T3-L1 cells, lymphocytes, monocytes, hepatocytes, isolated muscle cells, placental and liver membranes. In normal cells, in vitro, the antibodies mimic the changes seen in the patients' cells; the receptor binding affinity is decreased but the maximum binding capacity (R_0) is not significantly altered (Flier, et al., 1977a; Kahn, et al., 1977). The major kinetic effect of the antibodies in vitro appears to be to decrease the association rate rather than to increase the dissociation rate. The exact molecular mechanism by which they behave as competitive antagonists is unknown. It is interesting to note, however, that antibodies which impair receptor affinity in particulate membranes reduce the maximum binding capacity (R_0) when the membranes are solubilized (Harrison, et al., 1979d). This suggests that they may also alter the conformation or exposure of reactive sites by allosteric mechanisms.

The antibodies appear to be directed specifically to the insulin receptor. They do not alter the binding of a number of other hormones and growth factors tested and do not immunoprecipitate other receptors in solubilized membrane preparations (vide infra). In addition, we have not been able to demonstrate that the antibodies have any effect on insulin degradation either in intact cells or in membrane fractions suggesting that insulin degradation occurs at sites separate from the insulin binding site.

A number of lines of evidence favor the idea that the

underlying receptor (or at least its binding site) is normal
in patients with autoantibodies. Thus: 1) the binding
defect is reproduced by exposure of normal cells to antibody
in vitro; 2) cultured fibroblasts from affected patients
have normal binding; 3) elution of cell-bound antibodies by
acid-wash, or plasmapheresis, results in a return of binding
toward normal, and 4) binding to cells from patients in
remission is normal.

ASSAYS FOR RECEPTOR ANTIBODIES

Receptor antibodies have been measured directly by their
ability to inhibit insulin binding, immunoprecipitate the
solubilized insulin receptor, and mimic insulin-like
biological effects. In addition, the presence of the antibodies on cells may be inferred by the uptake of ^{125}I-protein
A or by the effect of an acid-wash to restore binding toward
normal. The binding inhibition and immunoprecipitation
assays are illustrated schematically in Figure 2.

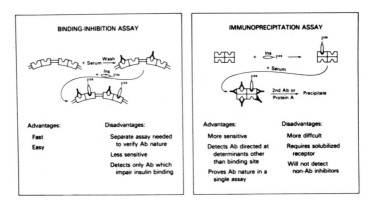

Figure 2. Assays for receptor antibodies

The immunoprecipitation assay potentially measures all receptor antibodies and not only those that happen to impair binding (Harrison, et al., 1979d). In practice, this assay is
more sensitive than the binding inhibition assay and in a
number of situations is the only means by which receptor
antibodies can be detected. It is also of interest that antibodies raised by immunization with partially-purified receptors may immunoprecipitate the receptor but not impair insulin
binding (Jacobs, et al., 1978).

Many of the naturally-occurring antibodies are directed at determinants close to the insulin binding site (Jarrett et al., 1976) and significant occupancy of the receptor by insulin impairs its immunoprecipitation (Harrison, et al., 1979d). However, solubilized receptors labeled with only a small tracer amount of ^{125}I-insulin can be precipitated quantitatively. This suggests that the receptor has more than one binding site or, that some antibodies also bind to determinants outside of the insulin binding region. The latter is almost certainly true since the antibodies are polyclonal and have been shown to be functionally heterogenous. Moreover, after destruction of the insulin binding activity with trypsin the antibodies still bind to solubilized receptors (Harrison, et al., 1979a) and induce insulin-like effects in whole cells (Kahn, et al., 1977). Recent studies show that the insulin receptor has a subunit structure (Lang, et al., 1979; Harrison, et al., 1979e) and therefore it seems reasonable to expect that the antibodies will recognize a variety of functionally-distinct components subserving cooperativity, affinity regulation and biological signal transduction, in addition to insulin binding.

INSULIN-LIKE EFFECTS OF RECEPTOR ANTIBODIES

The clinical state associated with insulin receptor autoantibodies has generally been one of severe insulin resistance consistent with the action of the antibodies to impair insulin binding. However, contrary to the expectation that the antibodies would behave as antagonists of insulin action it was found that their acute effect, in vitro was to mimic the actions of insulin. The insulin-like effects of the antibodies are listed in Table 2.

Table 2. INSULIN-LIKE EFFECTS OF RECEPTOR ANTIBODIES

Adipocytes

Stimulation of 2-deoxyglucose transport, glucose incorporation into lipid and glycogen, and oxidation to CO_2	Kahn, et al., 1977; Kasuga, et al., 1978
Stimulation of amino acid incorporation into protein	Kasuga, et al., 1978
Inhibition of lipolysis	Kasuga, et al., 1978
Activation of glycogen synthase	Lawrence, et al., 1978

Inhibition of phosphorylase
Activation of pyruvate dehydro-   R. Denton, personal
genase and acetyl CoA carboxylase   communication
Simulation of insulin's effect on   "   "
protein phosphorylation

3T3-Ll Fatty Fibroblasts

Stimulation of 2-deoxyglucose
transport and glucose oxidation   Karlsson, et al., 1978
to CO_2
Activation of lipoprotein lipase   Van Obberghen, et al., 1979

Muscle

Stimulation of 2-deoxyglucose
transport and glucose incorpora-   LeMarchand-Brustel, et
tion into glycogen   al., 1978
Activation of glycogen synthase   "   "

Liver

Stimulation of amino acid   A. LeCam, and P. Freychet,
(AIB) transport   personal communication

Placenta

Simulation of insulin's effects   L. C. Harrison, unpublish-
on protein phosphorylation   ed observation

The antibodies mimic not only membrane effects of insulin but
also intracellular effects independent of glucose transport
and, in addition, at least one long-term insulin effect,
namely, the stimulation of lipoprotein lipase activity in
3T3-Ll fatty fibroblasts. They do not, however, mimic the
long term growth effects of insulin (King, et al., 1979;
vide infra).

The bioactivity of the antibodies is dependent on their
bivalency (Kahn, et al., 1978a). While purified IgG and
F(ab')$_2$ inhibit insulin binding and mimic insulin's effects,
the monovalent F(ab') component only inhibits insulin binding (Figure 3). The bioactivity of the monovalent fragment
can, however, be restored by the addition of anti-F(ab')$_2$
antibody, indicating that bioactivity is dependent not only
on occupancy of the receptor, but also on cross-linking of

receptors or receptor subunits (Figure 4). There is evidence
that cross-linking may be a general requirement for activa-

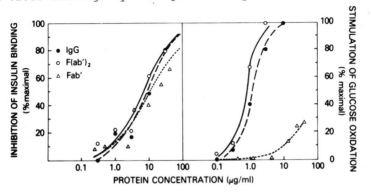

Figure 3. Comparison of the effects of intact IgG, F(ab')₂
and F(ab') on insulin binding and bioactivity.

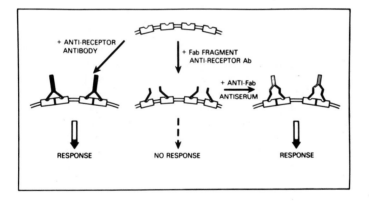

Figure 4. Crosslinking in receptor activation.

tion by antibodies, and possibly even by other ligands
including peptide hormones. IgE receptor-mediated mast cell
degranulation and histamine release requires cross-linking
of the IgE receptor with either IgE and second antibody,
antibodies to the receptor itself, or chemically cross-linked

IgE dimers (Metzger & Bach, 1978). It has also been shown
that bivalent, but not monovalent, antibodies will accelerate
the degradation of acetylcholine receptors in myasthenia
gravis (Drachman, et al., 1978). Whether insulin itself acts
by a cross-linking mechanism is speculative. Although the
circulating insulin is monomeric at physiologic concentrations
its local concentration at the cell membrane might be high
enough to induce self-association. (On the other hand, some
insulins e.g. guinea pig insulin, which do not dimerize in
solution still have intrinsic bioactivity.) In fact,
fluorescently-labeled analogues of insulin form microscopic-
ally-visible patches on the cell surface by rapidly diffus-
ing in the plane of the membrane, prior to capping and
internalization (Schlessinger, et al., 1978). However, the
physiological significance of this visible macro-aggregation
is unclear; the cross-linking that occurs with insulin
receptor antibodies or possibly with insulin itself must
initially be at a molecular level and most likely would
involve receptor subunits. Another piece of evidence in favor
of a cross-linking mechanism is that under certain conditions
the addition of insulin antibodies to insulin prebound at sub-
maximal concentrations can enhance insulin's action (Kahn,
et al., 1978a). Similar findings have recently been reported
for epidermal growth factor (EGF) (Schechter, et al., 1979).
Thus, an analogue of EGF with low biological activity was
shown to bind but not to redistribute into cell surface
patches; bivalent antibodies to EGF restored both bioactivity
and patch formation. Direct evidence for molecular cross-
linking in hormone action may be provided by elucidation of
the structure of receptors and by the study of reconstituted
receptors (and subunits). Finally, it should be noted that
agents which modify microtubules and microfilaments have no
effect on the bioactivity of either receptor antibodies or
insulin.

The studies on antibody bioactivity have several other
major implications. Firstly, they demonstrate that ligands
other than insulin which bind to the receptor mimic insulin's
actions. This was previously implied by the fact that some
lectins had insulin-like effects. However, the binding of
lectins is not restricted to sugars on the insulin receptor
alone; the specificity of the antibodies allows us to conclude that, contrary to traditional thinking, the nature of
the receptor interaction is the critical determinant, rather
than the nature of the ligand itself. The "information" for
insulin's action may therefore be "contained" within the

receptor. One might envisage that the role of the receptor is to maintain tonic inhibition of biological pathways, unless perturbed (? cross-linked). Secondly, the antibody studies imply that a specific degradation product of the insulin molecule is unlikely to be the mediator or "second messenger" of insulin's action.

The binding of insulin does not fulfill the assumptions for a simple thermodynamic equilibrium since a significant proportion of insulin is irreversibly bound (Kahn & Baird, 1978b), and is internalized to the site of lysosomes (Gorden, et al., 1979). We have also shown recently that part of the cell-associated insulin is covalently-coupled to the receptor (G. Saviolakis and L. C. Harrison, unpublished observation). The receptor antibodies are also internalized, with similar kinetics to insulin and, like insulin, are found to be preferentially associated with lysosomes (Carpentier, et al., 1979). It is presumed that internalization represents one possible degradative pathway for insulin and the receptor, but there is no direct evidence as yet that internalization is involved in the long-term effects of insulin such as enzyme induction. Specific binding sites for insulin are found on some intracellular organelles, particularly Golgi-endoplasmic reticulum (Bergeron, et al., 1978), but their role has not been established; they may simply be newly synthesized receptors en route to the cell surface.

The property of the monovalent receptor antibody to antagonise insulin at the receptor level has allowed the mechanism of insulin's mitogenic effects to be defined (King, et al., 1979). High concentrations of insulin stimulate thymidine uptake into DNA in fibroblasts but this effect is not mimicked by bivalent receptor antibody. When the cells are treated with monovalent receptor antibody to inhibit insulin binding the mitogenic effect of insulin persists. Since high concentrations of insulin cross-react with receptors for related growth factors, and since the binding to growth factor receptors is not inhibited by insulin receptor antibodies, **the mitogenic effects of insulin are probably mediated via its interaction with growth factor** receptors.

The insulin-like effects of the receptor antibodies in vitro present an apparent paradox since the donor patients are insulin-resistant and hyperglycemic, rather than hypo-glycemic. This discordance is not explained by species dif-

ferences since the antibodies have insulin-like effects in
both human and rodent adipocytes (Kasuga, et al., 1978b).
The major explanation appears to be that the bioactivity of
the antibodies is only short-lived (Karlsson, et al., 1979).
Hence, when cultured 3T3-L1 fatty fibroblasts are exposed to
receptor antibodies there is inhibition of insulin binding
and stimulation of glucose uptake and oxidation as seen in
normal adipocytes. However, this effect is maximal at two
hours and then decreases; glucose uptake returns to the
basal level and is then resistant to further stimulation by
either antibody or insulin (Figure 5). In the continued

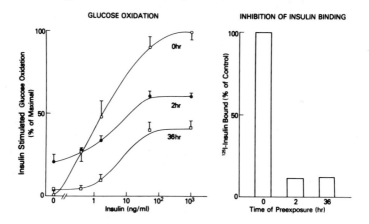

Figure 5. Effect on 3T3-L1 cells of pre-exposure to
receptor antibody (B-2).

presence of antibody there is a decreased sensitivity to
insulin because the antibody decreases receptor affinity.
However, in addition to decreased sensitivity the cells
also demonstrate decreased maximal responsiveness to insulin.
This has been termed "desensitization". The mechanism of
desensitization has not been precisely defined, but the
locus must be close to the binding site and early in the
pathway of insulin action since the activities of spermine
and Vitamin K_5, two agents which have insulin-like effects
without interacting with the receptor, are unaltered.
Desensitization is not affected by agents which modify
microtubules, microfilaments, or lysosomal function.

EXPERIMENTAL APPLICATION OF INSULIN RECEPTOR ANTIBODIES

The application of receptor antibodies as probes of

receptor function has been described. Two further examples
will further illustrate the utility of receptor antibodies.

Receptor Radioimmunoassay

The receptor can be measured in a radioimmunoassay by a
method which is in principle no different from any other
standard competitive binding assay (Harrison, et al, 1979a).
The solubilized insulin receptor is labeled with a tracer
amount of ^{125}I-insulin. A small fixed amount of ^{125}I-
insulin-receptor complex is then incubated at 4° with
receptor antibody and increasing amounts of unlabeled
receptor. The ^{125}I-insulin-receptor complex bound to antibody is subsequently precipitated by the addition of anti-
human IgG. The assay is sensitive to 0.1 nM insulin binding
sites and has a number of unique advantages. Firstly, it
measures the receptor independently of the insulin binding
function. Secondly, it uncovers immunological (and therefore structural) differences between insulin receptors.
Thus, although the insulin binding properties of the receptor
have been conserved throughout evolution and are virtually
identical in all tissues and species studied, equimolar
concentrations of insulin binding sites from different
species or from different tissues within the one species have
non-identical immunoreactivities. This is the first evidence
for heteorgeneity of insulin receptors. Finally, the
immunoassay has been applied to demonstrate that "down-regulation" of the insulin receptor in cultured lymphocytes,
(the loss of insulin binding after chronic exposure to
insulin) can be equated with loss of immunoreactive receptor
molecules.

Purification and Characterization of Receptors

Understanding the mechanism of receptor function will
ultimately require the purification of receptors and their
chemical and structural characterization. Several attempts
to purify the insulin receptor based on the use of affinity
chromatography with immobilized insulin have been reported
(Cuatrecasas, 1972; Jacobs, et al., 1977), but the purification achieved has only been a few percent and recoveries have
been too low to permit further characterization. Receptor
antibodies provide an alternative approach to purification.
We have obtained microgram quantities of purified receptor
by sequential affinity chromatography on wheat germ lectin
and receptor antibody (Harrison, et al., 1979e). The puri-

fied receptor is not associated with insulin degrading activity. In SDS-polyacrylamide gel electrophoresis it is resolved as two major components of molecular weight 82,000 and 35,000, and two minor components of molecular weight 66,000 and 55,000.

The antibodies have also been used to identify the insulin receptor from surface membranes of cultured lymphocytes labeled with ^{125}I and solubilized in Triton (Lang, et al., 1979). Analysis of the antibody-precipitated labeled membranes by SDS-polyacrylamide gel electrophoresis also demonstrated four components whose molecular weights were similar to those obtained by affinity chromatography. Moreover, the appearance of these components was suppressed by treatment of the solubilized membranes with unlabeled insulin, prior to the addition of antibody. These studies provide the first direct evidence for a complex subunit structure for the insulin receptor.

CONCLUSION

The studies of insulin receptor autoantibodies serve as a model for elucidating molecular mechanisms in immune disease and illustrate the importance of receptor antibodies as experimental probes. The characterization of the antibodies is based on the use of sensitive and specific functional assays for receptors. Cell surface receptors for peptide hormones, neurotransmitters, drugs, and antigens are prime candidates for immune-mediated disease and the application of the techniques described here may enlarge the domain of receptor diseases.

The existence of receptor autoantibodies implies a unified order of cellular recognition, covering the immune system and other systems (endocrine, neurologic, hematologic) whose functions are regulated by cell surface receptor interactions. The molecular mechanisms involved in hormone or neurotransmitter action are likely to be analogous to the interactions between antigens and antibodies, and to the regulation of the "immune response". Finally, it is conceivable that the existence of autoantibodies to peptide hormone receptors denotes, not a pathological breakdown of specificity between the immune and endocrine systems, but a failure to regulate a physiological system of "self" recognition.

REFERENCES

Aharonov A, Abramsky O, Tarrab-Hazdai R (1975): Humoral antibodies to acetylcholine receptor in patients with myasthenia gravis. Lancet ii:340.
Appel SH, Almon RR, Levy N (1975). Acetylcholine receptor antibodies in myasthenia gravis. N Engl J Med 293:760.
Bar RS, Harrison LC, Muggeo M, Gorden P, Kahn CR, Roth J (1979). Regulation of insulin receptors in normal and abnormal physiology in humans. Adv Int Med 24:23.
Bar RS, Gorden P, Roth J, Kahn CR, and De Meyts P (1976). Fluctuations in the affinity and concentration of insulin receptors on circulating monocytes of obese patients: effects of starvation, refeeding and dieting. J Clin Invest 58:1123.
Bar RS, Levis WR, Rechler MM, Harrison LC, Siebert CW, Podskalny JM, Roth J, Muggeo M (1978). Extreme insulin resistance in ataxia telangiectasia: Defect in affinity of insulin receptors. N Engl J Med 298:1164.
Bergeron JJM, Posner BI, Josefsberg Z, Sikstrom R (1978). Intracellular polypeptide hormone receptors: The demonstration of specific binding sites for insulin and human growth hormone in Golgi fractions isolated from the liver of female rats. J Biol Chem 253:4058.
Blackard WG, Gugelian PS, Small ME (1978). Down-regulation of insulin receptors in primary cultures of adult rat hepatocytes in monolayer. Endocrinology 103:548.
Carpentier J-L, Van Obberghen E, Gorden P, Orci L (1979). 125I-insulin receptor antibody binding to cultured human lymphocytes: morphological events are similar to the binding of 125I-insulin. Diabetes 28:345.
Cuatrecasas P (1972). Affinity chromatography and purification of the insulin receptor of liver cell membranes. Proc Natl Acad Sci (USA) 69:1277.
De Meyts P, Bianco AR and Roth J (1976). Site-site interactions among insulin receptors: characterization of negative cooperativity. J Biol Chem 251:1877.
Drachman DB, Angus CW, Adams RN, Michelson JD, Hoffman GJ (1978). Myasthenic antibodies cross-link acetylcholine receptors to accelerate degradation. N Engl J Med 298:1116.
Ehrlich P (1906). "Collected Studies on Immunity." New York: J Wiley & Sons.
Flier JS, Kahn CR, Roth J and Bar, RS (1975). Antibodies that impair insulin receptor binding in an unusual diabetic syndrome with severe insulin resistance. Science Wash., D.C. 190:63.
Flier JS, Kahn CR, Jarrett DB and Roth J (1976). Characteri-

zation of antibodies to the insulin receptor. A cause of insulin-resistant diabetes in man. J Clin Invest 58:1442.

Flier JS, Kahn CR, Jarrett DB and Roth J. Autoantibodies to the insulin receptor. Effect on the insulin receptor interaction in IM-9 lymphocytes. J Clin Invest 60:784.

Flier JS, Bar RS, Muggeo M, Kahn CR, Roth J, Gorden P (1978). The evolving clinical course of patients with insulin receptor autoantibodies: spontaneous remission or receptor proliferation with hypoglycemia. J Clin Endocrinol Metab 47:985.

Gavin JR, Roth J, Neville DM, Jr., De Meyts P and Buell DN (1974). Insulin dependent regulation of insulin receptor concentrations: A direct demonstration in cell culture. Proc Natl Acad Sci USA 71:84.

Gorden P, Carpentier J-L, Freychet P, LeCam A, Orci L (1978). Intracellular translocation of iodine-125-labeled insulin: direct demonstration in isolated hepatocytes. Science (Wash., D.C.) 200:782.

Harrison LC, Martin FIR and Melick (1976). Correlation between insulin receptor binding in isolated fat cells and insulin sensitivity in obese human subjects. J Clin Invest 58:1435.

Harrison LC, Flier JS, Itin A, Kahn CR, Roth J (1979a). Radioimmunoassay of the insulin receptor: New probe of receptor structure and function. Science (Wash., D.C.) 203:544.

Harrison LC, Muggeo M, Bar RS, Flier JS, Waldman T, Roth J, (1979b). Insulin binding defects induced by a serum globulin factor in ataxia telangiectasia. Clin Res 27:252A.

Harrison LC, Itin A (1979c). A possible mechanism for insulin resistance and hyperglycemia in NZO mice. Nature (London) 279:334.

Harrison LC, Flier JS, Roth J, Karlsson FA, Kahn CR (1979d). Immunoprecipitation of the insulin receptor: A sensitive assay for receptor antibodies and a specific technique for receptor purification. J Clin Endocrinol Metab 48:59.

Harrison LC, Itin A, Flier JS, Roth J (1979e). Major purification of the human insulin receptor using lectins and receptor antibody. Proc 61st Ann Meeting Endocrine Soc Anaheim, p 393.

Jacobs S, Chang K-j, Cuatrecasas P (1978). Antibodies to purified insulin receptor have insulin-like activity. Science (Wash., D.C.) 200:1283.

Jacobs S, Shechter Y, Bissell K, Cuatrecasas P (1977). Purification and properties of insulin receptors from rat liver membranes. Biochem Biophys Res Commun 77:981.

Jarrett DB, Roth J, Kahn CR, and Flier JS (1976). Direct

method for detection and characterization of cell surface receptors for insulin by means of ^{125}I-labeled autoantibodies against the insulin receptor. Proc Natl Acad Sci 73:4115.

Kahn CR, Neville DM, Jr, Roth J (1973). Insulin-receptor interaction in the obese-hyperglycemic mouse. J Biol Chem 248:244.

Kahn CR, Flier JS, Bar RS, Archer JA, Gorden P, Martin MM, and Roth J (1976). The syndromes of insulin resistance and acanthosis nigricans. Insulin-receptor disorders in man. N Engl J Med 294:739.

Kahn CR, Baird K, Flier JS and Jarrett Db (1977). Effects of autoantibodies to the insulin receptor on isolated adipocytes. Studies of insulin binding and insulin action. J Clin Invest 60:1094.

Kahn CR, Baird KL, Jarrett DB, Flier JS (1978a). Direct demonstration that receptor cross-linking or aggregation is important in insulin action. Proc Natl Acad Sci (USA) 75: 4209.

Kahn CR, Baird K (1978b). The fate of insulin bound to adipocytes: evidence for compartmentalization and processing. J Biol Chem 253:4900.

Karlsson FA, Van Obberghen E, Grunfeld C, Kahn CR (1979). Desensitization of the insulin receptor at an early post-receptor step by prolonged exposure to anti-receptor antibody. Proc Natl Acad Sci (USA) 76:809.

Kasuga M, Akanuma Y, Tsushima T, Suzuki K, Kosaka K, Kibata M (1978a). Effects of anti-insulin receptor autoantibody on the metabolism of rat adipocytes. J Clin Endocrinol Metab 47:66.

Kasuga M, Akanuma Y, Tsushima T, Iwamoto Y, Kosaka K, Kibata M, Kawanishi K (1978b). Effects of anti-insulin receptor autoantibodies on the metabolism of human adipocytes. Diabetes 27:938.

King GL, Kahn CR, Rechler MM, Nissley SP (1979). Direct demonstration that insulin and insulin-like growth factors produce their metabolic and growth effects via different receptors. Clin Res 27:486A.

Kosmakos FC and Roth J. Cellular basis of insulin-induced loss of insulin receptors. Endocrine Society, 58th Annual Meeting, June 23-25, San Francisco, Abstract 69, 1976.

Lang U, Kahn CR, Harrison LC (1979). The subunit structure of the insulin receptor of the human lymphocyte. Biochemistry (in press).

Lawrence JC, Jr, Larner J, Kahn CR, Roth J (1978). Antibodies to insulin receptor stimulate glycogen synthase in rat adipocytes. Mol Cell Biochm 22:153.

Le Marchand Brustel Y, Gorden P, Flier JS, Kahn CR and
Freychet P (1978). Anti-insulin receptor antibodies mimic
insulin binding and stimulate glucose metabolism in skeletal
muscle. Diabetologica 14:311.

Lindstrom JM, Seybold ME, Lennon VA Whittingham S, Duane DD
(1976). Antibody to acetylcholine receptor in myasthenia
gravis: prevalence, clinical correlates, and diagnositc
value. Neurology (Minneap) 26:1054.

Metzger H, Bach MK (1978). The receptor for IgE on mast
cells and basophils: Studies on IgE binding and on the
structure of the receptor. In Bach MK (ed): "Immediate
Hypersensitivity: Modern Concepts and Development,"
New York: Marcel Dekker, p 561.

Muggeo M, Flier JS, Abrams RA, Harrison LC, Deisserroth, AB,
Kahn CR (1979a): Treatment by plasma exchange of a patient
with autoantibodies to the insulin receptor. N Engl J Med
300:477.

Muggeo M, Kahn CR, Bar RS, Rechler MM, Flier JS, Roth J
(1979b): The underlying receptor in patients with anti-
receptor autoantibodies: Demonstration of normal binding
and immunologic properties. J Clin Endocrinol Metab 49:110.

Olefsky JM (1976): Insulin binding to adipocytes and
circulating monocytes from obese patients. J Clin Invest 57:
1165.

Roth J (1973): Peptide hormone binding to receptors: A
review of direct studies in vitro. Metabolism 22:1059.

Schechter Y, Hernaez L, Schlessinger, J, Cuatrecasas P (1979):
Local aggregation of hormone-receptor complexes is required
for activation by epidermal growth factor. Nature (London)
278:835.

Schlessinger J, Schechter Y, Willingham MC, Pastan I (1978):
Direct visualization of binding, aggregation, and internalization of insulin and epidermal growth factor on linking
fibroblastic cells. Proc Natl Acad Sci (USA) 75:2659.

Smith BR, Hall R: Thyroid-stimulating immunoglobulins in
Graves' disease. Lancet ii:427.

Van Obberghen E, Spooner PM, Kahn CR, Chernick SS, Garrison
MM, Karlsson FA, Grunfeld C (1979). Insulin-receptor antibodies mimic a late insulin effect. Nature (London) 280:500.

Venter JC, Fraser C, Harrison LC (1979). Autoantibodies to
the β_2-adrenergic receptor: a cause of β-adrenergic hyporesponsiveness in allergic rhinitis and asthma. (Submitted).

Pages 127—144, Membranes, Receptors, and the Immune Response
© 1980 Alan R. Liss, Inc., 150 Fifth Avenue, New York, NY 10011

REGULATION OF β-ADRENERGIC RECEPTOR DENSITY IN THE CONTROL
OF ADRENERGIC RESPONSIVENESS

Claire M. Fraser and J. Craig Venter

Department of Pharmacology and Therapeutics
SUNY at Buffalo, School of Medicine
Buffalo, NY   14214

INTRODUCTION

β-adrenergic receptors are lipoproteins which exist on
the surface of essentially all cells and modulate a wide
range of physiological events. β-adrenergic receptors demonstrate a marked stereoselectivity in binding adrenergic ligands and a sulfhydryl group appears to be involved in the
ligand binding site (Strauss and Venter, unpublished observations) in agreement with Ehrlich's receptor concept.
Advances in the molecular characterization of β-receptors and
the control of β-receptor responses at the cellular level
have provided some insight into the role of receptor density
in the regulation of physiological function. Disease states
such as asthma, hypertension and heart disease may in part be
related to variations in the concentration of β-adrenergic
receptors in specific organ or cell systems.

β-RECEPTOR CLASSIFICATION AND MOLECULAR CHARACTERIZATION

Adrenergic receptor substances which were postulated to
exist in the early 1900's (Dale, 1906; Langley, 1901)
were classified as alpha and beta in 1948 by Ahlquist
(Ahlquist, 1948). β-adrenergic receptors were further
classified into β_1 and β_2 sub-types by Lands et al., 1967.
In accordance with this pharmacological classification, β-
adrenergic receptors in cardiac muscle and adipose tissue
are defined as β_1 while those in airway smooth muscle, vas-
cular smooth muscle and liver are classified as β_2 (Furchgott, 1972). Support for β-receptor subclassification comes

from recent studies from this laboratory suggesting that a molecular heterogeneity exists in β-receptors isolated from various tissues. Differences in the detergent specificity and the stability of solubilized canine and hepatic β-receptors served as the impetus for investigation of other molecular parameters (Strauss et al., 1979). Subsequent studies demonstrated that the Stokes radii and apparent molecular weights of canine heart, liver and lung β-receptors differ substantially (Table 1). In addition, these receptor molecules exhibit a differential susceptibility to inactivation by sulfhydryl reagents such as dithiothreitol (DTT) (Table 2) (Strauss et al., submitted).

These observations are also supported by immunological evidence. Antibodies raised against partially purified [3H]-propranolol binding sites from dog heart block adenylate cyclase activation in heart membranes with no effect on adenylate cyclase activity in liver membranes (Wrenn and Haber, 1979). Conversely, autoantibodies to β-adrenergic receptors from the serum of asthma and allergic rhinitis patients block adrenergic ligand binding to lung β_2-receptors but not cardiac β_1-receptors (Venter et al., submitted).

TABLE 1

Molecular Parameters of Cardiac, Lung and Liver β-Adrenergic Receptors

Parameter	Heart	Lung	Liver
Stokes Radius a (nm)	4.2 ± 0.01 n = 9	5.8 ± 0.02 n = 4	5.8 ± 0.02 n = 6
Sedimentation coefficient $S_{20,W}$	3.69 ± 0.06 n = 10 (3.4 - 3.9)	3.78 ± 0.13 n = 8 (3.3 - 4.2)	3.67 ± 0.09 n = 13 (3.1 - 4.2)
Partial Specific Volume $\bar{V}$ g/ml	0.73	0.73	0.73
Molecular Weight (Mr)	65,000	91,000	90,000
Frictional ratio f/fo	1.6	2.0	2.0

(From Strauss et al., submitted)

Table 2

Molecular Subclassification of β-Adrenergic Receptors

Species	Cell or Tissue	IHYP Binding Inhibition by 1 mM DTT (%)	Stokes Radius (nm)	β-Receptor Subtype
Dog	Liver	0	5.8	β_2
Rat	Liver	0	-	β_2
Cat	Liver	0	-	β_2
Frog	Erythrocytes	-	5.8^a	β_2
Mouse	Lymphoma (S-49)	-	6.4^b	β_2
Dog	Lung	16 ± 6.4	5.8	β_2/β_1
Human	Lung (VA$_2$ Cells)	17 ± 6.0	5.8	β_2/β_1
Rat	Lung	32 ± 1.1	-	β_2/β_1
Rabbit	Lung	41 ± 2.0	-	β_1/β_2
Cat	Lung	43 ± 8.0	-	β_1/β_2
Dog	Adipocytes	41 ± 1.7	-	β_1/β_2
Rat	Glioma (C6 Cells)	44 ± 2.3	-	β_1/β_2
Turkey	Erythrocytes	35 ± 4.6	4.2	β_1/β_2
Rat	Heart	65 ± 6.1	4.8	β_1/β_2
Dog	Heart	80 ± 1.5	4.2	β_1

[a] Limbird & Lefkowitz 1978

[b] Haga et al 1977

(Data from Strauss et al submitted)

While there appear to be at least two distinct molecular forms of the β-receptor, some of the available data suggest that more than two forms may exist and that the cardiac β-receptor may differ from other β_1 receptors (Table 2). The data in Table 2 also indicate that while adrenergic ligand binding sites of β-receptors in a given species may not be identical, the β-receptor subtype in a particular tissue may be phylogenetically conserved.

The unique molecular nature of β-receptors in different tissues may allow for the selective regulation of β-receptor function; as in the interaction of lung but not cardiac β-receptors with circulating autoantibodies to β$_2$-receptors (Venter *et al.*, submitted).

RELATIONSHIP BETWEEN β-ADRENERGIC RECEPTOR DENSITY AND ADRENERGIC RESPONSIVENESS

We have shown that the modulation of β-receptor density on the cell surface can provide a substantial degree of control over the responsiveness of a particular cell or tissue to hormonal stimulation (Venter, 1980). The stoichiometry between β-receptor concentration and adrenergic responsiveness has, in part, been elucidated with the β-receptor affinity ligand, N-[2-hydroxy-3-(1-napthoxy)-propyl]-N-bromoacetylethylenediamine (NHNP-NBE) (Atlas *et al.*, 1976), which covalently modifies the β-adrenergic receptor at or near the catecholamine binding site (Venter, 1979).

NHNP-NBE can interact with β-receptors in intact cardiac muscle in a dose-related manner (Venter, 1979). The dose dependent inactivation of cardiac β-receptors by NHNP-NBE has been directly compared to NHNP-NBE modulation of the cardiac contractile response to isoproterenol. Figure 1 illustrates that increasing concentrations of NHNP-NBE shift the dose response curves for isoproterenol stimulated cardiac contractility to the right. Importantly, there is no reduction in the maximum responsiveness of the cardiac muscle provided that a sufficient concentration of isoproterenol is present.

The percentage of unoccupied β-receptors in the presence of increasing concentrations of NHNP-NBE was determined by radioligand binding with [^{125}I]-iodohydroxybenzylpindolol (IHYP) and is compared to the shift produced in the isoproterenol concentration required for a half-maximal contractile response (Table 3). These data indicate that isoproterenol can still produce a maximum contractile response in the heart by interacting with as few as 10% of the β-receptors present on the cell surface (Venter, 1979). These results demonstrate directly the existence of "spare" β-adrenergic receptors in the heart in relation to cardiac contractility. The same high efficiency coupling is also demonstrable for β-receptor mediated cyclic AMP production in the heart (Venter, 1979).

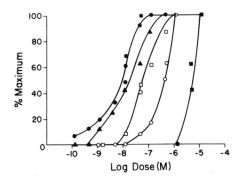

Figure 1

Log dose response curves for isoproterenol stimulated positive inotropic responses in cat papillary muscles following increasing concentrations of the covalent β-receptor antagonist, NHNP-NBE. Muscles were treated with 0.1 μM NHNP-NBE (closed triangles); 1.0 μM (open squares); 10 μM (open circles); and 100 μM NHNP-NBE for 10 minutes followed by extensive washing prior to isoproterenol testing. (From Venter 1979).

VA$_2$ cells, an SV40 transformed clone of human lung cells, provide a well characterized system with regard to IHYP binding and cyclic AMP production (Maguire *et al.*, 1975; Maguire *et al.*, 1976). As in cardiac muscle, the covalent β-receptor antagonist, NHNP-NBE, produces a dose-dependent loss of IHYP specific binding in these cells. Yet unlike the heart, irreversible inactivation of β-receptors in the VA$_2$ cells is accompanied by a concomitant stoichiometric loss of isoproterenol induced cyclic AMP production (Figure 2) (Venter, 1979).

These data from the VA$_2$ cells together with the data from the heart indicate that there are at least two types of coupling between β-receptors and adenylate cyclase, the high efficiency coupling found in cardiac muscle and the low efficiency or stoichiometric coupling observed in some cultured cell systems (Venter, 1979). There is evidence that tracheal smooth muscle cells may also display a high effi-

Table 3

Heart β-Receptor Occupation by NHNP-NBE vs Cardiac

Inotropic Responses to Isoproterenol

NHNP-NBE Concentration[a] (μM)	% Total β-Receptors Occupied[b]	Inotropic Response ED50 1-Isoproterenol (nM)[c]	% Control Maximum Response Achieved
CONTROL	0	9.8 ± 2.3 n = 7	100
0.1	0	22	100
1.0	43	70	100
10	69	500	100
100	90	5623	100

[a] Represents the final concentration of NHNP-NBE in cat papillary muscle baths for a 10 min incubation

[b] Calculated from IHYP binding data

[c] Determined from the mid-point of log dose response curves performed over 6 orders of magnitude range of isoproterenol concentrations

(From Venter, 1979)

ciency coupling between β-receptors and isoproterenol induced relaxation (Avner and Wilson, 1979). The cellular mechanisms which may allow for the expression of spare β-receptors have been discussed (Venter, 1980).

The high efficiency coupling between cardiac β-receptors and contractility allowing for the expression of spare β-receptors also provides a mechanism for the regulation of adrenergic responses. The above data with NHNP-NBE have illustrated that even with a substantial reduction in β-receptor density in the heart the maximum β-receptor mediated response can still be elicited provided sufficient catecholamine is available to the receptors. These data indicate that the density of cardiac β-receptors will determine the sensitivity of a given portion of the heart to catecholamines.

The β-receptor density in the heart varies substantially

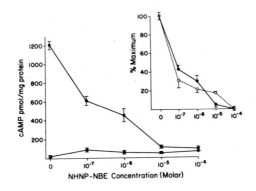

Figure 2

The inhibition of isoproterenol induced cyclic AMP formation in cultured cells in the presence of increasing concentrations of NHNP-NBE. VA$_2$ cells were assayed for cyclic AMP content in the non-stimulated state (lower curve) and in the presence of 10 μM isoproterenol (upper curve). Cells were preincubated for 10 min. with the indicated concentrations of NHNP-NBE and then washed three times. The inset illustrates the percent inhibition of the isoproterenol induced cyclic AMP production by NHNP-NBE (closed circles) and of IHYP specific binding to VA$_2$ membranes (open circles). (From Venter, 1979).

from one area to another, while the adenylate cyclase activity is much more constant. These data which suggest a variable ratio of β-receptors to adenylate cyclase throughout the heart are supported by the demonstration of corresponding variations in the sensitivity of different regions of the heart to catecholamine stimulated activation of adenylate cyclase (Venter, 1980).

The variations in β-receptor density may be of functional significance. For example, the sinoatrial node which is contained in or is surrounded by atrial myocardial cells, has eight times the density of β-receptors as the surrounding atrial muscle cells (Venter, 1980). From the dose response data in Figure 1 and Table 3, this receptor concentra-

tion difference could imply that the sinoatrial node might
elicit a maximal response to catecholamines before the threshold for the atria is exceeded. Mechanistically these
regional sensitivity differences could play an important
role in maintaining the heart in a normal functioning con-
dition (Venter, 1980).

REGULATION OF β-ADRENERGIC RECEPTOR DENSITY: POSSIBLE ROLE
IN DISEASE

β-receptor concentrations have been reported to be dependent on a number of contributing factors including the
rate of receptor synthesis and turnover (Fraser and Venter,
submitted), the cell cycle (Charlton and Venter, submitted),
cell density and/or cell to cell contact (Harden et al.,
1979; Fraser and Venter, submitted), receptor desensitization (Lefkowitz and Williams, 1978; Harden et al., 1979),
hormones such as thyroid hormone and glucocorticoids (Williams
et al., 1977; Fraser and Venter, submitted) and possibly by
circulating autoantibodies to β-receptors (Venter et al.,
submitted).

The rate of β-receptor synthesis and incorporation into
plasma membranes of human lung cells (VA$_2$, VA$_4$ and WI38 cells)
has recently been measured using NHNP-NBE (Fraser and Venter,
submitted). Following irreversible blockade of existing β-
receptors, new receptors appear in the membrane at a relatively constant rate of 2% of the initial density per hour
(Figure 3). The half-life of the β-receptors in this system
can be estimated to be on the order of 20-30 hours. Puromycin immediately blocks the incorporation of new β-receptors into the cell membrane demonstrating that active protein synthesis is required for the appearance of new β-receptor molecules.

These synthesis and turnover rates of the β-receptor
indicate that the half-life of the receptor in the cell membrane is relatively short. Therefore, factors which affect
the rate of β-receptor turnover may profoundly affect both
the density of β-receptors on the cell surface and the responsiveness of a particular organ or cell system.

There are several lines of evidence which suggest that
the physiological state of a tissue can influence the rate
at which specific membrane proteins turnover. For example,

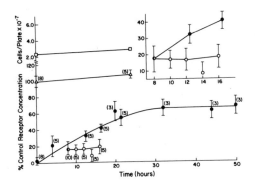

Figure 3

β-adrenergic receptor synthesis and incorporation rates into
VA₂ cell membranes. VA₂ cells were treated twice with 100
μM NHNP-NBE followed by extensive washing to remove unbound
ligand. β-receptor concentrations were measured in cell
membrane fractions as a function of time. Control synthesis rates (open triangles), synthesis rates in cells
treated with NHNP-NBE (closed circles), and synthesis rates
in cells treated with NHNP-NBE plus puromycin (0.1 mg/ml)
8 hours subsequent to NHNP-NBE treatment are indicated.
(From Fraser and Venter, submitted).

muscle denervation increases the turnover of the nicotinic
acetylcholine receptor (Berg and Hall, 1974) and this effect
can be blocked by direct electrical stimulation of the muscle (Lomo and Rosenthal, 1979). Circulating antibodies in
the sera of myasthenia gravis patients also accelerate degradation of the nicotinic acetylcholine receptor (Drachman
et al., 1978).

Various hormones have been shown to regulate the concentration of several membrane receptors. Gavin and co-
workers described a down-regulation of insulin receptor concentrations in lymphocytes exposed to low levels of insulin
(Gavin et al., 1974). This phenomenon of insulin regulation
of insulin receptor concentrations has been observed in a
number of species and appears to involve an energy dependent

increase in insulin receptor degradation (Kahn, 1976). Thyrotropin releasing hormone (TRH) receptor concentrations in
cultured rat pituitary cells decrease if cells are grown in
the presence of low concentrations of TRH or thyroid hormone
(Hinkle and Tashjian, 1975; Perrone and Hinkle, 1977) whereas hydrocortisone increases TRH receptor density in these
cells (Tashjian *et al.*, 1977).

Hydrocortisone produces a 100% increase in β-receptor
concentration in cultured human lung cells (VA$_2$, VA$_4$ and
WI38 cells) within a 24 hour period (Fraser and Venter,
submitted). The molecular mechanism responsible for this
increase in β-receptor concentration appears to be a glucocorticoid stimulated doubling in the rate of β-receptor synthesis and incorporation into lung cell membranes (Figure 4).

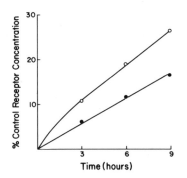

Figure 4

*β-adrenergic receptor incorporation rates into hydrocortisone
treated VA$_4$ cell membranes.* VA$_4$ cells were grown in the presence of 1 μM hydrocortisone for 18 hours prior to receptor
inactivation with 100 μM NHNP-NBE. β-receptor concentrations
were measured in intact cells as a function of time. The
rates of receptor synthesis and incorporation in control
cells (closed circles) and hydrocortisone treated cells
(open circles) are indicated. (From Fraser and Venter,sub-
mitted).

Glucocorticoids are commonly used in the treatment of asthma although their mechanism of action has not been established. The glucocorticoid induction of β-receptor synthesis rates in normal human lung cells suggests that their therapeutic effects in the treatment of asthma may involve the regulation of β-receptor concentrations.

Administration of thyroid hormone to rats results in an increased number of cardiac β-receptors (Williams et al., 1977). The effect of thyroid hormone in the heart is significant in terms of the increased sensitivity of the heart to catecholamines observed in hyperthyroidism such as in Graves' disease. Conversely, a decrease in cardiac responsiveness to catecholamines has been noted with hypothyroidism (Kunos et al., 1977) and supports the hypothesis that β-receptor density in the heart may play an important role in the control of cardiac function.

Another phenomenon involved in regulation of adrenergic responsiveness in a number of isolated cell systems is agonist induced desensitization of β-receptors (Lefkowitz and Williams, 1978; Harden et al., 1979). The molecular mechanisms of desensitization are not entirely clear. However, it has been reported that in vivo desensitization of tracheal smooth muscle to the actions of β-receptor agonists results from a reduction in the affinity of the receptor for agonists (Avner and Noland, 1978). Conolly and co-workers have suggested that desensitization of airway smooth muscle in asthmatics may occur as a consequence of prolonged use of isoproterenol-containing aerosols (Conolly et al., 1971). In contrast, isolated cardiac muscles display little, if any, tachyphylaxis when exposed repeatedly to agonists (Venter, 1980). The excess or spareness of β-receptors in the myocardium could possibly protect against the effects of desensitization.

There is increasing evidence that autoantibodies to membrane receptors can have substantial influence over receptor function. Autoantibodies to cell membrane receptors have been documented in a number of disease states in man. Antibodies to the nicotinic acetylcholine receptor have been implicated in myasthenia gravis (Patrick et al., 1973; Lindstrom et al., 1976), to the thyrotropin receptor in Graves' disease (Smith and Hall, 1974; and Manley et al., 1974) and to the insulin receptor in certain types of insulin resistant diabetes (Flier et al., 1975; Kahn et al., 1976;

Harrison *et al.*, 1978. See also Harrison, this volume).

Venter, Fraser & Harrison have recently identified auto-antibodies to β₂-receptors in the sera of asthma and allergic rhinitis patients. These autoantibodies precipitate soluble dog lung β-receptors in a dose-dependent manner in an indirect immunoprecipitation assay (Figure 5). At the

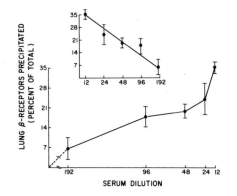

Figure 5

Immunoprecipitation of solubilized canine lung β-receptors with autoantibodies to β₂-adrenergic receptors. β-receptors in purified canine lung membranes were specifically labelled with IHYP, solubilized with 0.5% Triton X-100 and incubated with various dilutions of serum containing β-receptor anti-bodies. Precipitation of the labelled receptor antibody complexes was accomplished by the addition of an excess of anti-human IgG. The inset illustrates a semi-logarithmic plot of the immunoprecipitation data. (From Venter *et al.*, submitted).

lowest serum dilution tested, 30% of the solubilized lung β-receptors are specifically precipitated. Receptor precipitation is dependent on the addition of anti-human IgG (Venter *et al.*, submitted).

The β-receptor autoantibodies appear to be directed at

a determinants(s) in or near the ligand binding site of the receptor. Preincubation of membranes from dog lung, calf lung and human placenta with various dilutions of serum results in a concentration dependent reduction in IHYP specific binding to β-receptors compared to control serum (Figure 6). Pretreatment of the serum with anti-human IgG prior to

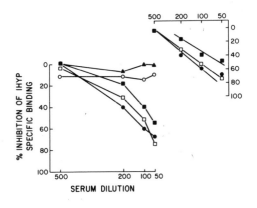

Figure 6

The effects of autoantibodies to $β_2$-adrenergic receptors on IHYP binding to membrane bound β-adrenergic receptors. Purified membranes from canine heart (open circles), canine lung (open squares), calf lung (closed circles) and human placenta (closed squares) were preincubated with the indicated dilutions of serum followed by determinations of IHYP specific binding to the β-receptors. Canine lung membranes were also preincubated with gamma globulin depleted serum (closed triangles). The inset illustrates a semi-logarithmic plot of the IHYP binding data. (From Venter *et al.*, submitted).

incubation with lung membranes completely abolishes its ability to inhibit IHYP specific binding to the receptor and confirms that the serum factor responsible for inhibition of IHYP specific binding is an IgG molecule. The autoantibodies have little or no effect on IHYP binding to dog heart β-receptors (Figure 6), consistent with the notion that heart and lung β-receptors are distinct molecular entities (Strauss et al., 1979). These data also support the idea that the adrenergic ligand binding site of the β-receptor within a given species may not be identical, but that β-receptor subtype in a particular tissue may be phylogenetically conserved (Strauss et al., submitted).

Receptor blockade by β-receptor antibodies could upset the balance between β-receptor mediated relaxation of airway smooth muscle and the opposing influence of other chemical mediators in the lung (Szentivanyi, 1968; Henderson et al., 1979). β-receptor autoantibodies may also reduce receptor density on smooth muscle cells by accelerating the rate of receptor degradation. Therefore, these autoantibodies could provide a molecular mechanism for β-adrenergic hyporesponsiveness observed in allergic rhinitis and asthma.

SUMMARY

Recent evidence strongly suggests that the density of β-adrenergic receptors in the heart and the lung may play a significant role in the tissue response to adrenergic stimulation. Thus, regulation of β-receptor density in a particular tissue may serve as an important mechanism in the control of adrenergic responsiveness. Variations in both cardiac and pulmonary β-receptor concentrations may be a major contributing factor to the etiology of clinical manifestations associated with some cardiovascular and respiratory disease states. Supported by grants from NIH #HL21329 and the American Heart Association.

REFERENCES

Ahlquist RP (1948). A study of the adrenotropic receptors. Am J Physiol 153: 586.

Atlas DM, Steer ML, Levitski A (1976). Affinity label for β-adrenergic receptor in turkey erythrocytes. Proc Nat Acad Sci USA 73: 1921.

Avner BP, Noland B (1978). In vivo desensitization to β-receptor mediated bronchodilator drugs in the rat: Decreased β-receptor affinity. JPET 207: 23.

Avner B, Wilson S (1979). Possible existence of "spare" β-receptors in rat tracheal smooth muscle. Proc West Pharmacol Soc 22: 177.

Berg D, Hall TW (1974). Fate of α-bungarotoxin bound to

acetylcholine receptors of normal and denervated muscle. Science 184: 473.

Charlton RR, Venter JC. Cell-cycle specific changes in β-adrenergic receptor concentrations in C6 glioma cells. Submitted for publication.

Conolly ME, Davies DS, Dollery CT, George CF (1971). Resistance to β-adrenoceptor stimulants (a possible explanation for the rise in asthma deaths). Brit J Pharmacol 43: 389.

Dale HH (1906). On some physiological actions of ergot. J Physiol London 34: 163.

Drachman DB, Angus CW, Adams RN, Michelson JD, Hoffman GJ (1978). Cross-linking of acetylcholine receptors by antibodies in myasthenia gravis. N Eng J Med 298: 1116.

Flier JS, Kahn CR, Roth J, Bar RS (1975). Antibodies that impair insulin receptor binding in an unusual diabetic syndrome with severe insulin resistance. Science 190: 63.

Fraser CM, Venter JC. The synthesis and regulation of β-adrenergic receptors in cultured cells. Submitted for publication.

Furchgott RF (1972). The pharmacological differentiation of adrenergic receptors. Hand Exp Pharmacol 33: 283.

Gavin JT III, Roth J, Neville DM, DeMeytes P, Buell DM (1974). Insulin-dependent regulation of insulin receptor concentrations: a direct demonstration in cell culture. Proc Nat Acad Sci USA 71: 84.

Haga T, Haga K, Gilman AG (1977). Hydrodynamic properties of the β-adrenergic receptor and adenylate cyclase from wild type and variant S49 lymphoma cells. J Biol Chem 252: 5776.

Harden TK, Foster SJ, Perkins JP (1979). Differential expression of components to the adenylate cyclase system during growth of astrocytoma cells in culture. J Biol Chem 254: 4416.

Harden TK, Su Y-F, Perkins JP (1979). Catecholamine-induced desensitization involves an uncoupling of β-adrenergic receptors and adenylate cyclase. J Cyclic Nucleotide Res 5: 99.

Harrison LC, Flier JS, Kahn CR, Jarrett DB, Muggeo M, Roth J (1978). Autoantibodies to the insulin receptor: Clinical and molecular aspects. In Rose NR, Bigazzi PE, Warner NL (eds): "Genetic Control of Autoimmune Disease," New York: Elsevier North-Holland p 61.

Henderson WR, Shelahmer JH, Reingold DB, Smith LJ, Evans R III, Kaliner M (1979). Alpha-adrenergic hyperrespon-

siveness in asthma. N Eng J Med 300: 642.
Hinkle PM, Tashjian AH Jr. (1975). Thyrotropin releasing
hormone regulates the number of its own receptors in
GH_3 strain of pituitary cells in culture. Biochem 14:
3845.
Kahn CR (1976). Membrane receptors for hormones and neurotransmitters. J Cell Biol 70: 261.
Kahn CR, Flier JS, Bar RS, Archer JA, Gorden P, Martin MM,
Roth J (1976). The syndromes of insulin resistance
and acanthosis nigricans. N Eng J Med 294: 739.
Kunos G, Vermes- Kunos I, Nickerson M (1974). Effects of
thyroid state on adrenoceptor properties. Nature 250:
779.
Lands AM, Arnold A, McAuliff JP, Ludvena FP, Brown TG (1967).
Differentiation of receptor systems activated by sym-
pathomimetic amines. Nature 214: 597.
Langley JN (1901). Observations on the physiological action
of extracts of the supra-renal bodies. J Physiol Lon-
don 27: 237.
Lefkowitz RJ, Williams LT (1978). Molecular mechanisms of
activation and desensitization of adenylate cyclase
coupled beta-adrenergic receptors. In George WJ,
Ignarro LJ (eds): "Advances in Cyclic Nucleotide Re-
search Vol. 9," New York: Raven Press, p 1.
Limbird LE, Lefkowitz RJ (1978). Agonist-induced increase
in apparent β-adrenergic receptor size. Proc Nat Acad
Sci USA 75: 228.
Lindstrom JM, Lennon VA, Seybold ME, Whittingham S (1976).
Experimental autoimmune myasthenia gravis and myasthenia
gravis: a biochemical and immunological approach. Ann
NY Acad Sci 274: 254.
Lomo T, Rosenthal J (1979). Control of acetylcholine sen-
sitivity by muscle activity in the rat. J Physiol
London 221: 493.
Maguire ME, Wilklund RA, Anderson HJ, Gilman AG (1976).
Binding of [^{125}I]-iodohydroxybenzylpindolol to putative
β-adrenergic receptors of rat glioma cells and other
cell clones. J Biol Chem 251: 1221.
Maguire ME, Sturgill TW, Anderson HJ, Minna JD, Gilman AG
(1975). Hormonal control of cyclic AMP metabolism in
parental and hybrid somatic cells. In Drummond GI,
Greengard P, Robison GA (eds): "Advances in Cyclic
Nucleotide Research Vol. 6," New York: Raven Press,
p 699.
Manley SW, Bourke JR, Hawker RW (1974). The thyrotropin
receptor in guinea-pig thyroid homogenate: interaction

with the long-acting thyroid stimulator. J Endocrinol 61: 437.

Patrick J, Lindstrom J, Culf B, McMillan J (1973). Studies on purified eel acetylcholine receptor and anti-acetylcholine receptor antibody. Proc Nat Acad Sci USA 70: 3334.

Perrone MH, Hinkle PM (1978). Regulation of pituitary receptors for thyrotropin-releasing hormone by thyroid hormones. J Biol Chem 253: 5168.

Smith BR, Hall R (1974). Thyroid-stimulating immunoglobulins in Graves' disease. Lancet 2: 427.

Strauss WL, Ghai G, Fraser CM, Venter JC (1979). Detergent solubilization of mammalian cardiac and hepatic β-adrenergic receptors. Arch Biochem Biophys 196: 566.

Strauss WL, Ghai G, Fraser CM, Venter JC. Hydrodynamic properties and sulfhydryl reagent sensitivity of β-adrenergic receptors: Molecular evidence for isoreceptors. Submitted for publication.

Szentivanyi A (1968). The β-adrenergic theory of the atopic abnormality in bronchial asthma. J Allergy 42: 203.

Tashjian AH Jr., Osborne R, Maina D, Knaian A (1977). Hydrocortisone increases the number of receptors for thyrotropin-releasing hormone on pituitary cells in culture. Biochem Biophys Res Comm 79: 333.

Venter JC (1979). High efficiency coupling between β-adrenergic receptors and cardiac contractility: Direct evidence for "spare" β-adrenergic receptors. Mol Pharm 16: 429.

Venter JC (1980). β-adrenergic receptors, adenylate cyclase and the adrenergic control of cardiac contractility. In Kunos G (ed): "Adrenoceptors and Catecholamine Action," New York: Wiley Interscience, in press.

Venter JC, Fraser CM, Harrison LC. Autoantibodies to the β_2-adrenergic receptor: A possible cause of β-adrenergic hyporesponsiveness in allergic rhinitis and asthma. Submitted for publication.

Williams LT, Lefkowitz RJ, Watanabe AM, Hathaway DR, Besch HR Jr. (1977). Thyroid hormone regulation of β-adrenergic receptor number. J Biol Chem 252: 2787.

Wrenn S, Haber E (1979). An antibody specific for the propranolol binding site of cardiac muscle. J Biol Chem 254: 6577.

Singer: I take it you have not done the studies to
             tell if these antibodies are agonists or
             antagonists?
Venter: That is correct. The highest titer we have is
             1:160. We are screening other patients for
             higher titers.

Singer: Do you see any correlation with autoantibody
             level and asthma?
Venter: I see definite correlation with autoantibody
             level and decreased beta-adrenergic respon-
             siveness. This is the first demonstration of
             an autoantibody to a beta receptor. The three
             that we found positive were out of 10-15
             patients. We have no idea of frequency in the
             population as a whole.

Singer: In monocytes, is the beta-adrenergic receptor
             beta-one or beta-two?
Venter: It is probably a beta-two subclass.

Pages 145—168, Membranes, Receptors, and the Immune Response
© 1980 Alan R. Liss, Inc., 150 Fifth Avenue, New York, NY 10011

ADAPTATION OF MEMBRANE-ASSOCIATED DETERMINANTS IS AN OUTGROWTH OF THEIR METABOLISM

Edward P. Cohen, M. D.

Department of Microbiology and Immunology
University of Illinois at the Medical Center
Chicago, IL 60612

SUMMARY
The quantity of receptors expressed by specialized cells for hormones, foreign antigenic substances, and other chemical stimuli diminishes after they associate with ligands, correlating with a specific reduction in the responsiveness of the cell to further stimulation. Ligand-induced adaptation of membrane receptors may be akin to antigenic modulation--the reversible disappearance of membrane-associated determinants stimulated by specific antibodies. Antigenic modulation has been studied extensively in the thymus-leukemia (TL) system of mouse leukemias. Antibody-induced changes in the quantities of TL antigens expressed by ASL-1 and RADA-1 cells, independently arising leukemia cell lines of strain A mice, are outgrowths of their metabolic turnover. After interacting with TL antibodies, the rate of TL antigen disappearance from the membrane increases while the rate of antigen synthesis remains unchanged. Antiserum with specificities for two membrane-associated determinants of ASL-1 cells, TL and a tumor-associated antigen, leads to modulation of TL antigens alone; the tumor antigen persists. Selectivity of modulation is taken as an indication that complex cellular controls govern the affect of antiserum on the expression of membrane antigens. To detect the presence of regulatory controls governing the expression of membrane determinants, stable somatic hybrids of ASL-1 murine leukemia cells and LM(TK)⁻ cells, a sustained mouse cell line, were prepared and antiserum affects on membrane antigen expression were investigated. The metabolic half-lives of each of three antigen deter-

minants investigated was distinct from the others examined.

The hybrid cells have lost their capacity to modulate TL antigens. TL antigens of hybrid cells, unlike those of parental ASL-1 cells, continue to be expressed in the presence of high titers of TL antiserum. Similarities between antigenic modulation and down regulation exist, among which are the fate of receptor-ligand complexes, changes in their metabolism after binding to ligand, and the dependence of the reactions upon continued sources of cellular energy.

INTRODUCTION

Hormones and antigenic substances are examples of ligands whose affects on responsive cells depend upon interactions with appropriate preexistent receptors. Extensively described alterations in cellular physiology occur after hormone interaction with preexistent complementary receptors, including changes in cell metabolism, stimulation of cell division, and the synthesis and secretion of specialized products. Antibody formation is initiated after antigenic materials interact with immunoglobulin-like receptors on suitably differentiated lymphoid cells. In this instance, the extraordinarily large number and diversity of agents capable of eliciting an immune response serves to emphasize the wide specificity of membrane-bound receptor molecules formed by lymphoid cells of the organism. They are believed to be clonally restricted, reflecting the nature of the antibody response itself.

After hormone stimulation, previously responsive cells are refractory to further stimulation (16,22,42); in the case of antibody synthesis, exposing lymphoid cells to antibodies to the antigen receptors themselves leads to diminished or absent responses (29,30). Through what cellular mechanisms are the biological affects of such ligands controlled? The available evidence indicates that diminished reactivity correlates with decreases in the quantities of receptors present. This effect, namely, the reduction in the quantity of specific receptors on the surfaces of insensitive cells following exposure, termed "down regulation", has been described for insulin receptors (16,42), β adrenergic receptors (23,37), acetylcholine receptors of mouse muscle cells (19,45), growth hormone receptors (33), antigen receptors (29,30) and others (Table 1).

It is conceivable that the cellular mechanisms leading to reductions in receptor number are akin to those leading to reductions in the quantities of thymus-leukemia (TL) antigens following exposure to TL antiserum. TL antigens are membrane-associated glycoproteins associated with the surface membranes of muscle thymus cells and leukemias (6,31).

We determined that changes in the quantities of TL antigens occurred as an outgrowth of their metabolism. As other cellular components, membrane-associated determinants undergo a metabolic "turnover", i.e., they are synthesized and degraded spontaneously (48,49). We considered two general models to explain ligand-induced affects upon the quantities of receptors present, one of which involves changes in the rate at which receptors disappear from the membrane and other changes in the rate at which receptors are synthesized and inserted into the membrane:

1.   During adaptation, controls governing the rate of receptor turnover may be altered so that they are removed more rapidly than previously. Under this scheme, the rate of receptor disappearance may exceed the rate of replacement until a new steady state is reached at low or absent receptor levels.

Membrane-associated receptors are "shed" from the membrane to the surrounding medium (7), in some instances in association with cytoskeletal actin (28). Adaptation may occur by a "shedding" of receptors from the membrane to the medium as a consequence of their combination with specific ligand. Membrane determinants as mammary tumor (7), H-2 (28), and TL antigens of murine leukemia cells and others are "shed" spontaneously from the cell (49). The usual rate of receptor metabolism may be unaffected by their combination with ligand; however, the receptors may be "loosely" bound to the membrane, allowing them to be "pulled" off after their association with ligand. Antibody-induced "shedding" has been described for the virally-specified determinants of cells infected with measles virus (39) and for acetylcholine receptors of mouse muscle cells (29). Not every determinant is effected this way.

Hormone receptors of various cell types and TL antigenic determinants of murine leukemia cells are traced intracellularly after association with ligand (43).

2. During adaptation, controls governing the rate of receptor synthesis may be altered, leading to a diminution in their rate of synthesis. The "usual" rate of disappearance of receptor may continue as before, leading to a progressive reduction in the quantities of receptors present. Alternatively, the ligand might "trigger" an enzyme-mediated change in membrane-associated complementary antigens and receptors. Such a modification could result in a molecule whose structure is altered in such a way that the new form no longer combines with the specific external ligand.

Conceivably, the ligand might lead to the cessation, in the case of glycoprotein receptors, of receptor glycosylation, preventing insertion into the membrane. Thy-1 (-) mutants of mouse myeloma cells have been described with such a defect (47). There is no evidence, however, that diminution in the quantity of one determinant affects the quantity or rate of metabolic turnover of another independently arising determinant (10). Incubation of TL(+) cells in medium with antibodies to TL antigens has no affect upon the metabolism of H-2^a antigens of the same cells (12).

Some of these possible mechanisms were investigated by my colleagues and me, along with other laboratory groups (13,43).

The Metabolism of Membrane-Associated Macromolecules in the Presence (and Absence) of Specific Antiserum.
As other membrane-associated glycoproteins, antigens which are exposed to the external milieu may be labeled "externally" with ^{125}I in the presence of lactoperoxidase. Intracytoplasmic constituents are not labeled by this procedure. Antigens in the process of biosynthesis may be labeled by incubating viable cells under growth conditions in medium to which ^{3}H-fucose has been added (36).

Detergent-solubilized hydrophobic macromolecules retain their antigenic specificity in the detergent solution and may be selectively immunoprecipitated with specific antiserum. The metabolic turnover of membrane determinants is investigated by extracting radioactively-labeled cells with nonionic detergents as nonidet P-40 (NP-40) and determining the specific activity of immunoprecipitates raised at equivalence with specific antiserum. The biosynthetic rate of membrane-associated glycoproteins is determined by incubating the cells for defined periods in medium containing ^{3}H-fucose followed by extraction with NP-40 and recovery of the antigens by selective immuno-precipitation. The rate of antigen degradation is esti-mated by labeling the cells with ^{125}I followed by incu-bation for varying periods and recovery by immunoprecipi-tation of remaining antigens from NP-40 cell extracts. These techniques have been described in detail previously (48,49).

Using this approach, we investigated the affect of specific antiserum on the rate of synthesis and the rate of degradation of several determinants of murine leukemia cells. The results we obtained are summarized in Table 2; they indicate the following:

1. The metabolic half-life of TL antigens of RADA-1 cells, a radiation-induced leukemia cell line of strain A mice, incubated in medium free of TL antibodies, is 16 hours. The half-life of TL antigens of RADA-1 cells incubated in medium containing TL antiserum shortens to 4 hours.

The shortened half-life of TL antigens of modulating cells results from a more rapid rate of antigen disappear-ance from the membrane than replacement (Fig. 1b, 1d). This is the case in analogous experiments involving differing antiserum concentrations with specificities for various determinants of the TL antigen complex. The biosynthetic rate of TL antigens is unaffected by exposing the cells to TL antiserum; the rate of antigen synthesis is indistinguishable in cells incubated in the presence, or absence, of TL antiserum (Fig. 1a, 1c). TL antigen-anti-body complexes have been traced to intracytoplasmic endo-cytic vacuoles (43). Analogous results have been obtained for ASL-1 cells, an independently arising leukemia cell line of the same mouse strain.

2. TL antigens, like other membrane-associated determinants, are "shed" from the cells to the surrounding medium, in an antigenically intact form. They may be recovered by immunologic means from the medium. The rate of "shedding" of TL antigens from ASL-1 cells exposed to TL antiserum and undergoing modulation is not detectably different than that of non-modulating cells (48,49).

3. The half-life of H-2^a antigens of ASL-1 cells is approximately 26 hours; it is distinctly different than that of TL antigens of the same cell types. The metabolic half-life of H-2^a antigens is unaffected by incubating the cells in medium containing H-2^a antiserum. H-2^a antigens of these cells do not undergo modulation.

4. Incubating ASL-1 cells in medium containing H-2^a antiserum has no affect upon the rate of turnover of TL antigens; TL antibodies have no affect upon the rate of turnover of H-2^a antigens. The half-lives of each appear to be controlled independently of each other (35).

During the course of our investigations, we detected a tumor-associated antigen of ASL-1 cells using antisera appearing in syngeneic mice injected with inactivated ASL-1 cells (48,49). The rate of metabolism of the tumor-associated antigen of ASL-1 cells is distinct from that of TL and H-2 antigens formed by the same cells. Its half-life of 44 hours is unaffected by exposing the cells to specific antiserum. Unlike TL, the tumor antigen fails to modulate.

Exposing the cells to sera containing antibodies to both TL and the tumor-associated antigen leads to a progressive reduction in the expression of TL antigens with no detectable effects upon the expression of the tumor antigen (Fig. 2). That only one of two membrane-associated antigens undergoes modulation in the presence of antibodies to both is an indication that modulation is not 'simply' the result of the combination of antigens and antibody on the surface of the cell, but that more complex cellular mechanisms likely are involved.

The Expression of Membrane-Associated Antigens by Somatic Hybrids of TL(+) and TL(-) Murine Cells.
The presence in differentiated cells of regulatory control mechanisms governing various aspects of specialized functions may be revealed in studies of somatic hybrid cells prepared by fusing parental cells engaged in unique, specialized activities. After fusion, the regulatory controls operative in one parental cell affect analogous functions of the other (18,25). Fusion of nonneoplastic antibody-forming cells of mouse origin with immunoglobulin-producing mouse myeloma cells, as an example, leads to persistence of immunoglobulin synthesis (40,41). Fusion of parental lymphoid cells, only one of which is forming

immunoglobulins, leads to cessation of antibody formation (9). Similar controls appear to be operative in the formation of membrane determinants (1,8,14,26,27).

To detect the presence of regulatory factors affecting the expression of membrane-associated antigenic determinants, and their metabolic half-lives, we prepared hybrids of ASL-1 cells [TL 1,2,3 (+), H-2^a (+), Thy 1.2 (+) and tumor antigen (+)] and LM(TK)$^-$ cells [H-2^k (+), TL(-), Thy 1.2 (-) tumor antigen (-)], and analyzed clonal isolates of hybrid cells for their expression of several membrane-associated antigens, their metabolism, as well as their expression in the presence of specific antiserum. The hybrid cells formed in approximately equal proportions the H-2 antigens of both parental cell types along with a hybrid karyotype consisting of approximately 85 characteristic mouse chromosomes including the identification of "marker" chromosomes originating in each parental source.

TL 1,2,3 antigenic determinants and the tumor-associated antigen of ASL-1 cells are actively formed and expressed by ASL-1 x LM(TK)$^-$ hybrid cells (34). Thy 1.2 antigens' membrane-associated determinants, associated with ASL-1 but not LM(TK)$^-$ cells, are absent in fused cells (21,34).

ASL-1 x LM(TK)$^-$ and RADA-1 x LM(TK)$^-$ hybrid cells, unlike the parental cells from which they are derived, fail to modulate TL antigens. Hybrid cells exposed for prolonged periods to high titers of TL antiserum, conditions in excess of that required to stimulate the modulation of parental cells, remain sensitive to fresh TL antiserum and complement. After antibody exposure, the cells retain TL antigens on their surface membranes as detected by their positive staining characteristics in fluorescent antibody tests, immunoprecipitation of TL antigens from NP-40 cell extracts of the cells (Fig. 3), as well as their capacity to reduce, by absorption, TL antisera of known titers. Sensitivity to TL antibodies and complement persists. The attempts to stimulate modulation of the hybrid cells include exposing the cells for up to 22 hours to each of several different preparations of TL antiserum at five-fold higher concentrations than required to modulate ASL-1 cells (parental cells, under similar conditions, convert in 6 hours to TL antibody and C resistance), as well as the use of indirect methods involving the addition of rabbit antimouse immunoglobulins.

Metabolism of Membrane Antigens of Hybrid Cells.
The metabolic turnover rate of TL antigens is different
in hybrid than parental cells. These differences may be
taken as a likely indication that cellular control
mechanisms govern not only the expression of TL antigens
but their rate of metabolism as well.

The half-life of TL antigen expression of ASL-1 cells
is 18 hours; the half-life of TL antigens expressed by 13
different clonal isolates of ASL-1 x LM(TK)⁻ hybrid cells
ranges between 28 and 32 hours. Unlike ASL-1 cells, the
metabolic half-life of TL antigens of hybrid cells failing
to undergo antigenic modulation is not affected by exposing
the cells to TL antiserum (Table 2). In all, twenty-five
clones of hybrid cells have been investigated in this
analysis. None underwent antigenic modulation; in no
instance is there an indication that TL antiserum affects
either the expression or the metabolic turnover rate of TL
antigens of hybrid cells.

Each of the clones of hybrid cells investigated forms
the tumor-associated antigens of ASL-1 cells. Its metabolic half-life, like that of TL antigens, is different in
hybrid than parental cells. The half-life of the tumor-
associated antigen of hybrid cells is approximately 36
hours, less than its half-life of 44 hours in parental
cells. Its metabolic half-life is unaffected by incubating either parental or hybrid cells in medium containing
specific antiserum. It does not undergo modulation.

The metabolic half-life of H-2ᵃ antigens of ASL-1 or
RADA-1 parental and their respective hybrid cells,
approximately 26 hours in all instances, is equivalent.
Like the tumor-associated antigen of ASL-1 cells, the
half-life of H-2ᵃ antigens is unaffected by incubating
the cells in medium containing H-2ᵃ antiserum. H-2ᵃ
antigens of these cell types fail to undergo modulation.
These results are a possible indication that the metabolic
turnover rates of analogous membrane-associated determinants of parental and hybrid cells as well as their
persistence in the presence of specific antiserum reflect
the existence of complex cellular controls governing not
only membrane determinant expression but their rates of
metabolism as well.

Modulation of the Membrane-Antigen Specified by Epstein-Barr Virus.

Human lymphoid cells productively infected with Epstein-Barr Virus (EBV) form, in addition to various intracytoplasmic virally-specified determinants, a characteristic membrane-associated antigen (EBV-MA). EBV-MA, like other antigens associated with productive infection, is specified by the virus. Unlike membrane- associated determinants specified by information contained in the cellular genome, e.g., $H-2^a$, TL, the presence of EBV-MA results from information provided by external, i.e., viral, sources.

To determine if virally-specified determinants of productively infected cells undergo antigenic modulation, general lines of EBV-containing cells, forming EBV-MA, were exposed to EBV-MA antiserum. The expression of EBV-MA was detected by fluorescent-antibody methods, as described in the relevant figure legends.

Selected human sera from healthy adult volunteers contain EBV-MA antibodies and stain productively infected EBV(+) cell lines (Table 3). Human neonatal (cord blood) cells fail to stain under similar conditions as do Raji cells in which EBV is latent.

The proportion of positively staining cells exposed to EBV-MA antiserum gradually diminished over a 24-hour period of incubation until by 48 hours, all cultures were negative (Table 4). In a manner analogous to that described for the modulation of TL antigens, positively staining cells gradually reappeared after antiserum removal (Table 2).

Could these results be explained by antibody-dependent selective destruction of EBV(+) cells? This question was investigated by determining the proportion of stained cells in acetone-fixed (to reveal intracytoplasmic, virally-specified determinants) and unfixed cells. The results (Table 5) indicate that the proportion of cells which stain remains the same if fixed preparations are examined. EBV-MA antibody and complement fail to kill EBV(+) cells.

The gradual disappearance of cells expressing EBV-MA in the presence of EBV-MA antiserum, followed by their reappearance after antiserum removal, strongly suggests that such virally-specified determinants undergo antigenic modulation.

Antigenic Modulation--A Possible Model for Ligand-
Induced Adaptation of Receptors.

Is the mechanism leading to reductions in the quantities of hormone receptors an aftermath of hormone stimulation analogous to that leading to the modulation of
membrane antigens? The precise answer has not been determined; however, the two phenomena have many features in
common. After their association on the cells' surface,
antigen-antibody complexes of cells undergoing modulation
may be traced intracellularly to endocytic vacuoles where
they are degraded (43). Their re-expression is inhibitable
by chemical agents affecting protein synthesis (44).
Complexes of thyrotropin-releasing hormone and its receptor
are traced after association to endocytic vacuoles where
they are degraded to constituent amino acids (20). Low
density lipoprotein receptors of human cells binding low
density lipoproteins are internalized (2). Glucocorticoid
receptors of mouse fibroblasts are endocytosed after their
association with hormone; in this instance, they are
"recycled" within 30 minutes to the surface membrane of the
cell and new protein synthesis is not required (3).

The rate of disappearance of TL antigens of ASL-1
leukemia cells from the membrane is accelerated if the
cells are incubated in medium containing TL antibodies.
The metabolic half-life of "exposed" TL antigens on the
cells' surface is shortened as a result. The rate of
disappearance of acetylcholine receptors is accelerated and
their half-life of expression is shortened in cells incubated in medium containing specific ligands; the process is
energy dependent (45).

The quantity of TL antigens expressed by TL(+) leukemia
cells is reduced if the cells are exposed, either in vitro
or in vivo (in pre-immunized recipients), to TL antibodies.
The quantity of receptors for several physiologically-
active ligands, as insulin, is reduced as a consequence of
exposing the cells to the relevant ligand (Table 1).

Immunoglobulin-like receptors for antigen on the
surface membranes of the cells are believed to be one means
through which cells recognize foreign antigenic substances,
stimulating humoral immunity. The receptors for antigen,
like TL, undergo modulation, converting cells previously
responsive to antigen to cells which are "inert" insofar as
antigenic stimulation is concerned.

Both modulation and down regulation lead to diminished quantities of specific cell surface determinants; both phenomena correlate with alterations in the "usual" cellular responsiveness to external stimuli. Genetic controls regulating the consequences of receptor-ligand interaction appear to be critical determining factors.

TABLE 1

Examples of membrane-associated determinants
whose expression is modified by specific ligand

Classi-fication	Determinant	Ligand	Cell type	Reference
	Insulin receptor	Insulin	Various mammalian	(16,42)
	Thyrotropin-releasing hormone	Thyrotropin-releasing hormone	Rat	(38)
Hormone receptors	Growth hormone	Growth hormone	Human	(33)
	Choriogonado-tropin receptor*	Choriogonado-tropin	Human	(11)
	Thyrocalci-tonin receptor*	Thyrocalci-tonin	Human	(46)
	Epidermal growth factor receptor	Epidermal growth factor	Mouse	(11)
Neuro-transmitter	Acetylcholine receptor	Acetylcholine; antibodies to the receptor	Mouse	(19,29)

TABLE 1 (Continued)

Examples of membrane-associated determinants
whose expression is modified by specific ligand

Classifi-cation	Determinant	Ligand	Cell type	Refer-ence
	Thymus-leukemia		Mouse	(6,31, 48,49)
	Immunoglobulin-like		Mouse	(29,30)
	Gross leukemia associated		Mouse	(5)
	Forssman		Mouse	(15)
Antigenic substances	Mammary tumor virus associated		Mouse	(7)
	Paramecium specific		Paramecia	(38)
	Friend virus associated		Human	(17)
	Burkitt's lymphoma associated		Human	(4)
	Melanoma associated		Human	(4)
Unclassified	Glucocorticoid receptor	Glucocorticoids	Mouse	(3)
	β-adrenergic receptor	Catecholamine agonists	Mammalian and non-mammalian	(32)
	α-adrenergic receptor	Epinephrine*	Mammals	(32)
	Low density lipoprotein receptor	Low density lipoproteins	Human	(2)

*Postulated

TABLE 2

Metabolic half-life of several membrane-associated
determinants of parental and hybrid murine cells

Determinants	Cell type	Antiserum	Half-life, hours
TL 1,2,3*	ASL-1	$(-)^+$ $(+)^{++}$	18 9
	ASL-1 x LM(TK)$^-$	$(-)$ $(+)$	28-32** 28-32**
	RADA-1	$(-)$ $(+)$	16 4
	RADA-1 x LM(TK)$^-$	$(-)$ $(+)$	28-32*** 28-32***
H-2^a	ASL-1	$(-)$ $(+)$	26 26
	ASL-1 x LM(TK)$^-$	$(-)$ $(+)$	26** 26**
H-2^k	ASL-1 x LM(TK)$^-$	$(-)$ $(+)$	26** 26**
Tumor-associated	ASL-1	$(-)$ $(+)$	44 44
	ASL-1 x LM(TK)$^-$	$(-)$ $(+)$	34-38** 34-38**

TABLE 2 (Continued)

Metabolic half-life of several membrane-associated
determinants of parental and hybrid murine cells

Determinants	Cell type	Antiserum	Half-life, hours
Tumor-		(-)	46
associated	RADA-1	(+)	46
		(-)	34-38***
	RADA-1 x LM(TK)⁻	(+)	34-38***

⁺In the absence of specific antiserum.

⁺⁺In the presence of specific antiserum.

*Shared by individual molecules (48,49).

**Based on an analysis of 14 colonies.

***Based on an analysis of 11 colonies.

TABLE 3

Staining of surface membranes of EBV(+) cells
by selected human sera

Serum	Proportion cells positive				
	Daudi	Maku	HR-1	Raji	Raji (after IUDR)
E.P.C.	25 ± 2	6 ± 1	5 ± 2	< 1	10 ± 1
W.L.	35 ± 1	6 ± 2	8 ± 1	< 1	5 ± 1
R.S.	40 ± 1	6 ± 1	9 ± 2	< 1	7 ± 1
V.vS.	22 ± 2	7 ± 1	8 ± 1	< 1	6 ± 1
K.Z.	34 ± 1	2 ± 1	5 ± 1	< 1	5 ± 1
M.P.	25 ± 1	5 ± 1	8 ± 1	< 1	6 ± 1
D.D.	22 ± 2	7 ± 2	8 ± 1	< 1	8 ± 2
M.A.T.	28 ± 3	8 ± 1	7 ± 1	< 1	7 ± 1
J.E.	25 ± 1	6 ± 2	5 ± 1	< 1	6 ± 1
T.P.*	32 ± 3	8 ± 1	6 ± 1	< 1	10 ± 2

Various lines of EBV(+) cells were removed from tissue culture incubation, washed two times with cold PBS and incubated at 4° for 30 minutes in medium containing a 1:10 dilution of serum from healthy human donors. After incubation, the cells were washed and incubated for 30 minutes at 4° with a 1:50 dilution of fluorescein-conjugated goat antihuman IgG. After washing, the cells were suspended in PBS and observed at room temperature in a Leitz Microscope equipped with an ultraviolet light source. Productive viral infection was induced in Raji cells during incubation at 37° for three days in medium containing 30 µg/ml IUDR (Calbiochem). Incubation was continued for three additional days after IUDR removal before the cells were examined for positive membrane fluorescence.

*Serum from a patient in the recovery phase of infectious mononucleosis.

TABLE 4

The membrane-associated antigen of EBV-infected cells
undergoes antigenic modulation

With EBV-MA antiserum (hrs)	Proportion cells positive		
	Daudi	HR-1	Maku
0	35	10	18
3	38	NT*	NT
6	25	NT	NT
24	10	< 1	2
48	< 1	< 1	< 1
96	< 1	< 1	< 1
After EBV-MA antiserum removal (hrs)			
48	22	11	15

*Not tested.

Various EBV(+) cells were incubated in medium to which a
1:50 dilution of human serum containing EBV-MA antibodies
was added. At varying intervals, the cells were examined
by fluorescence microscopy, as described in the legend to
Table 3, for the presence of EBV-MA(+) cells.

TABLE 5

The membrane-associated antigen of EBV-infected
Daudi cells undergoes antigenic modulation

	Proportion of viable cells positive			
	After antiserum addition			After antiserum removal
Serum	0	24	48 (hours)	96 (hours)
E.P.C.	30	20	0	25
W.L.	25	22	0	22
R.S.	25	5	0	15

	Proportion of acetone-fixed cells positive			
Serum	0	24	48 (hours)	96 (hours)
E.P.C.	28	28	35	25
W.L.	31	32	27	28
R.S.	26	24	27	22

Daudi cells were removed from tissue culture incubation,
washed, and incubated in medium supplemented with a 1:50
dilution of EBV-MA(+) human serum. The proportion of cells
showing positive membrane fluorescence was determined as
described in the legend to Table 1. Aliquots of the cell
suspension taken after acetone fixation were tested at the
same times for the presence of intracellular virally-
specified antigens.

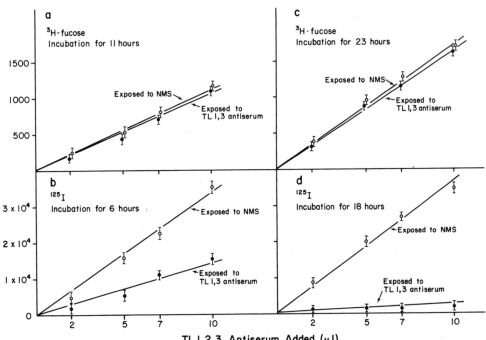

Figure 1. Solubilization and immunoprecipitation of [3H] fucose-labeled (a and c) or 125I-labeled (b and d) membrane antigens of RADA-1 cells preincubated in medium containing TL 1,2,3, antiserum or normal mouse serum (NMS) for 2 or 6 hours. For cells labeled with 3H, [3H] fucose was present throughout the entire period of incubation. After washing, the cells were extracted with NP-40 and TL antigens released from the cells were immunoprecipitated with various amounts of TL 1,2,3 antiserum (23).

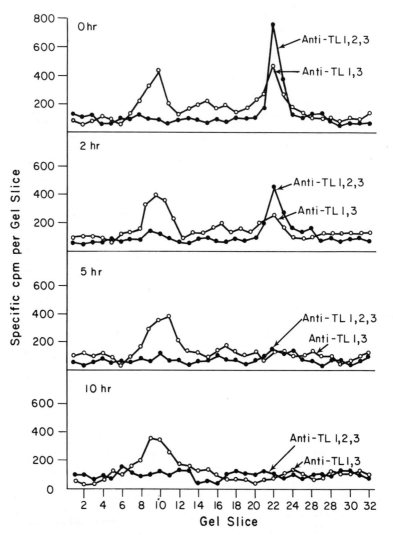

Figure 2. Nonidet P-40 extracts of ^{125}I-labeled RADA-1
cells undergoing modulation. SDS-polyacrylamide
gel electrophoresis of the immunoprecipitates
formed with TL 1,2,3 antiserum (containing
antibodies for TL antigens) or TL 1,2,3
antiserum (containing antibodies for TL and the
tumor-associated antigen) (10).

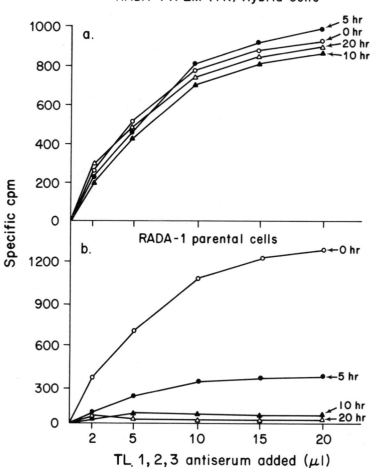

Figure 3. Recovery of TL antigens from the surface
membranes of RADA-1 or RADA-1 x LM(TK)⁻ hybrid
cells at varying periods after antiserum
exposure.

REFERENCES

1. Allison DC, Meier P, Majeune M, Cohen, EP (1975).
   Cell 6:521
2. Anderson RGW, Brown MS, Goldstein, JL (1977).
   Cell 10:351.
3. Aronow L (1978). Fed Proc 37:162
4. Aoki T, Geering G, Beth E, Old LJ (1972). In Nakahara
   W, Nishioka K, Hirayama T, Ito Y (eds): "Recent
   Advances in Human Tumor Virology and Immunology,"
   Univ, Tokyo Press, p. 425.
5. Aoki T, Johsnon PA (1972). J Natl Cancer Inst 49:183.
6. Boyse EA, Stockert E, Old LJ (1967). Proc Natl Acad
   Sci (USA) 58:954.
7. Calafat J, Hilgers J, Van Blitterswijk WJ, Verbeet M,
   Hageman PC (1976). J Natl Cancer Inst 56:1019.
8. Cerni C (1977). Oncology 34(5):216.
9. Coffino P, Knowler B, Nathanson SG, Scharff MC (1971).
10. Cohen EP, Liang W (1976). J Supramol Struc Suppl
    #1:89.
11. Das M, Fox CF (1978). Proc Natl Acad Sci 75:2644.
12. Davies DAL, Alkins BJ, Boyse EA, Old LJ, Stockert E,
    (1969). Immunology 16:669.
13. Esmon NL, Little JR (1976). J Immunol 117:919.
14. Fellous M, Kamoun M, Wiels J, Dausset J, Clements G,
    Zeuthen J, Klein G (1977). Immunogenetics 5(5):423.
15. Franks D, Daniel MR, Gurnes BW, Combs RRA (1964).
    Exptl Cell Res 36:310.
16. Gavin JR, Roth J, Neville DM, DeMeyts P, Buell DN
    (1974). Proc Natl Acad Sci 71:84.
17. Genovesi EV, Mark PA, Wheelock EF (1977). J Exp Med
    146:520
18. Harris H (1970). "Cell Fusion." Cambridge, MA:
    Harvard Univ. Press, p ?
19. Heinemann S, Bevan S, Kullberg R, Linsdtrom J, Rice J
    (1977). Proc Natl Acad Sci 74:3090.
20. Hinkle PM, Tashijian AH (1975). Biochemistry 14:3845 .
21. Hyman R, Kelleher RJ (1975). Som Cell Genetics 1:335.
22. Kahn CR, Neville DM Jr, Roth J (1973). J Biol Chem
    248:244
23. Kebebian JW, Zatz M, Romero JA, Axelrod J (1975). Proc
    Natl Acad Sci 42:3735
24. Kirschner MA, Widner JA, Ross GH (1970). J Clin
    Endocrinol Metab 30:504
25. Klebe RJ, Chen T, Ruddle FH (1970). Proc Natl Acad Sci
    (USA) 66:1220

26. Klein G, Clements G, Zeuthen J, Westman A (1976). Int J Cancer 17(6):715.
27. Klein G, Terasaki P, Billing R, Honig R, Jondal M, Rosen A, Zeuthen J, Clements G (1977). Int J Cancer 19(1):66.
28. Koch GLG, Smith MJ (1978). Nature 273:274.
29. Kohler H (1975). Transplant Rev 27:24.
30. Kohler H, Richardson BC, Smyk S (1978). J Immunol 120:233.
31. Lamm MG, Boyse EA, Old LJ, Lisowska-Bernstein G, Stockert E (1968). J Immunol 101:99.
32. Lefkowitz RJ (1978). Fed Proc 37:123.
33. Lesniak MA, Roth J, Gordon P, Gavin JR (1973). Nature New Biol 241:20.
34. Liang W, Cohen EP (1975). Proc Natl Acad Sci 72:1873.
35. Liang W, Cohen EP (1976). Som Cell Genetics 2:291.
36. Liang W, Cohen EP (1977). J Natl Cancer Inst 58:1079.
37. Mukherjee C, Caron MG, Lefkowitz RI (1975). Proc Natl Acad Sci 72:1945.
38. Nanny DL (1968). Ann Rev Gen 2:121.
39. Rustigian R (1966). J Bacteriol 92:1805.
40. Schwaber J (1975). Exp Cell Res 93:343.
41. Schwaber J, Cohen EP (1973). Nature 244:444.
42. Soll AH, Goldfine ID, Roth J, Kahn CR, Neville DM Jr (1974). J Biol Chem 249:4127.
43. Stackpole CW, Jacobson JG, Lardis MP (1974). J Exp Med 140:839.
44. Stall AM, Knopf PM (1978). Cell 14:33.
45. Stanley EF, Drachman DB (1978). Science 200:1258.
46. Tashijian AJ Jr, Melvin KEW (1968). New Eng J Med 279:279.
47. Trowbridge IS, Hyman RI, Mazauskas C (1978). Cell 14:21.
48. Yu AC, Cohen EP (1974). J Immunol 112:1285.
49. Yu AC, Cohen EP (1974). J Immunol 112:1296.

Harrison: What is the maximum degree of down regulation for TL antigens?

Cohen: We find that cells convert to antibody complement resistance <u>before</u> TL antigens disappear from their surface membranes. Eventually, the antigens reach undetectable levels of expression using methods as sensitive as ^{125}I-labeling.

Session III.
Developmental Aspects of
Cell Recognition

Pages 171—188, Membranes, Receptors, and the Immune Response
© 1980 Alan R. Liss, Inc., 150 Fifth Avenue, New York, NY 10011

EMBRYONIC CELL RECOGNITION: CELLULAR AND MOLECULAR ASPECTS

A. A. Moscona

Laboratory for Developmental Biology
Cummings Life Science Center
University of Chicago, Chicago, Illinois 60637

INTRODUCTION

The aim of this article is to introduce the non-embryo-
logist to the problem of embryonic cell recognition and its
significance in development. Since the term cell recognition
is more widely familiar in the context of immunological
phenomena, I shall start by comparing immunological and
embryonic cell recognition.

Immunological recognition is a systemic defense mechanism for safeguarding the genotypic integrity and individual-
ity of the organism against foreign intrusion. It depends on
the activities of a highly specialized class of cells, the
lymphocytes; their differentiation endows them with the
capacity to produce antibodies and to multiply when stimulated by foreign antigens. There is no evidence that immunological recognition is, in itself, essential for embryonic
morphogenesis and development. Embryonic cell recognition,
on the other hand, is a morphogenetic mechanism expressed by
practically every cell in the embryo at some stage of development. It serves for mutual identification - positive and
negative - among embryonic cells, and enables them to sort
out according to classes and types, to associate and to
become arranged into tissue-forming patterns.

Each of these recognition mechanisms can express a very
large spectrum of cognitive specificities. Lymphocytes are
capable of recognizing a practically unlimited variety of
foreign antigens by means of a correspondingly large range

of specific antibodies. In the case of embryonic cells, the
fact that the numerous types and sub-types become selectively
assorted and aggregated into tissues and organized within
tissues suggests a corresponding versatility of their recognition mechanism. There has been considerable progress
toward analysis of genetic control of immunological recognition (Marx, 1978). The genetic basis of embryonic cell
recognition is unknown, but it is not unreasonable to look
for principles similar to those involved in control of antibody diversity. In fact, it has been hypothesized that both
these recognition mechanisms have an evolutionary relatedness
Burnet, 1971; Bennett et al., 1972); they may have evolved
from the mechanism of cell surface-mediated recognition
between mating types in microorganisms and could be akin to
some of the processes involved in the recognition-interaction
between sperm and egg (Moscona, 1963; Monroy and Rosati,1979).

The aim of our work has been to isolate from embryonic
tissue cells macromolecules specifically involved in embryonic cell recognition and selective cell aggregation. From
the surface membrane of neural retina cells of chick embryos,
we have obtained a glycoprotein which, according to the
evidence at hand, represents a component of the mechanism
responsible for self-recognition and histotypic association
of these cells (Moscona, 1975). Preparations with similar
biological activity have been obtained also from other neural
tissues of chick and mouse embryos (Moscona, 1974; Hausman
et al., 1976). The term cognin has been suggested to designate cell membrane proteins that function specifically in
embryonic cell recognition and morphogenetic cell affinities
(Moscona et al., 1975; Moscona, 1975).

RECOGNITION AND SORTING OUT OF CELLS IN THE EMBRYO

The early embryo consists, by and large, of a cluster
of multiplying cells and, in order to construct tissues and
organs the cells must become spatially segregated and sorted
out into distinct groupings and patterns. Most tissues
arise from "precursor" cells that originate away from their
final destinations; these cells migrate, singly or in co-
horts, to their definitive locations and assemble there into
primordia of tissues and organs. Well known examples are
the translocations of primordial germ cells, lymphopoietic
and erythropoietic cells, neural crest cells (Fig. 1). The
precision of this complex reshuffling and sorting out of
cells has implied that embryonic cells possess surface

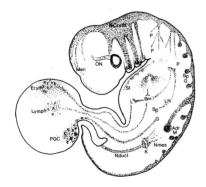

Fig. 1.   Diagrammatic representation of some of the cellular
traffic involved in the formation of tissues and organs
during vertebrate embryogenesis. The diagram combines events
taking place at different stages of development. The "pathways" connect the original sites of cells with their destinations; they do not accurately depict the actual routes of
the cells. The progenitors of erythroid cells (Eryth)
originate in the yolk-sac endoderm and are transported by
the circulation to the subsequent sites of erythropoiesis
(L, liver; Bm, bone marrow). The progenitors of lymphoid
cells are transported to the bone marrow (Bm), thymus (Thy),
lymph nodes (LN), and spleen (Sp). The primordial germ
cells (PGC) migrate from the yolk sac to the germinal ridges
and colonize the gonads (G). Cells from the neural crest
(NCrest) migrate in swarms or individually, and give rise to
a variety of structures, among them meninges (Men), carti-
lages of the embryonic skull (Mx, Md), pigment cells (P),
spinal ganglia (SpG), and adrenal medulla (AdrM). Axons
that grow out of retinal ganglion cells form the optic nerves
(ON), which advance toward the visual centers in the brain.
The nephric ducts (Nduct) elongate toward aggregations of
nephric mesenchyme cells (Nmes) to form the kidney rudiments
(K). The sternum (St) is formed by mesenchymal cells that
migrate from the dorsal region of the embryo. The heart (H)
arises from aggregations of cells originating in the "heart-
forming territory." The translocations of cells involved in
histogenesis of the nervous system are not included here.
(From, Moscona and Hausman, 1977).

mechanism for mutual identification and selective attachment. It is now generally held that the specificity of these mechanisms evolves progressively, coordinately with cell differentiation. I have suggested that, as cells in the embryo diversify into different classes and types, their surfaces become differentially encoded with patterns of molecular labels that display outwardly their changing phenotypic identities and determine their cognitive interactions and histogenetic affinities.

Embryonic cell recognition can be classified into three major categories summarized in Table 1.

TABLE 1

1. Germ Layer-Specific Cell Recognition: results in segregation of early embryo cells into the three germ layers: ectoderm, mesoderm and endoderm.

2. Tissue-Specific Cell Recognition: reflects surface differences between cell populations that constitute the different tissues in the embryo; it enables cells that have the same histological identity to group together into a tissue-forming assemblage.

3. Cell Type-Specific Recognition: reflects differences in surface characteristics of the various cell types that make up a single tissue; determines positioning and organization of individual cells within the tissue framework.
   a) Homotypic cell recognition: results in associations between cells of the same type (e.g., myoblast-myoblast; chondrocyte-chondrocyte).
   b) Allotypic cell recognition: results in the association of similar, but non-identical cell types (e.g., neuron A – neuron B).
   c) Heterotypic cell recognition: results in the association of different, but functionally affiliated cell types (e.g., neuron-glia; neuron-muscle; "homing" of cells to heterologous locations, as in early erythropoiesis, lymphopoiesis or primordial germ cells migration).
   d) Surface domain recognition: (a sub-category of b and c) suggests that different areas of a single cell surface may have different cognitive affinities, thereby enabling the cell to associate simultaneously with other cell types (e.g., neuron A ← neuron B → muscle).

Subdividing cell recognition into various classes points out some of its inherent complexity, but it also breaks down the problem into more defined questions. In this respect, especially valid is the distinction between tissue and cell type-specific levels of recognition. Our work has been concerned mainly with tissue-specificity, since we expected it to be more amenable to experimental analysis by available methods.

TISSUE-SPECIFIC CELL RECOGNITION

a) Antigenic Differences. Early in this work, the possibility arose that tissue-specific cell recognition might depend on cell-surface components different and characteristic for each tissue. Indications to this effect were provided by the finding of tissue-specific surface antigens on cells from different embryonic tissues. Rabbits were immunized with cell suspensions prepared from various tissues of the chick embryo, such as neural retina cells or liver cells, and the resulting antisera were extensively absorbed with heterologous cells. Such absorbed antisera were found to contain antibodies which bound to the cell surface, but only to the kind of cells used as the immunogen (Moscona and Moscona, 1962; Goldschneider and Moscona, 1972). The retina antiserum reacted only with the surface of retina cells, and did not bind to liver cells; the liver-specific antiserum bound to the surface of hepatocytes, but not of retina cells (Goldschneider and Moscona, 1972). These, and similar results with other tissues demonstrated the existence of antigenically distinct tissue-specific cell-surface determinants. Findings consistent with this conclusion were reported also by others (Fischman et al., 1976; Friedlander and Fischman, 1977).

The role of such tissue-specific cell-surface determinants, especially whether they are involved in cell recognition, could not be established by these studies. To examine this question it was obviously necessary to isolate tissue-specific cell-surface constituents and to determine in an appropriate test system their effects on morphogenetic cell associations.

b) Aggregation in Vitro of Dissociated Embryonic Cells. The test system used by us is based on morphogenetic aggregation of cell suspensions freshly obtained from tissues of

avian or mammalian embryos. Under suitable in vitro conditions the cells can be made to reaggregate into multicellular
complexes within which they reconstruct their characteristic
tissue pattern. This system makes it possible to investigate
in detail how cells associate into tissues, and it can also
be used for testing the effects of preparations derived from
the cell surface on morphogenetic cell associations.

If an embryonic tissue such as neural retina (from 10-
day chick embryo) is briefly exposed to a solution of pure
trypsin in a buffer, the enzyme cleaves intercellular bonds,
degrades cell-surface and intercellular proteins, and increases the internal "fluidity" of the cell membrane; the
cells detach from one another and can be dispersed into
suspension. When the cell suspension is gently swirled on
a shaker at 37°C, the cells regenerate surface components
lost in the dissociation and reaggregate into progressively
larger clusters. Within these aggregates the cells move
about and become spatially sorted out, establishing contacts
with matching partners; in 24 hrs the cells reconstruct their
characteristic tissue architecture (reviewed in: Moscona,
1974). Reaggregated embryonic retina cells reform retino-
typic tissue; heart cells reconstruct cardiac tissue; brain
cells restitute brain-like tissue, etc. The process illustrates the expression of type-specific cell affinities,
i.e., the capacity of the various cells that make up a given
tissue to choose among alternative partners and to associate
so as to construct their histotypic pattern.

Tissue-specific cell affinities can also be readily
demonstrated in this experimental system by combining in
suspension cells from different tissues of the same embryo.
As the cells reaggregate they segregate in accordance with
their tissue-identities, so that the cells of each tissue
assemble into distinct groupings. A large number of such
binary cell combinations have been examined, using variously
labeled cells, and the results have been uniformly consistent
with a mechanism for tissue-specific cell recognition
(Moscona, 1974). This mechanism is not strictly species-
specific; in combinations of mouse and chick embryo cells
from the same kind of tissue, the cells recognize their histotypic homology and jointly form a hybrid, bispecific tissue.
This is not entirely surprising; considering that cell
recognition is essential for embryonic morphogenesis, it is
conceivable that its molecular mechanism might have arisen
early in vertebrate evolution and has been conserved without

drastic changes.

SPECIFIC CELL-CELL LIGANDS: A WORKING HYPOTHESIS

Based on our and other work, a working hypothesis has been proposed for investigating the mechanism of embryonic cell recognition (Moscona, 1962, 1974, 1975). It has evolved from Sperry's views (1943, 1950) about the nature of neuronal specification, and Weiss' (1947) concept of "molecular ecology" of cell surfaces. According to this hypothesis, embryonic cell recognition (differential cell affinities) is mediated by interactions of cell-surface components which can selectively link cells and which function as recognition sites and specific intercellular ligands. The selectivity of cell recognition is determined by a combination of two conditions: the molecular characteristics of individual ligand sites, and the patterns of ligand organization, i.e., their topographic-spatial arrangement on the cell surface. It is assumed that these ligand-patterns can differ characteristically depending on cell type, domain of the cell surface, and the state of cell differentiation, and that this accounts for type-specific sorting out and alignment of cells. Thus, when two cells meet, positive recognition and morphogenetic affinity will result if their juxtaposed surface areas possess topographically matching patterns of biochemically complementary (interacting) ligands. A high degree of pattern matching and ligand complementarity would result in high affinity interactions between cells; different degrees of pattern mismatch would result in correspondingly lower affinities and potentially unstable cell contacts. Negative cell recognition could be the outcome of biochemical non-complementarity of ligands, or of non-matching ligand patterns. Experimentally, the ligands can be disrupted with trypsin and the cells separate; aggregation and histotypic association of the cells require regeneration of the ligand sites and their organization into a pattern characteristic for the given cell. In the early stages of cell aggregation this pattern may still be randomized, and this could account for the initial non-selective adhesions of the different cell types.

Such a dual system combining qualitative-biochemical diversity of ligands and topographic-quantitative diversity of ligand patterns could endow cells with a sufficiently versatile cognition mechanism to accommodate tissue-specific cell affinities and the various kinds of type-specific cell recognition. The hypothesis suggested that tissue-specific cell affinities (i.e., the segregation and grouping of cells according to tissue-identities) might be due to qualitatively different ligands predominating in different tissues (a possibility consistent with the tissue-specific cell-surface antigens referred to above). On the other hand, type-specific cell recognition (sorting out and histotypic organization of various cells within a tissue) might depend largely on matching and alignment by cells of their specific ligand patterns. Accordingly, cells in a given tissue might be expected to share the same kind of tissue-specific ligands; however, it is not excluded that a single tissue may contain still other kinds of ligands, perhaps on different surface domains of cells, especially in areas of allotypic and heterotypic cell contacts (see Table 1).

Implicit in these views was the prediction that it should be possible to isolate from embryonic tissues materials with the functional features of the postulated tissue-specific cell ligands. Addition of such a material to freshly trypsinized cells would supply the cells with "instant" ligands which, by binding to the cell membrane should markedly enhance morphogenetic cell reaggregation; the cells would form larger aggregates at a faster rate than the controls. However, the essential conditions are that the effect of this material should be tissue-specific and conducive to tissue reconstruction. Compliance with these conditions would be consistent with the functional characteristics expected of tissue-specific cell ligands and would strongly support the validity of the cell-ligand hypothesis.

PREPARATIONS WITH CELL-LIGAND ACTIVITY

Preparations with cell-ligand activity have been obtained from several tissues of chick and mouse embryos (Moscona, 1974; Hausman and Moscona, 1975, 1976). Also Edelman and co-workers (Rutishauser et al., 1976; Brackenbury et al., 1977) using another bioassay, isolated cell-binding materials from chick embryo cells. The first crude preparation was obtained from neural retina cells of chick embryos (Moscona, 1962; Lilien and Moscona, 1967; McClay and Moscona, 1974); when it was added to suspensions of retina cells it caused a striking enhancement of cell aggregation resulting in aggregates that were markedly larger than the controls (Fig. 2). Most importantly, the effect was tissue-specific, in that this material did not enhance the aggregation of cells from tissues other than the retina. And furthermore, the reaggregated cells became histologically organized. Therefore, the conditions described above have been met. Preparations with tissue-specific cell-aggregating activity were obtained also from embryonic cerebrum and optic tectum (Moscona, 1974; Hausman et al., 1976). The isolation of such materials from non-neural tissues has not yet been rigorously investigated.

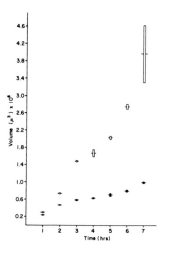

Fig. 2. Kinetics of aggregation of neural retina cells (from 10-day chick embryo). Open bars: the effect of the cell-aggregating glycoprotein on the rate of aggregation and of increase in volume of aggregates. Solid bars: controls. The bars represent standard deviation for 100 aggregates obtained from paired cultures.

Purification and characterization of retina cognin. In subsequent work, cell membranes obtained from retinas of 10-day chick embryos were used for isolating the cell-aggregating material (Hausman and Moscona, 1976). The purified membranes were extracted with butanol in buffer; the aqueous phase was fractionated and the activity was finally localized by isoelectric focusing in a peak at pH 4. Electrophoresis of this purified material on polyacrylamide gels with or without SDS resulted in a single band. Further analysis showed it to be a glycoprotein, with the carbohydrate representing less than 15% of the total (Tables 2, 3). All tests so far indicate that this material is homogeneous; but we cannot completely rule out the possibility of minor contaminants, or of heterogeneities of the kind often found in glycoproteins. In solution this material has a molecular weight of 50,000 ± 6,000 and does not appear to form multimers. However, it is possible that, at the cell surface it associates with similar or other membrane components into complexes which represent the functional cell ligands.

TABLE 2

Amino-acid and carbohydrate composition of retina-specific cell-aggregating factor, the retina cognin (From Hausman and Moscona, 1975).

Amino acid	No. of residues/mol	Amino acid or sugar	No. of residues/mol	
Lys	31	Val	34	
His	12	Met	3	
Arg	13	Ile	15	
	56	Leu	40	
Asp	47	Tyr	10	
Glu	55	Phe	10	
	102	Trp	ND	
Thr	23			112
Ser	22			
Pro	25			
Gly	24	GlcN	10	
Ala	40	Man	10	
Cys	ND	Gal	10	
	134	Sialic acid	1-2	
				32

TABLE 3

Some Characteristics of Retina Cognin

50,000 $\pm$ 6,000 M.W.	Binds to cells at 37° and 4°C
pI 4	Expression of activity (after
Sedimentation value 3.3	binding to cell surface) requires:
Stoke's radius 36 $\pm$ 1	protein synthesis
f/f$^\circ$ 1.3	optimal temperature microfilaments
Carbohydrate content 10-15%	calcium
Labels metabolically with ^{14}C-amino acids and ^{3}H-glucosamine	Antiserum to retina cognin prevents aggregation of retina cells.

This glycoprotein rapidly binds from solution to the surface of freshly dissociated retina cells at 37° and at 4°C. Its binding capacity is not destroyed by modification of the carbohydrate portion with neuraminidase, galactose oxidase, beta-galactosidase or periodate; however, it is possible that, after binding to the cell surface the carbohydrate is "repaired". Binding is not prevented by pretreatment of cells with cytochalasin; therefore, intactness of microfilaments is not essential for this step, but is required later on (see below). Binding may involve reaction with a "receptor" and subsequent insertion of the glycoprotein into the cell membrane; however, these possibilities have not yet been clarified.

Binding is followed by expression of cell-aggregating activity; this requires protein synthesis, optimal temperature, integrity of microfilaments, and calcium. The requirement for protein synthesis suggests that still other membrane proteins, which had been removed by cell trypsinization, may be involved in the formation of the functional cell-ligand complex; a possible candidate is the large molecular weight protein obtained from retina cells by Edelman's group (Brackenbury et al., 1977) and implicated in cell adhesion. The temperature requirement also may reflect the need for protein synthesis; in addition, it suggests that membrane fluidity and lateral rearrangement of membrane components are required for the characteristic function of the cognin. Microfilaments may be involved in anchoring cell ligands and in stabilizing their topographic pattern on the cell surface.

Tissue-specific cell-aggregating preparations obtained from other embryonic neural tissues have not yet been biochemically characterized; preliminary results indicate that, in these cases as well, activity is associated with protein-carbohydrate complexes. It is of interest that the effects of these tissue-specific preparations are not species-specific; this is consistent with the trans-species effectiveness of the cell recognition mechanism, as discussed above.

Taken as a whole, the information from these embryonic systems (and also from cell aggregation studies in sponges and slime molds) points to the existence of a class of cell-surface proteins that function in the mechanism of cell recognition and morphogenetic cell associations. The term cognins has been proposed for proteins with this particular function (Moscona et al., 1975; Moscona, 1975). As suggested above, cell-ligands are considered to represent complexes of cognin molecules; their specificities as determinants of cell affinities would depend on their composition, steric configurations, and topography on the cell surface. (Some authors refer to cell-recognition molecules as lectins, a ubiquitous term for sugar-binding proteins; its use in the present context could lead to needless confusion).

STUDIES WITH ANTISERUM TO RETINA COGNIN

The retina cognin is antigenic in rabbits. The antibodies react specifically with the cognin in solution and prevent it from binding to retina cells, and from enhancing their aggregation. Addition of this antiserum (gamma-globulin fraction, or FAB fragments) to suspensions of retina cells inhibits their normal aggregation: the antibodies bind to cognin molecules as they regenerate on the cell surface and block their function. This result further substantiates the role of cognin in cell associations. Aggregation of non-retina cells is not inhibited by this antiserum.

We have used this antiserum for immunolabeling the cell surface, to visualize by scanning electron microscopy (SEM) regeneration of cognin-containing sites on retina cells. The cells were treated with the anti-cognin rabbit gamma-globulin; they were then exposed to a suspension of polystyrene latex

microbeads precoated with anti-rabbit goat gamma-globulin
(GAR). The beads attached to cognin-antibody sites present
on the cell surface and labeled them. The cells were examined by SEM (for details see: Ben-Shaul et al., 1979).
Three kinds of cell preparations were used: 1) Retina cells
immediately after dissociation with trypsin; their surface
was expected to be depleted of cognin and therefore unable
to bind to label. 2) Dissociated retina cells, incubated
for several hours in serum-free culture medium to allow
cognin regeneration; these cells were expected to bind the
label. 3) Trypsin-dissociated embryonic liver cells, incubated for several hours; assuming specificity of the antiserum for retina cognin, liver cells were not expected to
label.

The results were consistent with the above expectations
(Fig. 3).

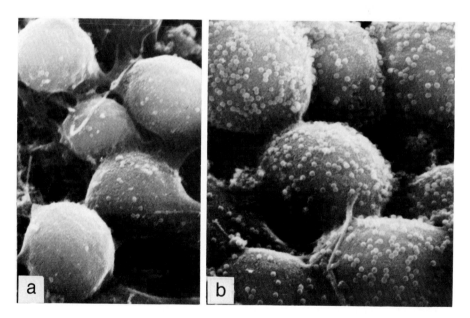

Fig. 3. Scanning electronmicrographs of dissociated retina
cells (10-day chick embryos) labeled with immunolatex microbeads for detection of cognin sites on cell surface (see text
for details). a) Freshly trypsinized cells showing only background level of labeling; x 5,000. b) Labeling after incubation
of the cells for 6 hrs to allow cognin regeneration; x 15,000.

Freshly dissociated retina cells did not label above background level; however in the course of incubation for up to
6 hrs, they showed progressively increasing capacity for
label binding, indicative of cognin appearance on their
surface. These results agree with other evidence concerning
timing of cognin regeneration on the cell surface, and coincident with acquisition by the cells of aggregation competence (Hausman and Moscona, 1979). Liver cells did not label
with antiserum to retina cognin neither immediately after
their dissociation, nor after prolonged incubation. Therefore, the antigen (retina cognin) is not detectable on the
surface of liver cells.

The tissue-specificity of the binding of retina cognin
to cells was examined by immunolabeling in the following
experiments. Freshly trypsinized retina cells were exposed
to a solution of retina cognin at $4^{\circ}C$; they were then treated
for immunolabeling of cognin (as above) and examined by SEM.
As expected, the cells showed heavy labeling due to the presence of bound cognin on the cell surface. In contrast,
similarly treated liver cells showed no labeling, thus
demonstrating that retina cognin binds preferentially to the
surface of retina cells.

The immunolabeling procedure was applied also to the
question of age-dependent changes in the capacity of trypsin-
dissociated retina cells to regenerate cognin on the cell
surface. Earlier studies have indicated that this capacity
declined with embryonic age of the cells. It has long been
known that cells dissociated from retinas of older embryos
were less capable of morphogenetic reaggregation than cells
from younger embryos (Moscona, 1962); this suggested that,
following completion of tissue morphogenesis, cognin production declined rapidly. In fact, attempts to isolate cognin
from cell membranes of late embryonic retinas were unsuccessful (Hausman and Moscona, 1976) suggesting that, after the
tissue had achieved its definitive cellular organization,
the cognitive mechanisms required for setting it up were no
longer active.

Cells were dissociated from retinas of younger and older
embryos and were incubated for up to 24 hrs to allow cognin
regeneration; they were then treated for immunolabeling of
cognin and examined by SEM. While cells from younger retinas
labeled as expected, the amount of labeling declined with
embryonic age; retina cells from embryos older than 14 days

showed essentially no regeneration of labeling sites (Ben-
Shaul et al., 1979)*. The temporal pattern of this decline
closely corresponded to the age-dependent decrease in aggregation competence of these cells.

COMMENTS AND DISCUSSION

The above labeling studies and related work on cell
immunolysis by antiserum to retina cognin (Hausman and
Moscona, 1979)*have provided semi-quantitative information
about the presence or absence of retina cognin on the embryonic cells at various developmental stages (Ben-Shaul et al.,
1979). Significant procedural improvements will be required
for the next major step: quantitative mapping of the spatial
distribution of cognin sites on different types of retina
cells and on various areas of their surface. Such studies
should make it possible to determine if there are distinct
and characteristic topographic patterns of cognin sites on
different cell types in the retina, how they are modulated
during cell differentiation, and how they change with normal
cell function and in pathological states. This information
will be essential for advancing the analysis of cell recognition from the level of tissue specificities to that of
cell-type specificities, i.e., to differences between
individual cells in a tissue.

The hypothesis outlined here suggests that cells in
different tissues are characterized by biochemically different cognins, and that such differences might be involved in
tissue-specific cell grouping and cell affinities. Purification of cognins from several embryonic tissues and
comparative studies on their biochemical characteristics
might help to determine if their differences can account for
tissue-specific cell affinities. However, the hypothesis
does not exclude the possibility of partial sharing of
similar cognin molecules by cells in related tissues (for
example, in neural retina and optic tectum); in fact, there
is suggestive evidence that this may be the case (Ben-Shaul
et al., 1979). Nor is it excluded that cells within a single
tissue may possess more than one molecular variant of cognin.

The hypothesis proposes that multimers of cognin
molecules constitute the cell-ligands which are the functional entities in morphogenetic cell-cell associations. A test
of this assumption would require isolation from embryonic

---

*In press, Develop. Neuroscience

cell membranes of such complex entities. The methods used so far have not been suitable for this purpose, and a direct approach to this question has yet to be attempted.

Assuming a structural complexity of cell-ligands, their specific function would be dependent on their composition, steric configuration, and patterning on the cell surface. Therefore, the basis for embryonic cell affinities is unlikely to be as simple as has been sometimes imagined. Several hypothetical possibilities have been envisaged for "cross-linking" of embryonic cells and a number of diagramatic schemes have been published by others. These have depicted various modes of association between glycoprotein and protein molecules, involving non-enzymatic or enzyme-mediated processes. However, a realistic reappraisal of the nature of embryonic cell recognition, and an updated definition of this problem call for a temporary lull in model-building and place a premium on fact-finding.

REFERENCES

Bennett D, Boyse EA, Old LJ (1972). Cell surface immuno-genetics in the study of morphogenesis. In Silvestri LG (ed): "Cell Interactions: Proceedings of the Third Lepetit Colloquium," Amsterdam: North Holland, p 247.

Ben-Shaul Y, Hausman RE, Moscona AA (1979). Visualization of a cell surface glycoprotein, the retina cognin, on embryonic cells by immunolatex labeling and scanning electron microscopy. Develop Biol 72:89.

Brackenbury R, Thiery JP, Rutishauser U, Edelman GM (1977). Adhesion among neural cells of the chick embryo: 1. An immunological assay for molecules involved in cell-cell binding. J Biol Chem 252:6835.

Burnet FM (1971). "Self-recognition" in colonial marine forms and flowering plants in relation to the evolution of immunity. Nature 232:230.

Fischman DA, Doering JL, Friedlander M (1976). Muscle development in vitro: regulation of cell fusion and serological analysis of the myogenic cell surface. In Ebert JD, Marois M (eds): "Tests of Teratogenicity in Vitro," Amsterdam: North Holland, p 233.

Friedlander M, Fischman DA (1977). Surface antigens of the embryonic chick myoblast: expression on freshly trypsinized cells. J Supramolecular Structure 7:323.

Goldschneider I, Moscona AA (1972). Tissue-specific cell surface antigens in embryonic cells. J Cell Biol 53:435.

Hausman RE, Knapp LW, Moscona AA (1976). Preparation of tissue-specific cell-aggregating factors from embryonic neural tissues. J Exp Zool 198:417.

Hausman RE, Moscona AA (1975). Purification and characterization of the retina-specific cell-aggregating factor. Proc Natl Acad Sci USA 72:916.

Hausman RE, Moscona AA (1976). Isolation of retina-specific cell-aggregating factor from membranes of embryonic neural retina tissue. Proc Natl Acad Sci USA 73:3594.

Hausman RE, Moscona AA (1979). Immunologic detection of retina cognin on the surface of embryonic cells. Exp Cell Res 119:191.

Lilien JE, Moscona AA (1967). Cell aggregation: its enhancement by a supernatant from cultures of homologous cells. Science 157:70.

Marx JL (1978). Antibodies (II): another look at the diversity problem. Science 202:412.

McClay DR, Moscona AA (1974). Purification of the specific cell-aggregating factor from embryonic neural retina cells. Exp Cell Res 87:438.

Monroy A, Rosati F (1979). The evolution of the cell-cell recognition system. Nature 278:165.

Moscona AA (1962). Analysis of cell recombinations in experimental synthesis of tissues in vitro. J Cell Comp Physiol 60:65, Suppl 1.

Moscona AA (1963). Studies on cell aggregation: demonstration of materials with selective cell-binding activity. Proc Natl Acad Sci USA 49:742.

Moscona AA (1974). Surface specification of embryonic cells: lectin receptors, cell recognition and specific cell ligands. In Moscona AA (ed): "Cell Surface in Development" New York: John Wiley & Sons, p 67.

Moscona AA (1975). Embryonic cell surfaces: mechanisms of cell recognition and morphogenetic cell adhesion. In McMahon D, Fox F (eds): "Developmental Biology - Pattern Formation, Gene Regulation," New York: W A Benjamin, p 19.

Moscona AA, Hausman RE (1977). Biological and biochemical studies on embryonic cell-cell recognition. In Lash JW, Burger MM (eds): "Cell and Tissue Interactions," New York: Raven Press, p 173.

Moscona AA, Hausman RE, Moscona M (1975). Experiments on embryonic cell recognition: in search for molecular mechanisms. In Raoul Y (ed): "Proceedings 10th FEBS Meeting," Amsterdam: North Holland, Vol 38, p 245.

Moscona AA, Moscona MH (1962). Specific inhibition of cell aggregation by antiserum to suspensions of embryonic cells. Anat Rec 142:319.

Rutishauser U, Thiery JP, Brackenbury R, Sela BA, Edelman GM (1976). Mechanisms of adhesion among cells from neural tissues of the chick embryo. Proc Natl Acad Sci USA 73:577.

Sperry RW (1943). Visuamotor coordination in the newt after regeneration of the optic nerve. J Comp Neurol 79:33.

Sperry RW (1950). Neuronal specificity. In Weiss P (ed): "Genetic Neurology," Chicago: University Chicago Press, p 232.

Weiss P (1947). The problem of specificity in growth and development. Yale J Biol Med 19:235.

ACKNOWLEDGMENT

The original work referred to in this manuscript has been supported by Research Grant HD01253 from the National Institute of Child Health and Human Development.

Pages 189—202, Membranes, Receptors, and the Immune Response
© 1980 Alan R. Liss, Inc., 150 Fifth Avenue, New York, NY 10011

TERMINAL DEOXYNUCLEOTIDYL TRANSFERASE AND LYMPHOCYTE
DIFFERENTIATION

F. J. Bollum[1] and Irving Goldschneider[2]

[1]Department of Biochemistry, Uniformed Services
University of the Health Sciences, Bethesda, MD
[2]Department of Pathology, University of Connecticut
Health Center, Farmington, CT

INTRODUCTION

A major part of current information about lymphocyte
differentiation stems from analysis of a variety of surface
markers. The presence of surface immunoglobins, the Thy-1
system, the Lyt system and many others all provide rather
dependable classifications for lymphocyte sub-populations.
Surface markers are especially useful since they provide a
basis for fluorescence sorting of viable cells as well as
population analysis. The limitations of surface marker
analysis arise from the indefinite nature of the substance
being analyzed. With the exception of immunoglobulin
markers, the chemical composition, structure, and (in most
cases) contribution to lymphocyte function is usually unknown. For these reasons surface marker systems are often
quite species specific and cannot be used across species
barriers without additional biochemical knowledge.

The enzyme called terminal deoxynucleotidyl transferase
(TdT) has now been shown to be quite useful in the analysis
of lymphocyte differentiation. TdT is different from surface markers in all aspects, thus providing independent
though complimentary information. TdT differs from surface
markers by virtue of being an intracellular protein, by
being known as a homogeneous substance, and by possessing
enzyme activity. The enzyme activity consists of an unusual
kind of deoxynucleoside triphosphate polymerization that
proceeds in the absence of any known template, and may be
responsible for some form of DNA diversification in primitive
lymphocytes. Last, but by no means least, measurements of

TdT by enzyme activity or immunoreactivity can be used in a wide variety of species, indicating a rather unique generality within animals possessing well-defined immune systems. This latter quality is somewhat reminiscent of the immunoglobulins themselves.

In this report we summarize our current biochemical and biological studies on TdT in experimental systems. Analysis for the presence of TdT is also useful for diagnostic work on human leukemias (Bollum, 1979), that is not the subject of this discussion. Although biochemical experiments do not yet clearly delineate the activity of TdT in DNA metabolism, the biological experiments now demonstrate a most pervasive influence of TdT$^+$ cells during development of the immune system.

STRUCTURE OF TERMINAL TRANSFERASE

TdT was purified to homogeneity from calf thymus gland (Chang and Bollum, 1971) and shown to have a molecular weight of 32,400 daltons by equilibrium centrifugation. Electrophoresis in acrylamide gels containing Na-dodecylsulfate demonstrated that the homogeneous protein contained peptide chains of approximately 24K and 8K. Calf thymus is the richest source of enzyme available in quantities useful for protein chemistry.

Antiserum against homogeneous bovine TdT developed in rabbits (Bollum, 1975b) exhibits exceptionally good cross-reaction with enzyme from humans, rodents and chickens. The immunoadsorbent purified rabbit anti-TdT also cross-reacts with enzyme positive human, rodent, and chicken cells, permitting cytological and biochemical studies with this reagent in several systems.

The structure of TdT in human and mouse lymphoblastoid cell lines was examined by immunoprecipitation of extracts from cells labelled with radioactive amino acids. Only cell lines known to be positive by assay for enzyme activity produced a radioactive immunoprecipitate (Human 8402, Molt 4, CEM-10, NALM-1 and Mouse P-1798), while enzyme negative lines (Human 8392, CEM-23) were negative for immunoprecipitate. Analysis of the immunoprecipitates by fluorography of SDS gels demonstrated a single 58K peptide (Bollum and Brown, 1979). The immunoprecipitate was shown to contain TdT activity. These results are important for all later studies since they demonstrate the absolute specificity of the immuno-adsorbent purified antibody used in all of our cytological studies. The 58K protein discovered in these investigations may represent the native form of TdT. The 32K from (24K + 8K) isolated from calf thymus may be a degraded product. These findings may eventually be helpful in comparative structural analysis of the 58K and 32K forms.

A high molecular weight form of TdT has been isolated from acute leukemia patient material (Deibel and Coleman, 1979). The possible existence of a high molecular weight form in calf thymus has been suggested (Johnson and Morgan, 1976) and our current work confirms this suggestion. The resolution of these structural differences into a common form remains a problem of continuing interest. Isolation and translation of TdT messenger RNA will be most helpful in this regard.

IS TERMINAL TRANSFERASE ACTIVE IN VIVO?

A specific TdT product has never been identified or isolated from cells. One might wonder what would happen in a randomly dividing population of TdT$^+$ cells arrested in DNA synthesis. Such cells should contain replication forks having free 3-OH' groups, possibly subject to the action of TdT in the presence of an unbalanced mixture of dNTP's. A number of authors (Carson et al., 1979; Wortman et al., 1979) have noted the selective deoxynucleoside toxicity of cultured TdT$^+$ T cells as opposed to TdT$^-$ B cells. Deoxyguanosine is especially toxic to T cells, and we (A. Green and F. J. Bollum, unpublished, 1979) reasoned that this could be due to addition of dGMP residues to replication forks, followed by failure of the repair system. Deoxyguanosine sequences are known to be resistant to the action of some endo- and exonucleases (Lefler and Bollum, 1969) because of aggregation structures.

The toxicity of 300µM deoxyguanosine was examined in a number of T and B lines. Viability and DNA content were measured by fluorescent flow cytology. The results in Table 1 show that deoxyguanosine kills most T cell (TdT$^+$) lines while B lines (TdT$^-$) remain viable.

Table 1: Deoxyguanosine Toxicity in B and T Cells

Cell Line	Description	TdT	dGuo Toxicity
8402	Lymphoblastoid T (Human)	+	+
8392	Lymphoblastoid B (Human)	-	-
Molt 4 R	Lymphoblastoid T (Human)	+	+
NALM-1	Lymphoblastoid Pre-B (Human)	+	+
K-562	Lymphoblastoid B (Human)	-	-
CEM-10	Lymphoblastoid Cloned T (Human)	+	+
CEM-23	Lymphoblastoid Cloned? (Human)	-	+
X63	Myeloma B (Mouse)	-	-
C3XB6F1	Thymus (Mouse)	+	+

In these experiments all cells were grown in RPMI 1640 with 10% fetal calf serum. Deoxyguanosine was present at 300µM for 16 hours and was removed by medium change. Positive toxicity was scored as less than 50% viable cells 24 hours after deoxyguanosine removal.

DNA analysis shows simple arrest in B lines with no cell death and permanent DNA arrest, followed by cell death, in most T lines. Since this generality did not hold in the cloned lines CEM-23 (TdT$^-$) we still cannot attribute deoxyguanosine toxicity solely to presence of TdT. CEM-23 has other abberant characteristics and so further analysis will be required for final interpretation of these experiments.

ONTOGENETIC STUDIES ON TERMINAL TRANSFERASE

The development of TdT in cells of the lymphohemopoietic system has been most intensively studied by immunofluorescent cytology in bird and rodent embryos. The avian system shows the greatest apparent simplicity (Fig. 1). TdT$^+$ cells first

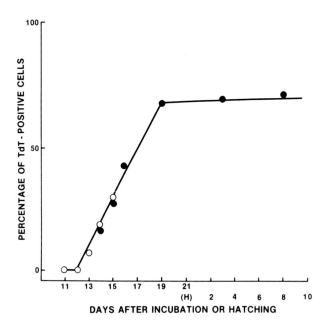

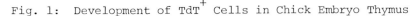

Fig. 1: Development of TdT$^+$ Cells in Chick Embryo Thymus

appear in the thymus of 12-day chick embryos and increase to a plateau at 18 days in ovo, at which time about 70% of the thymocytes (most cortical thymocytes) react with antibody to TdT (Sugimoto and Bollum, 1979). Rare positive cells are found in Bursa and in blood, but no significant "second compartment" or transient populations have been found. The developing rodent shows a time-adjusted similarity in TdT$^+$ cells in the thymus, but a second compartment and transient populations are observed.

In mice and rats TdT$^+$ cells are found first in thymus, appearing at about 18 days in utero. This population increases to about 70% (most cortical thymocytes) by 10 days after birth. The second compartment of TdT$^+$ cells arises in the bone marrow shortly after birth and rises to a stable plateau of 2-4% of bone marrow lymphocytes at 15-20 days post-partum (Gregoire et al., 1979). The thymus (first compartment) and bone marrow (second compartment) are referred to as stable populations of TdT$^+$ cells (Fig. 2). They

STABLE POPULATIONS

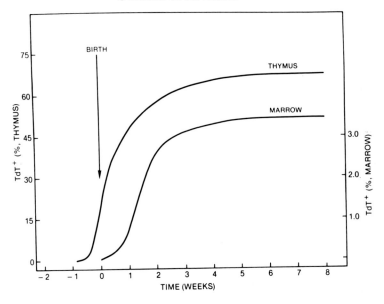

Fig. 2: Development of Stable TdT$^+$ Cell Populations in Rat Thymus and Marrow

persist into early adulthood and perhaps throughout life.

The most significant recent finding on TdT$^+$ cells concerns the transient populations that appear in various secondary lymphoid organs. The appearance and disappearance of TdT$^+$ cells in spleen, with a maximum population (about 0.5%) around 21 days after birth, was noted in our initial study in rats (Gregoire et al., 1979). The TdT positivity of this population persists for several weeks and then disappears. Dr. Ryuhei Sasaki discovered a sweeping transient of TdT$^+$ cells in rat peripheral blood, arising around 3 days after birth (Bollum, 1979; Sasaki and Bollum, 1979). This population shows an abrupt maximum (up to 10% of lymphocytes) at 10-12 days (Fig. 3), then disappears. Lymphocytes in

TRANSIENT POPULATIONS

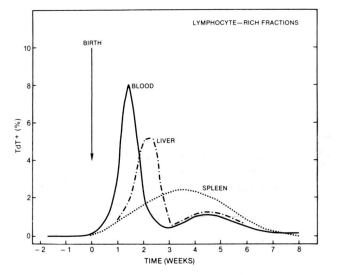

Fig. 3: Development of Transient TdT$^+$ Cell Populations in Rat Blood, Liver, and Spleen

adult rat blood are normally negative. Other transients have been observed in liver and lung, but kidney, heart, and other non-hematopoietic organs do not show these effects.

Where are these transient cells coming from and where do they go? The first question can be answered at least partly. The second question and a third --- what do they do? --- still elude us.

The source of the transient populations has been examined in the mouse for obvious reasons. Normal mice (NIH/Swiss, nu/+) exhibit the same general development of stable populations and transient populations observed in rats. Nude mice

(NIH/Swiss, nu/nu) exhibit all populations except the transient population that appears in the peripheral blood of
nu/+ litter mates. Thus the blood population originates
primarily in the thymus, whereas bone marrow, spleen, liver
and lung TdT+ cells arise from other sources. Earlier experiments had previously demonstrated the presence of bone
marrow TdT by enzyme assay in nude mice (Hutton and Bollum,
1977), and a source independent of thymus was suggested. We
(Goldschneider and Bollum, unpublished, 1979) have now analyzed the sources of transient populations of TdT+ cells in
mice using surface markers. The blood population is found to
be post-thymic and other transients are pre-thymic, providing
independent confirmation of the nude mouse experiment. We
would not like to claim 100% "post-thymic" lymphocytes in
blood and 0% post-thymic in other sources, but 90% and 5% are
good numbers from either type of experiment.

WHAT CELL LINEAGES EXPRESSES TdT?

The prevalence of TdT+ cells in thymus cortex immediately
associates this marker with T-cell precursors. This is true
in all systems where other suitable markers are available --
such as Thy 1, E-rosettes, etc. But how about the bone marrow
TdT+ cells, are they related only to T cells? The answer is
no, if one is willing to accept immunoglobulin markers as
being confined to B-lineage cells. The human cell line NALM-1
(Fig. 4) is TdT+ and CyIgμ+ (Minowada et al., 1979). In

**anti-TdT-
FITC** **anti-IgM-
TRITC**

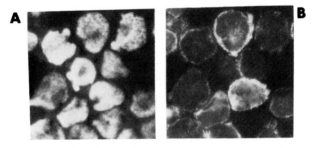

Fig. 4: Double Immunofluorescence of NALM-1 Cells
A. Anti-TdT-FITC
B. Anti-IgM-TRITC

normal human bone marrow it is also possible to show a minor TdT[+] population expressing CyIgμ[+] (Janossy et al., 1979). This is the phenotype for pre-B cells, and a wealth of evidence now demonstrates TdT presence in B-lineage cells (cf. Bollum, 1978) as originally suggested (Bollum, 1975a).

WHERE DO WE GO FROM HERE?

The problem concerning the biochemical and immunological function of TdT[+] cells and/or their progeny still remains, although TdT is now clearly related to lymphocyte differentiation. We know that TdT[+] cells in bone marrow and thymus (Fig. 5) can be destroyed by hydrocortisone derivatives and

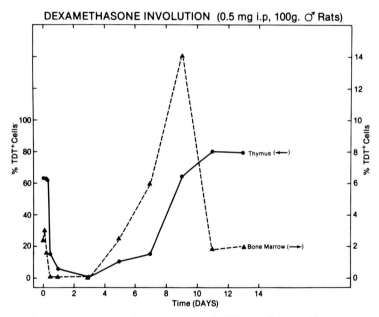

DEXAMETHASONE INVOLUTION (0.5 mg i.p, 100g. ♂ Rats)

Fig. 5: Dexamethasone Involution of Rat Thymus and Bone Marrow

that rapid regeneration from progenitor cells occurs (Gregoire et al., 1979; Bollum, 1975a). Others have shown thymosin induction of TdT[+] activity in bone marrow

(Pazmino et al., 1978). We have extended these studies
(I. Goldschneider, A. F. Ahmed, F. J. Bollum, and A. L.
Goldstein, unpublished, 1979) to show that coordinate induction of TdT$^+$ and Lyt antigens can occur in bone marrow and
spleen cells (Table 2). All of these findings provide further

Table 2:   Percent TdT$^+$ Spleen and Bone Marrow Cells
Expressing Lyt Antigens* after Incubation
with Thymosin

Treatment	Cell Fractions Examined	Spleen nu/+	nu/nu	Bone Marrow nu/+	nu/nu
Untreated	Total	0	0	0	0
Spleen Extract	A - D	0	0	0	0
Thymosin Fr. 5	A - D	99	74	85	
Thymosin α1	A - D	95	70	55	

*Determined by double immunofluorescence

correlation between presence of TdT and lymphocyte differentiation; they indicate that pursuit of the meaning of this correlation may provide new mechanistic insights. We need to
isolate TdT$^+$ cells, study their differentiation in isolation,
and examine function in the differentiated elements.

CELL SEPARATION STUDIES

Rat bone marrow cells sorted on 0° scatter for size show
that most TdT$^+$ cells are in the 10.4μ population (I. Goldschneider, D. Metcalf, F. Battye, T. Mandel, and F. J. Bollum,
unpublished, 1979). An enrichment of about 5-fold is obtained
on the first sort. The enriched population is then stained
for Thy-1 and sorted again on intensity of Thy-1 fluorescence.
Judicious selection on this sort provides 87% pure TdT$^+$ cells
at about 14% yield, an overall enrichment of about 20-40 fold.
These populations will be useful for future studies on the
properties of TdT$^+$ cells.

DISCUSSION

Early observations on the unique distribution of TdT activity in thymus (Chang, 1971) and bone marrow (Coleman et al., 1974) have now been confirmed by immunocytochemistry in several species. Cytochemical analysis demonstrates that these stable populations develop early in ontogeny and persist in adult life. Transient populations have now been observed in secondary lymphoid organs in rodents and these findings show some correlation with the development of immunocompetence. The TdT^+ populations can be regulated by lympholytic steroids and certain thymic hormones. The presence of TdT can be demonstrated in primitive T cells and in cells that are phenotypically pre-B ($CyIg\mu^+$). All of these observations are consistent with a relation of TdT to cells connected to cellular and humoral immunity.

The most mysterious aspect of TdT relates to its ability to polymerize deoxynucleotides. No other enzyme activity has been demonstrated for homogeneous TdT. No similar deoxynucleotide polymerizing enzyme has been demonstrated in animals lacking an immune system. In order to participate in sequence diversification TdT would have to operate on DNA molecules in some manner. The discovery of new forms of TdT with almost double the molecular weight of the previously known forms suggests a search for new or modified catalytic activities in these forms.

Irrespective of the final action that will be ascribed to TdT, it provides a generally useful marker for lymphocyte differentiation. This use is providing new insights into differentiation and migration of TdT^+ lymphocytes in the immunopoietic system.

ACKNOWLEDGEMENTS

The research reported in this report is supported by Public Health Service Grants CA-23262 (F. J. Bollum) awarded by the National Cancer Institute and AI-09649 and AI-14743 (I. Goldschneider) awarded by the National Institute of Allergy and Infectious Diseases.

Mouse thymocyte line C3XB6Fl was generously provided by Dr. J. N. Ihle, Frederick Cancer Research Center, Frederick, Maryland.

REFERENCES

Bollum FJ (1975a). Terminal deoxynucleotidyl transferase: Source of immunological diversity. Karl August Forster Lectures, Akad Wiss U Lit (Mainz), Steiner Verlag, pp 1-47.

Bollum FJ (1975b). Antibody to terminal deoxynucleotidyl transferase. Proc Nat'l Acad Sci USA 72:4119.

Bollum FJ (1978). Terminal deoxynucleotidyl transferase: Biological studies. In Advances in Enzymology, Meister A (ed). Wiley Interscience, NY, pp 347-374.

Bollum FJ (1979). Terminal deoxynucleotidyl transferase as a hematopoietic marker. Blood, in press.

Bollum FJ, Brown M (1979). A high molecular weight form of terminal deoxynucleotidyl transferase. Nature 278:191.

Carson DA, Kaye J, Matsumoto S, Seegmiller JE, Thompson (1979). Biochemical basis for the enhanced toxicity of deoxyribonucleosides toward malignant human T cell lines. Proc Nat'l Acad Sci USA 76:2430.

Chang LMS (1971). Development of terminal deoxynucleotidyl transferase activity in embryonic calf thymus gland. Biochem Biophys Res Commun 44:124.

Chang LMS, Bollum FJ (1971). Deoxynucleotide polymerizing enzymes of calf thymus gland V. Homogeneous terminal deoxynucleotidyl transferase. J Biol Chem 246:909.

Coleman MS, Hutton JJ, DeSimone P, Bollum FJ (1974). Terminal deoxynucleotidyl transferase in human leukemia. Proc Nat'l Acad Sci USA 71:4404.

Deibel MR, Coleman MS (1979). Purification of a high molecular weight human terminal deoxynucleotidyl transferase. J Biol Chem 254:8634.

Gregoire KE, Goldschneider I, Barton RW, Bollum FJ (1979). Ontogeny of terminal deoxynucleotidyl transferase positive cells in lymphohemopoietic tissues of rat and mouse. J Immunol 123:1347.

Hutton JJ, Bollum FJ (1977). Terminal deoxynucleotidyl transferase is present in athymic nude mice. Nucleic Acid Research 4:457.

Janossy G, Bollum FJ, Bradstock KF, McMichael A, Rapson N, Greaves MF (1979). Terminal transferase positive human bone marrow cells exhibit the antigenic phenotype of common acute lymphoblastic leukemia. J Immunol 123:1525.

Johnson D, Morgan AR (1976). The isolation of a high molecular weight terminal deoxynucleotidyl transferase from calf thymus gland. Biochem Biophys Res Commun 72:840.

Lefler CF, Bollum FJ (1969). Deoxynucleotide polymerizing enzymes of calf thymus gland III. Preparation of poly N-acetyl deoxyguanylate and polydeoxyguanylate. J Biol Chem 244:594.

Minowada J, Koshiba H, Janossy G, Greaves MF, Bollum FJ, (1979). A Philadelphia chromosome positive human leukaemia cell line (NALM-1) with pre-B characteristics. Leukemia Research 4:in press.

Pazmino NH, Ihle JN, Goldstein AL (1978). Induction in vivo and in vitro of terminal deoxynucleotidyl transferase by thymosin in bone marrow from athymic mice. J Exp Med 147: 708.

Sasaki R, Bollum FJ (1979). Transient populations of terminal transferase positive (TdT$^+$) cells in neonatal rat blood and liver. Fed Proc 38:4502.

Sugimoto M, Bollum FJ (1979). Terminal deoxynucleotidyl transferase (TdT) in chick embryo lymphoid tissues. J Immunol 122:392.

Wortman RL, Mitchell BS, Edwards NL, Fox IH (1979). Biochemical basis for differential deoxyadenosine toxicity to T and B lymphoblasts: Role for 5'-nucleotidase. Proc Nat'l Acad Sci USA 76:2434.

Hood: If you think TdT operates in the rearrangement of Ig genes, why is there asymmetric distribution of TdT in B and T lymphocytes? And why is there a late appearance in ontogeny of TdT if the function is related to DNA processing?

Bollum: We do not know. It is partly a matter of how to measure a marker. Is cytoplasmic IgM a good marker? We have only a single marker we can use, so the asymmetry may be more apparent than real.

Hood: What diversity patterns would you expect after TdT processing?

Bollum: The diversity is either on the chromosomes, or not. If not on the chromosomes, then it will be hard to find. How does the enzyme work? It works best in test tubes, and on small substrates.

Silverstein: Can you tell us about TdT expression among the cells that resist hydrocortisone treatment?

Bollum: The pluripotential stem cell is not sensitive to hydrocortisone. Other cells regenerate from the pluripotential stem cell.

Pages 203—214, Membranes, Receptors, and the Immune Response

MATURATION OF B-CELL CLONES

John J. Fung, Kristine Gleason, Ronald Ward and
Heinz Köhler
La Rabida-University of Chicago Institute and
Department of Pathology and Biochemistry
E. 65th Street at Lake Michigan
Chicago, Illinois   60649

INTRODUCTION

The developing immune response in inbred mice appears to
be an exceptionally suited experimental system to study the
processes and mechanisms in maturation. The reasons for this
are multiple and become more evident by drawing a simplify-
ing analogy to observations in developmental biology. One
can picture each individual clone of immunocompetent cells as
a mini-organ which undergoes several discrete maturation steps
before it reaches the full response potential. Though the
cells of these clones are circulating and do not engage in the
long-lasting physical contacts found between cells in organs,
the interactions between cells of different clones are in-
tense, relying mainly on soluble mediations, such as immunoglobulins or factors. Only recently, it became possible to
analyze these clonal maturation processes through the development of specific clonal markers for cells and through new
assay systems which probe the activities and responses of
single clones. The chief advancements were made using idiotypes as clonal markers (Köhler et al, 1977) and the organ
cultures system pioneered by Klinman (Klinman, 1972). The
splenic foci assay system allows repeated sampling of responsive B-cells derived from a single precursor cell over a
considerable time span. Thus, the response kinetics and any
maturational changes can be analyzed at the level of individual clones.

Of the several experimental systems which had been used
for studying B-cell ontogeny--in vivo and in vitro responses,

in adoptive transfers--the splenic foci assay appears to be the best suited to detect most of the developmental stages in B-cells (Teale et al, 1978). Changes in clonal profiles, changes in clone size, susceptibility to tolerance induction or anti-idiotype suppression, changes in isotypes and homing preference can all be observed conveniently with this technique at the level of individual clones. Furthermore, factors provided by the environment can be controlled by manipulating the donor of the organ fragments through T-cell priming or T-cell mediated suppression. Thus, key mechanisms occurring in ontogeny can be investigated, such as establishment of clonal dominance, tolerance induction, idiotype suppression or the role of T-cells in maturation.

Recently we have begun to use the splenic foci system to study the maturation of T-independent and T-dependent responses to phosphorylcholine (PC) (Köhler, 1975). These studies allowed us to identify functional markers which seem to define different developmental stages of B-cells. Furthermore, we began to compare the ontogeny of idiotype-defined clones in the response to (1-3)-dextran with that of clones responding to PC. From these studies it became apparent that there exists a temporal hierarchy in the maturation of different idiotypes responding to different antigens.

THE RESPONSE OF NEONATAL AND ADULT BONE MARROW CELLS AFTER ADOPTIVE TRANSFER

The onset of responsiveness to three T-independent antigens was investigated after adoptive transfer into syngeneic, lethally irradiated recipients. In the appearance of the response to PC, the T15 idiotype was used, and in the response to (1-3)-dextran, J558 and M104E were used as idiotypic clonal markers. 800r-irradiated BALB/c mice received syngeneic neonatal liver cells or adult bone marrow cells. Groups of reconstituted hosts were immunized with three antigens, TNP-Ficoll, PnC and (1-3)-dextran in the second, third and eighth weeks after reconstitution. The PFC response to TNP-, PC- and Dextran-SRBC was measured 5 days later. As seen in Tables 1 and 2, a distinct response pattern can be recognized. The pattern of the appearance of responsiveness is identical for neonatal liver cells and adult bone marrow cells indicating a similar type of stem cell, giving rise to these PFC responses. The response to TNP-Ficoll appears first after reconstitution, followed by the response to dextran. The response to

TABLE 1

RESPONSE IN RECIPIENTS OF 10[7] NEONATAL LIVER CELLS

RESPONSE[a]	WEEKS AFTER RECONSTITUTION[b]		
	Two	Three	Eight
ANTI-TNP	0, 0, 0, 0, +, 0, +	++, ++, ++, ++	+++, +++, +++, +++, +++, ++, ++, ++
ANTI-PC	0, 0, 0, 0, 0, 0, +	+, 0, +, 0, +, 0, +, 0, 0, 0, 0, +, 0, 0, 0, +	+, +, +, +, 0, 0, 0, +, +
ANTI-DEX.	0, 0, 0, 0, 0, 0, +	+, +, 0, 0, +, ++, ++, +, +, +, 0, 0	++, +, ++, ++, ++, ++, +++

a) Balb/c mice were X-radiated with 800r and reconstituted with 10[7] neonatal syngeneic liver cells.

b) The reconstituted hosts were immunized with TNP-Ficoll, dextran B1355 and C-polysaccharide at different times after reconstitution. The primary PFC response to the three antigens was measured five days after immunization:

0 = <1,000 PFC/spleen; + = 1,000-10,000 FPC/spleen; ++ = 10,000-100,000 PFC/spleen; +++ = >100,000 PFC/spleen

TABLE II

RESPONSE IN RECIPIENTS OF 10[7] ADULT BONE MARROW CELLS

RESPONSE	WEEKS AFTER RECONSTITUTION		
	Two	Three	Eight
ANTI-TNP	+, +, +, 0, +, +, +	+, +, +, +, ++, +, 0, +, +, +, +	++, +++, ++, +++, ++
ANTI-PC	+, +, +, 0, 0, 0, 0	0, 0, 0, +, +, +, 0, 0	+, +, 0, +, +
ANTI-DEX.	+, 0, 0, 0, 0, ++, +	0, +, +, +, +, +, 0	++, ++, ++, ++, ++

For experimental details, see Table 1.

TABLE 3

CLONOTYPE ANALYSIS OF INDIVIDUAL MICE RENCONSTITUTED WITH 10^7 NEONATAL LIVER CELLS OR 10^7 ADULT SPLEEN CELLS

	PFC/Spleen: Anti-PC (x10^-2)	% T15	PFC/Spleen: Anti-Dex (x10^-2)	% J558	% M104E
Three (Neonatal Liver Cells)	3	N.D.[c]	218	37	64
	3	N.D.	143	58	24
	0	N.D.	56	50	50
Eight	17	N.D.	344	24	15
	23	64	39	N.D.	N.D.
	49	61	535	N.D.	N.D.
	0	N.D.	345	73	0
	1	N.D.	1109	71	56
	87	89	824	N.D.	N.D.
Three (Adult Spleen Cells)	95	N.D.	46	N.D.	N.D.
	28	N.D.	76	31	39
	31	N.D.	44	N.D.	N.D.
Eight	357	N.D.	245	21	25
	85	85	166	13	22
NORMAL RESPONSE	148	90	354	28	2
	808	99	236	6	3
	452	95	114	12	78
	568	77	430	7	18

(Left axis label: WEEKS AFTER RECONSTITUTION WITH:)

a) Lethally radiated (800r) Balb/c mice were reconstituted with 10^7 neonatal or adult syngeneic cells. 3 or 8 weeks after reconstitution the mice were immunized with C-polysaccharide or dextran B1355.

b) The primary PFC response to PC and dextran was measured 5 days after immunization. Clonotype analysis was done with plaque inhibition by homologous anti-T15, anti-J558 and anti-M104E. As controls the PFC response and clono-types of normal adult Balb/c to PC and dextran are shown.

c) N.D. = Not done.

PC emerges last. In some reconstituted animals the response
to PC is absent, even eight weeks after reconstitution.
Clonotype analysis of individual animals confirms and extends
these observations (Table 3). In every reconstituted animal
that produced a substantial anti-PC response, the clonotype
was T15-dominant. In contrast, the relative amounts of J558
and M104E idiotypes is highly variable in normal and reconstituted responses. This lack of consistent idiotype pattern in
the anti-dextran response is seen already three weeks after
reconstitution with neonatal liver cells. Thus, the individual idiotype pattern for anti-dextran response must be
already determined very **early** in ontogeny, at least before
the third week after **r**econstitution with neonatal liver cells.
This early fixation of idiotype pattern is in contrast to the
T15 anti-PC response where we failed to detect the T15 clonal
dominance which is typical for the adult response in the third
week after reconstitution. From the data in Table 3, it is
also evident that the precursor for the three idiotypes, T15,
J558 and M104E are assorted independently in the transfers,
indicating that the cell dose of 10^7 cells used for reconstitution is limiting. This independent assortment argues
against any substantial contribution of host cells in the
reconstituted responses.

FUNCTIONAL AND TOPOGRAPHICAL DIFFERENCES AS DIFFERENTIATION
MARKERS

Klinman's splenic foci assay was used to search for functional and topographical differences in neonatal cells. Neonatal liver and spleen cells from 6-day-old and adult mice
were assayed in splenic fragments taken from hemocyanin-primed
animals (Table 4). The number of precursors for PC-Hy and
TNP-Hy in cells from adult mice is in agreement with Klinman's
data (Sigal et al, 1975). Spleen cells from day 1 animals
have no detectable precursors for anti-PC, but day 6 animals
contain a small number of PC-specific precursors. In contrast, day 1 liver cells have PC-precursors, while day 6
livers contain much less. The absolute frequency for liver-
derived precursors cannot be calculated at this point since
we do not know the homing efficiency for neonatal liver cells.

These findings demonstrate that the first PC-specific precursors emerge in the neonatal liver already at the time of
birth. However, the T15 clone in these early responses is not
yet dominant. Six days later the first precursors for PC

TABLE 4

ANALYSIS OF PC- AND TNP-PRECURSORS IN ADULT AND NEONATAL BALB/c

DONOR CELLS[a] FROM:	# CELLS ANALYZED (x 10^{-7})	# PC-PRECURSORS[b] PER 10^6 B-CELLS	% T15 IDIOTYPE	# TNP PRECURSORS[b] PER 10^6 B-CELLS
SPLEEN CELLS				
Adult animals	62	32.4 ± 13.7	79	215.7 ± 28.3
Day 1 animals	18	0	--	N.D.
Day 6 animals	16	6.67 ± 2.39	65	74.0 ± 17.3

	# OF FOCI ANALYZED	# OF PC-POSITIVE FOCI[c]		TNP-POSITIVE FOCI
LIVER CELLS				
Day 1 Animals	1728	26 (1.5%)	23	9.4%
Day 6 Animals	960	5 (.5%)	N.D.	3.7%

a) Balb/c mice were primed with hymocyanin 6-8 weeks prior to use. 2 x 10^7 syngeneic donor cells were given to these mice 4-6 hours after X-radiation (1400r). 18 hours later, spleen fragments were cultured and immunized with PC-hemocyanin or TNP-hemocyanin.

b) Culture supernatants from splenic fragments were assayed for anti-PC, T15 idiotype and anti-TNP antibodies by RIA.

c) Since the homing efficiency of liver cells is not known, the data are expressed as percentage of positive foci from the total number of fragments analyzed.

appear in the spleen and here the T15 clonal dominance is already established. Thus, we can describe a maturation sequence for T-dependent PC-specific precursors: PC^+T15^- precursors in the neonatal liver $\longrightarrow PC^+T15^+$ in day 6 spleen. The migration of PC precursor from liver to spleen is coupled with the maturation of clonal dominance.

Susceptibility to tolerance induction has been used as a functional criteria for maturity of B-cells (Metcalf et al, 1976; Cambier et al, 1976). We have used this marker together with the susceptibility to anti-idiotype suppression. The interesting finding here is that tolerization and idiotype suppression become effective at different stages of maturity (See Table 5). The T15 clone in the day 1 liver which is not dominantly expressed, cannot be suppressed by anti-T15 while it is sensitive to suppression six days later in the spleen. PC precursors in both organs, however, can be tolerized by PC-rabbit-Ig. Adult precursors are resistant to tolerization but still partially suseptible to idiotype suppression. Thus, the susceptibility to tolerization is the earliest functional marker in this system defining an immature progenitor cell type which precedes the more mature progenitor which is also sensitive to idiotype suppression. This interpretation is in agreement with Klinman's finding of the reversal of anti-idiotype suppression by idiotype in early neonatal cells (Accolla et al, 1976; Strayer et al, 1975).

The analysis of PC-precursors in neonatally idiotype suppressed mice (Strayer et al, 1975) reveals the presence of day 1 liver cell types. The total number of precursors in these animals, which are unresponsive in vivo, is close to normal adult levels and the T15 clone is also dominant. However, these precursors are susceptible to tolerance induction to the same extent as neonatal liver and spleen cells. They are also partially suppressable by anti-idiotype though less so than neonatal cells. These characteristics of precursors in neonatally suppressed animals clearly labels them as immature cells similar to cells found in neonatal animals.

Another marker in B-cell ontogeny is the appearance of T-dependent and T-independent responses to the same antigen. The temporal hierarchy is still under discussion (Cambier et al, 1977; Kettman et al, 1979; Quintans et al, 1979). By the criteria of susceptibility to anti-idiotype suppression and tolerization, the T-independent precursors to PC resemble an immature cell type. The data in Table 6 show that

TABLE 5

DIFFERENTIAL TOLERIZATION OF IMMATURE B-CELL PRECURSORS
FOR T-DEPENDENT ANTI-PC RESPONSES

	DONOR CELLS:[a]	TOLEROGEN[b]	CLONES/10^6 TRANSF. CELLS	% CONTROL RESPONSE	% T15
EXPERIMENT ONE	DAY 1 LIVER	-- PC-Rabbit-Ig Anti-T15 10^{-2} Anti-T15 10^{-3}	.10 .03 .08 .10	100 30 80 100	25 N.D. 33 25
	DAY 6 SPLEEN	-- PC-Rabbit-Ig Anti-T15 10^{-2} Anti-T15 10^{-3}	.18 .08 .05 .10	100 44 28 56	69 33 25 50
	NEON. SUPPRESSED ADULT (120 days old)	-- PC-Rabbit-Ig Anti-T15 10^{-2} Anti-T15 10^{-3}	.28 .10 .13 .20	100 36 46 71	64 25 60 73
	NORMAL ADULT	-- PC-Rabbit-Ig. Anti-T15 10^{-2} Anti-T15 10^{-3}	.45 .38 .20 .32	100 84 44 71	74 80 55 69
EXPERIMENT TWO	NEON. SUPPRESSED ADULT (230 days old)	-- PC-Rabbit-Ig Anti-T15 10^{-2} Anti-T15 10^{-3}	.72 .30 .50 .58	100 42 69 81	76 N.D. N.D. N.D.
	NORMAL ADULT	-- PC-Rabbit-Ig Anti-T15 10^{-2} Anti-T15 10^{-3}	.87 .80 .60 .75	100 92 69 87	83 N.D. N.D. N.D.

a) Recipient Balb/c mice, primed with hemocyanin 6-8 weeks
before, were given 1400 r and 2 x 10^7 syngeneic cells
4-6 hours later.

b) Tolerization and immunization of splenic foci were done
according to Metcalf and Klinman (1976). PC-Rabbit-Ig was
added at a final concentration of 5 x 10^{-7} M. The idiotype binding capacity of anti-T15 was 100 µg/ml.

TABLE 6

DIFFERENTIAL TOLERIZATION OF ADULT B-CELL PRECURSORS
FOR T-DEPENDENT AND T-INDEPENDENT ANTI-PC RESPONSES

ANTIGEN	TOLEROGEN[a]	CLONES/10^6 TRANSF. CELLS	% CONTROL RESPONSE	% T15 IDIOTYPE
	--	.45	100	74
	PC-Rabbit-Ig	.38	84	80
PC-Hy	Anti-T15 10^{-2}	.20	44	55
	Anti-T15 10^{-3}	.32	71	69
	--	.40	100	N.D.
PnC	PC-Rabbit-Ig	.03	7.5	"
	Anti-T15 10^{-2}	.00	0	"
	Anti-T15 10^{-3}	.03	7.5	"
PC-Hy	--	.93	100	N.D.
+	PC-Rabbit-Ig	.33	35	"
PnC	Anti-T15 10^{-2}	.18	19	"
	Anti-T15 10^{-3}	.28	30	"

a) Tolerization and immunization of splenic fragments done
as described in Table 5. The concentration of the T-
independent antigen PnC was 1 µg C-polysaccharide per
fragment.

TABLE 7

B-CELL MATURATION SCHEME

MARKER FUNCTION	CELL TYPE	DIFFERENTIATION STEP
OMNIPOTENT	STEM CELL	IDIOTYPE
TOLERIZABLE	PROGENITOR I	COMMITMENT
SUPPRESSIBLE BY ANTI-IDIOTYPE	PROGENITOR II	(Network-Driven Maturation)
RESPONDING IN FOCI	PRE B-CELL I	CLONAL EXPANSION
RESPONDING IN VIVO	PRE B-CELL II	(Antigen-driven Maturation)

T-independent precursors, responding to PnC in splenic fragments from non-primed animals, are totally suppressed by
tolerogen and anti-idiotype. From these findings one would
predict that T-independent precursors to PC appear late in
ontogeny and remain in a rather immature state for long times
in adult mice.

TENTATIVE SCHEME FOR B-CELL MATURATION

Based on the discussed functional markers for maturity
of B-cells we will attempt to draw a tentative flow sheet
for B-cell maturation. (See Table 7.) Stem cells, not yet
committed to the expression of an idiotype, would have to be
labeled as omnipotent. The first maturation steps are most
clearly detectable in splenic foci. With these early neonatal cells no responses in vivo can be demonstrated. For
this reason we have labeled these cells as progenitors (Kaplan et al, 1978). Early progenitors (Progenitor I) are
tolerizable but resistant to anti-id suppression (Progenitor
II). Indirect experimental evidence and reasoning led us to
the speculation that these maturation events are driven by
network interaction (Köhler et al, 1978). The next step in
ontogeny is the acquisition of the adult-type idiotype pattern: in the response to PC the establishment of the T15
clonal dominance, or in the anti-Dex response the individually different balance of J558 and M104E idiotypes. An
interesting intermediate in these pre-B-cell forms are the
cells which are unresponsive in vivo but fully responsive in
foci (Pre-B-cell I). The mature Pre-B-cell can be triggered
in foci and in the animal (Pre-B-cell II). It can be expected
that antigen is an important factor in these final maturation
steps which occur in the transition from Pre-B-cell I to
Pre-B-cell II.

SUMMARY

The maturation of B-cells was investigated in adoptive
transfers and splenic foci. Anti-idiotypic antigens were
used to identify clones responding to PC and dextran. A
distinct temporal hierarchy of responsiveness could be observed in which the anti-TNP response appears first, followed
by anti-dextran and anti-PC. Tolerance induction and anti-
idiotype suppression were used as markers for maturing B-
cells responding in splenic foci. A differential

susceptibility to these manipulations establishes two types of progenitor cells. A scheme for the maturational steps of B-cells is proposed.

ACKNOWLEDGEMENT

The skillful help of Ms. Sue Smyk is gratefully acknowledged. The research was supported by USPHS grants AI 11080 and AI10242. JJF is supported by training grant T32-9MO 7281, KG by A107090, and RW by 5T329MO7183.

REFERENCES

Acolla RS, Gearhart PJ, Sigal NH, Cancro MP, Klinman NR (1976). Eur J Immunol 7:876.
Cambier JC, Kettman JR, Vitetta ES, Uhr JR (1976). J Exp Med 144:293.
Cambier JC, Vitetta ES, Uhr JW, Kettman JR (1977). J Exp Med 145:778.
Kaplan DR, Quintans J, Köhler H (1978). Proc Natl Acad Sci US 75:1967.
Kettman JR, Cambier JC, Uhr JW, Ligler F, Vitetta ES (1979) Immunol Rev 43:69.
Klinman NR (1972). J Exp Med 136:241.
Köhler H (1975). Transpl Rev 27:26.
Köhler H, Rowley DA, Du Clos T, Richardson B (1977). Federation Proc 36:221.
Köhler H, Kaplan DR, Kaplan R, Fung J, Quintans J (1979). In "Cells of Immunoglobulin Synthesis," Academic Press, p. 357.
Metcalf ES, Klinman NR (1976). J Exp Med 143:1327.
Quintans J, McKearn JP, Kaplan D (1979). J Immunol 122:1750.
Sigal NH, Gearhart PJ, Klinman NR (1975). J Immunol 68:1354.
Strayer DS, Lee WMF, Rowley DA, Köhler H (1975). J Immunol 114:728.

Bona: Models on the sequential expression of V genes
            do not fit with the maturation scheme you have
            proposed. For one thing, why do you think
            there are such large differences in the
            functional activity of liver B cells and spleen
            B cells?

Kohler: If we look at a neonatal liver and a neonatal
            spleen, we see that the liver is larger and
            contains more B-cell precursors. The liver
            is more mature in terms of B-cell precursors.
            B cells will migrate from the liver to the
            spleen and apparently undergo maturation
            processes during this time.

Quintans: How do you expect the neonatal day 1 liver cell
            to be susceptible to anti-idiotype?

Kohler: The finding is that there are a few T15 precur-
            sors in day 1 liver. Only approximately 25% of
            the anti-PC foci are T15 positive. And these
            T15 positives are resistant to anti-idiotype
            suppression.

Quintans: Are you suggesting that T15 positive cells
            appear later in ontogeny than T15 negative
            cells?

Kohler: Not exactly. The data indicate that the T15
            dominance appears later, at about day 5, but
            the T15 precursors are already present by day 1.

Session IV.
Genetic Aspects of
Idiotype Expression

Pages 217—230, Membranes, Receptors, and the Immune Response
© 1980 Alan R. Liss, Inc., 150 Fifth Avenue, New York, NY 10011

ANTIGEN BINDING VARIANTS OF THE S107 MOUSE MYELOMA CELL
LINE

Wendy D. Cook, Stuart Rudikoff*, Angela M.
Giusti, Donald J. Zack, Terry Kelly and Matthew
D. Scharff

Department of Cell Biology
Albert Einstein College of Medicine
1300 Morris Park Avenue
Bronx, New York   10461

                    and

*Laboratory of Cell Biology
National Cancer Institute
National Institutes of Health
Bethesda, Maryland

INTRODUCTION

Idiotypic serological markers which distinguish the
variable regions of individual antibodies have been extremely
useful in studying the organization and expression of immunoglobulin genes. A number of studies have suggested a relationship between the sequence of the hypervariable regions
of the immunoglobulin polypeptide chains and idiotype (Capra
and Kehoe, 1975; Givol, 1979). This has lead to the feeling
that, at least in most immunoglobulins, specificity and idiotype are closely related (Capra and Kehoe, 1975; Givol, 1979).
On the other hand, studies with levan binding myelomas
(Lieberman et al., 1977; Vrana et al., 1978; 1979) as well as
others (Potter, 1977) reveal dissociations between sequence,
idiotype, and specificity (Marshak-Rothstein et al., 1979).
In addition, there are some perplexing and provocative reports
of idiotype positive non-antigen binding immunoglobulins
(Cazenave et al., 1974; Oudin and Cazenave, 1971) and even
of an idiotype positive immunoglobulin with altered specificity (Sigal, 1977).

We have attempted to learn more about the genetic control of variable region structure and to examine the relationship between antigen binding and idiotype by generating
a family of antigen binding variants of a single mouse myeloma cell line. We were prompted to initiate these studies
because of our previous finding that somatic cell variants
with changes in immunoglobulin expression and structure occur
frequently in cultures of mouse myeloma cells (Scharff,
1975). Such variants arise spontaneously at a rate of 10^{-3}/
cell/generation and at a higher rate with mutagenesis (Baumal
et al., 1973). This genetic instability appears to be restricted to the immunoglobulin genes since in these same
cells other traits, such as drug resistance, mutate at the
expected low frequencies of $10^{-5} - 10^{-7}$ (Baumal et al., 1973;
Margulies et al., 1976). While it was tempting to try to
relate the genetic instability of mouse myeloma cells to the
somatic generation of antibody diversity, all of the initial
structural variants had changes in their constant rather than
in their variable regions (Adetagbo et al., 1977; Scharff et al.,
1975). Since this might have resulted from the methods used
for detecting variants, we decided to look more directly for
variable region variants.

We chose to study the S107 cell line which secretes a
phosphocholine (PC) binding IgA K immunoglobulin of the T-15
idiotype (Cohn et al., 1969; Potter and Lieberman, 1970).
This idiotype is the predominant one elicited in BALB/C
mice when they are immunized with PC bound on a variety of
carriers (Lee et al., 1974). The complete amino acid sequence of the S107 heavy chain variable region and part of
the sequence of the S107 light chain variable region have
been determined (Barstad et al., 1974; Rudikoff and Potter,
1976). There is equally extensive sequence data on a number of other PC binding mouse myeloma proteins (Kabat et
al., 1976a). Computer analysis (Kabat et al., 1976b) and
x-ray diffraction (Padlan et al., 1976) have provided considerable insight into the folding and contact residues of
the PC-binding proteins.

IDENTIFICATION OF ANTIGEN BINDING VARIANTS

Antigen binding variants were identified and their
spontaneous frequency determined using a modification of the
techniques we had used for studying constant region variants
(Coffino et al., 1972). S107 cells grow well in tissue

culture and can be cloned with a high efficiency in soft agarose. A fresh clone was recloned and PC attached to the protein carrier, keyhole limpet hemocyanin (KLH), was over-layed in agarose. The S107 immunoglobulin was secreted into the agar surrounding the clone and the PC-KLH precipitated with the antibody to form a visible antigen-antibody precipi-tate around almost all of the clones. In a number of in-dependent experiments, between 0.1 and 1% of the clones were not surrounded by a visible precipitate (Cook and Scharff, 1977) (Table 1). Such unstained clones could have lost the ability to synthesize, assemble, or secrete the antibody or

Table 1

Frequency of Variant Clones

Subclone	Overlay	Unstained/ Stained	%
	PC-KLH	10/1105	.91
S107.3.4S3			
	Anti-IgA	4/1339	.29

they could have been secreting an immunoglobulin with a de-creased affinity for PC-KLH. In order to determine the frequency of clones which were no longer secreting the S107 immunoglobulin, an aliquot of the same cells which had been analyzed with antigen were cloned in separate dishes and overlayed with rabbit antibody against mouse IgA. As can be seen in Table 1, such non-secreting variants do arise but they only represent about a third of the non-antigen binding variants. We have shown in previous studies that other cell lines also generate both loss and structural variants (Scharff et al., 1975).

In order to confirm and extend this observation, a num-ber of variant clones were recovered from the agar and ex-amined both serologically and biochemically. It is worth pointing out that mouse myeloma cells provide an unusual somatic cell genetic system both because of the high fre-quency of variants and because the variant gene product is made in such large amounts that it can be easily recovered

and characterized. The presumptive variant clones were recloned to ensure cellular homogeneity and then their intracellular and secreted immunoglobulins were examined by agar
diffusion with both antibody against IgA and with the antigen PC-KLH. As would be expected from the results shown in
Table 1, approximately 30% of the variants did not produce
serologically identifiable IgA. The other 70% of the variants synthesized and secreted IgA. None of these secreted
IgA molecules reacted with PC-KLH in agar diffusion (Table
2). This decrease in antigen binding was confirmed when the
variants were injected into BALB/c mice and the IgA purified
from the resultant ascites fluid. This is illustrated in
Table 2 for one first generation antigen binding variant, U_1.
The purified variant (U_1) and parental (S107.3.4) proteins
were also examined for their ability to hemagglutinate PC-
Sheep red blood cells (PC-SRBC). This first generation
variant did agglutinate PC-SRBC but at a much lower titer
than the S107 parent (Table 2). This was confirmed when the
U_1 variant was examined in a solid phase radioimmunoassay
(Cook and Scharff, 1977) for its ability to compete with the
S107 parent for binding to PC-KLH (Table 2). In addition to
low antigen binding variants like U_1 we have characterized
one 1st generation variant (U_4, Table 2) which does not
agglutinate PC-SRBC and competes very poorly with S107 for
PC-KLH in the radioimmunoassay (Cook, 1979).

These findings suggested that the S107 cell line frequently generates variants producing immunoglobulins with
changes in antigen binding. Since equal amounts of purified
protein were used in the assays depicted in Table 2, the
decrease in antigen binding could not have been due to decreased synthesis of immunoglobulin by the variant. Since
IgA is secreted in its polymerized form by S107, a defect in
polymerization could have resulted in a decrease in avidity.
However, as shown by SDS gel analysis and chromatography of
undenatured material on S300 Sephacryl, the U_1 variant (and
all of the others to be described) secrete the same relative proportion of polymers as S107.

Table 2

Antigen Binding Characteristics of 1st, 2nd and 3rd Generation Variants

Generation (clone)	agar diffusion Anti-IgA	PC-KLH	HA titer[a] PC-SRBC	RIA[b] PC-KLH (%)
Parent (S107.3.4)	+	+	8192	100
1 (U$_1$)	+	−	128	9
1 (U$_4$)	+	−	0	>1
2 (S$_3$S$_1$)	+	+	512	26
3 (U$_{10}$)	+	−	0	<0.25

a) 250 µg of purified antibody was used as starting material

b) Competition between parental and variant antibody was examined by attaching PC-KLH to a polyvinyl plate. A fixed amount of endogeneously labelled S107 protein plus varying amounts of unlabelled parental or variant protein were added to each well.

$$\text{relative binding} = \frac{\text{ng of parent required for 50\% inhibition of binding of label}}{\text{ng of variant required for 50\% inhibition of binding of label}}$$

Neither U$_4$ nor U$_{10}$ reached an end point.

IDENTIFICATION OF 2nd AND 3RD GENERATION VARIANTS

The first generation low antigen binding variant U_1 (Table 2) was recloned and overlayed with PC-KLH. The vast majority of the subclones were not surrounded by visible antigen-antibody precipitate. However, some clones did secrete immunoglobulin which reacted with PC-KLH. In a number of independent experiments, the frequency of such second generation variants with increased binding was similar to the frequency of first generation variants (Cook and Scharff, 1977). So far these have all turned out to be phenotypic revertants in that none are identical to the parent. As can be seen in Table 2, a representative 2nd generation variant, S_3S_1, binds PC-SRBC and PC-KLH better than the 1st generation variant U_1 from which it is derived but less well than the S107.3.4 parental clone. When the S_3S_1 2nd generation variant was overlayed with PC-KLH, a third generation non-antigen binding variant, U_{10}, was obtained. We have not been able to detect significant binding of U_{10} protein to either PC-KLH or PC-SRBC (Table 2). Furthermore, neither U_{10} nor the 1st generation variant, U_4, bind to PC-Sepharose columns.

We have attempted to identify revertants to higher antigen binding amongst the U_4 and U_{10} non-antigen binding variants. If they exist, their frequency is lower than 1/80,000. Since the U_4 and U_{10} proteins have little or no affinity for PC-KLH or PC-SRBC, it is possible that revertants do arise but that their binding is still to low to be detected.

As already mentioned, all of the variants described in Table 2 synthesize the same amount of IgA as the S107 parent and form the same relative amounts of polymers (Cook and Scharff, 1977; Cook et al., 1979). SDS gel analysis also shows that the heavy and light chains of these variants and of the S107 parent are the same size (Cook, 1979).

HAPTEN BINDING

In the studies described above, we have shown that the variant proteins of S107 have a decreased binding for PC-KLH or PC-SRBC. Equilibrium dialysis (Colowick, 1969) and hapten induced fluorescence enhancement (Jolley & Glaudemans, 1974) have been used to assess their affinity for hapten alone. As expected, the first and third non-antigen binding variants, U_4 and U_{10}, do not show detectable binding for PC by one or both of these assays. However, when the first generation low antigen binding variant U_1, the second generation variant S_3S_1, and S107.3.4 proteins were examined using the fluorescent enhancement assay, their association constants did not differ significantly (Cook, 1979). At the moment we are not certain how to interpret this apparent discrepancy between the binding of PC attached to a carrier and free hapten. It is possible that the radio-immunoassay, which is a competition assay, and hemagglutination are more sensitive to small changes in binding than hapten binding assays. It is also possible that the antigen binding sites of U_1 and S_3S_1 are partially blocked so that hapten bound to carrier cannot enter the site while free hapten can. Further studies with hapten attached to linkers may resolve this issue.

SEROLOGICAL CHARACTERIZATION

The S107 protein is of the T-15 idiotype which has been studied extensively in many laboratories. Two types of antibodies have been made against this idiotype: 1) antibodies that specifically react with the T-15 idiotype have been produced in rabbits or other species by immunizing with S107, TEPC 15, or HOPC 8 proteins and absorbing with non T-15 PC-binding IgA myelomas such as McPC603, TEPC 167, and M511 (Potter and Lieberman, 1970) and 2) hapten binding-site specific antibodies have been produced by binding rabbit antisera to a column bearing S107 proteins and then eluting the column with PC. Those antibodies that are competed off by hapten react with antigenic determinants in or near the hapten binding site and compete with hapten for those sites (Claflin and Davis, 1975). We have also generated monoclonal antibodies that are T-15 variable region specific by immunizing rats with the S107 protein and fusing the spleen cells with mouse myeloma cells. These homogeneous antibodies do not inhibit antigen binding and are therefore not binding-site specific.

Radioimmunoassays have been carried out with all of these antisera. All of the variants bind less well to binding-site specific antibody than the S107 parent (Table 3). When the parent and U_1 were compared with non site-specific rabbit and anti-variable region antibody, they were indistinguishable. Similarly, our T-15 specific monoclonal antibody does

Table 3

Relative binding[1]
rabbit

Generation		Site Specific (%)	Variable Region (%)	Mono-Clonal (%)
Parent	(S107.3.4)	100	100	100
1	(U_1)	9	100	100
1	(U_4)	20[2]	nd	100
2	(S_3S_1)	18	27	100
3	(U_{10})	<0.1	nd	100

1) relative binding =

$$\frac{\text{ng of parent required for 50\% inhibition of binding of label}}{\text{ng of variant required for 50\% inhibition of binding of label}}$$

Neither U_4 nor U_{10} reached an end point.
2) This figure is from a separate experimental determination and should not be compared with the other variants in this column.

not distinguish between any of the variants tested. These results suggest that the variants differ from S107 in conformation in or near the binding site but that other parts of the variable region are very similar in all of the proteins.

TRYPTIC PEPTIDE ANALYSIS

In order to determine if the changes in antigen binding and serology were associated with changes in the amino acid sequence of the heavy or light chains of the variants, we have analyzed the tryptic peptides of all of the variants described above except the first generation non-antigen binding variant U_4 which is a recent isolate. Variant cells were incubated with either ^{14}C-lysine or arginine, their heavy and light chains were purified from the medium, mixed with purified ^{3}H-labelled parental heavy or light chains, digested with trypsin, and the double labelled samples were analyzed by ion exchange chromotography (Weitzman & Scharff, 1976). The polypeptide chains of each variant were separately compared with the chains of their immediate parent (Table 4).

Table 4

Presence of Peptide Map Differences

Generation (pro- teins compared)	L chain labelled with		H chain labelled with	
	Lysine	Arginine	Lysine	Arginine
P vs 1st ($S107$ vs U_1)	−	−	−	+
1st vs 2nd (U_1 vs S_3S_1)	−	−	−	+
2nd vs 3rd (S_3S_1 vs U_{10})	−	?	−	+

All of the reproducible and significant differences were in the arginine containing peptides of the heavy chain. In each case, the variant differed from its immediate parent by one or two tryptic peptides. In addition, there was a questionable peptide difference in an arginine containing peptide of the light chains of the 3rd generation variant, U_{10}, and its immediate parent, S_3S_1.

DISCUSSION

We have described the frequent and spontaneous occurrance of somatic cell variants of the S107 cell line which produce immunoglobulins with changes in their ability to bind antigen. These changes in antigen binding are associated with changes in the serology of the hapten binding rate and in the tryptic peptides of the heavy chain. The obvious expectation is that these variants have changes in the amino acid sequence of their heavy chain variable regions. However, more detailed characterization of some of these variants suggests that the changes in antigen binding may be more complex than anticipated. First of all, two of the variants do not bind PC at all. This is surprising, since the 7 PC binding myelomas differ from each other at a number of residues in the 2nd and 3rd hypervariable regions of the heavy chain but continue to bind PC quite well (Padlan et al., 1976). Secondly, some of the variants have decreased binding for PC-KLH and PC-SRBC but the same affinity for free hapten. Thirdly, even though the 3rd generation U_{10} variant differs from its immediate parent by peptide analysis, we have been unable so far to find any amino acid substitutions in its heavy chain variable region. This raises the possibility that the loss of antigen binding in this variant is due to a change in the constant region which either alters the folding of the binding site or affects the association of heavy and light chains. Constant region variants do arise both in the S107 and in other myeloma cell lines.

The peculiar properties of some of these variants, the high frequency of both antigen binding and constant region variants in mouse myeloma cells, and the fact that abnormal cells are being studied makes it difficult to determine the relevance of these findings to the normal generation of antibody diversity. It is possible that constant region variants arise frequently in normal cells but are selected against while variable region changes are selected for by antigen. It is also possible that the instability is due to the unusual structure of the immunoglobulin genes (Seidman et al., 1978). While further studies are required to resolve these issues, this system has allowed us to generate variant proteins which have interesting dissociations between idiotype and antigen binding.

ACKNOWLEDGEMENTS

WDC is supported by a scholarship from the Young Men's Philanthropic League. AMG is an immunology trainee supported by training grant CA 09173 from the National Institutes of Health. DJZ is a medical scientist trainee supported by grant 5T32GM7288 from the National Institute of General Medical Sciences. This work was supported by grants from the National Institutes of Health (AI 10702 and AI 5231) and the National Science Foundation (PCM77-25635).

REFERENCES

Adetugbo K, Milstein C, Secher DS (1977). Molecular analysis of spontaneous somatic mutants. Nature 265:299.

Barstad P, Rudikoff S, Potter M, Cohn M, Konigsberg W, Hood L (1974). Immunoglobulin structure: amino terminal sequences of mouse myeloma proteins that bind phosphorylcholine. Science 183:962.

Baumal R, Birshtein BK, Coffino P, Scharff MD (1973). Mutations in immunoglobulin-producing mouse myeloma cells. Science 182:164.

Capra JD, Kehoe JM (1975). Hypervariable regions, idiotypy and the antibody-combining site. Adv Immunol 20:1.

Cazenave PA, Ternynck L, Avrameas S (1974). Similar idiotypes in antibody-forming cells and in cells synthesizing immunoglobulins without detectable antibody function. Proc Natl Acad Sci USA 71:4500.

Claflin JL, Davie JM (1975). Specific isolation and characterization of antibody directed to binding site antigenic determinants. J Immunol 114:70.

Coffino P, Baumal R, Laskov R, Scharff MD (1972). Cloning of mouse myeloma cells and detection of rare variants. J Cell Physiol 79:429.

Cohn M, Notani G, Rice SA (1969). Characterization of the antibody of the C-carbohydrate produced by a transplantable mouse plasmacytoma. Immunochemistry 6:111.

Colowick SP, Womack FC (1969). Binding of diffusible molecules: rapid measurement by rate of dialysis. J Biol Chem 224:774.

Cook W, Dharmgrongartama B, Scharff MD (1979). Variable and constant region variants of mouse myeloma cells. In Pernis B, Vogel HJ (eds):"Cells of Immunoglobulin Synthesis", New York: Academic Press, p. 99.

Cook WD (1979). Antigen binding variants in a mouse myeloma cell line. Doctoral Thesis.

Cook WD, Scharff, MD (1977). Antigen binding mutants of mouse myeloma cells. Proc Natl Acad Sci USA 74:5687.

Givol D (1979). The antibody combining site. In Lennox ES (ed):"International Review of Biochemistry: Defense and Recognition II B, Vol. 23, Structural Aspects", Baltimore: University Park Press, p 71.

Jolley ME, Glaudemans CPJ (1974). The determination of binding constants for binding between carbohydrate ligands and certain proteins. Carbohydrate Research 33:377.

Kabat EA, Wu TT, Bilofsky H (1976a). "Variable regions of immunoglobulin chains." Cambridge, Ma.: Bolt Beranek and Newman, Inc.

Kabat EA, Wu TT, Bilofsky H (1976b). Attempts to locate residues in complementarity-determining regions of antibody combining sites that make contact with antigen. Proc Natl Acad Sci USA 73:617.

Lee W, Cosenza H, Kohler H (1974). Clonal restriction of the immune response to phosphorylcholine. Nature 247:55.

Lieberman R, Vrana M, Humphrey W, Chien CC, Potter M (1977). Idiotypes of inulin binding myeloma proteins localized to vauluable region light and heavy chains: genetic significance. J.Exp Med 146:1294.

Margulies DH, Kuehl WM, Scharff MD (1976). Somatic cell hybridization of mouse myeloma cells. Cell 8:405.

Marshak-Rothstein A, Siekevitz M, Mudgett-Hunter M, Margolies M, Gefter M (1979). Hybridoma proteins expressing the predominant idiotype of the anti-azophenylaisenate response of the A/J mouse. Proc Natl Acad Sci USA in press.

Oudin J, Cazenave PA (1971). Similar idiotypic specificities in immunoglobulin fractions with different antibody functions or even without detectable antibody function. Proc Natl Acad Sci USA 68:2616.

Padlan EA, Davies DR, Rudikoff S, Potter M (1976). Structural basis for the specificity of phosphorylcholine binding immunoglobulins. Immunochemistry 13:945.

Potter M (1978). Antigen-binding myeloma proteins of mice. Immunol 25:141.

Potter M, Lieberman R (1970). Common individual antigenic determinants in five of eight BALB/c IgA myeloma proteins that bind phosphorylcholine. J Exp Med 132:737.

Rudikoff S, Potter M (1976). Size differences among immunoglobulin heavy chains from phosphorylcholine-binding proteins. Proc Natl Acad Sci USA 73:2109.

Scharff MD (1975). The synthesis, assembly, and secretion of immunoglobulin: a biochemical and genetic approach. Harvey Lectures 69:125.

Scharff MD, Birshtein BK, Dharmgrongartama B, Frank L, Kelly T, Kuehl WM, Margulies D, Morrison SL, Preud'homme JL and Weitzman S (1975). The use of mutant myeloma cells to explore the production of immunoglobulins. In "Molecular Approaches to Immunology," New York: Academic Press, p. 109, Smith EE, Ribbons DW (eds).

Seidman JG, Leder A, Nav M, Norman B, Leder P (1978). Antibody diversity: the structure of cloned immunoglobulin gene suggests a mechanism for generating new sequences. Science 202:11.

Sigal N (1977). Novel idiotype and antigen-binding characteristics in two anti-dinitrophenyl monoclonal antibodies. J Exp Med 146:282.

Vrana M, Rudikoff S, Potter M (1978). Sequence variation among heavy chains from insulin-binding myeloma proteins. Proc Natl Acad Sci USA 75:1957.

Vrana M, Rudikoff S, Potter M (1979). The structural basis of a hapten-inhibitable κ-chain idiotype. J Immunol 122: 1905.

Weitzman S, Scharff MD (1976). Mouse myeloma mutants blocked in the assembly, glycosylation and secretion of immunoglobulin. J Mol Biol 102:237.

Claflin: Could you comment on the relative differences in the analogues to the variants?

Scharff: Taking three analogues, we find that their relative binding differs for the variants but the order of effectiveness is the same.

Kabat: Could the lack of differences in binding constant be due to the insensitivity of your techniques? The competition assays are more sensitive to small differences than equilibrium dialysis.

Scharff: Yes. Our techniques cannot detect two-fold differences. Techniques other than equilibrium dialysis or fluorescence amplification might conceivably be more valid, but presently the discrepancy between antigen and hapten binding is not resolved.

Hood: What did you say about the difference in the light chains?

Scharff: All have identical light chains by peptide maps, except possibly U_4 and U_{10}. V_H on the H chain may be different, also. If they are different, peptide maps will be significant.

Kohler: Could the difference in the peptide map be due to the association of carbohydrate with the protein?

Scharff: Conceivably. However, there is no carbohydrate in the variable region of the heavy chain.

Hood: We have not found any carbohydrate in the light chain U region through residue 88.

Pages 231—247, Membranes, Receptors, and the Immune Response

STUDIES OF GENETIC CONTROL AND MICROHETEROGENEITY OF AN
IDIOTYPE ASSOCIATED WITH ANTI-P-AZOPHENYLARSONATE
ANTIBODIES OF A/J MICE

A.R. Brown*, P. Estess**, E. Lamoyi*, L. Gill-
Pazaris*, P.D. Gottlieb† J.D. Capra**, A. Nisonoff*

*Rosenstiel Research Center, Brandeis University
Waltham MA;**Department of Microbiology,University
of Texas, Southwestern Medical School, Dallas,
Texas; †Center for Cancer Research and Department
of Biology, Massachusetts Institute of Technology,
Cambridge, MA.

Strain-specific idiotypes can serve as genetic markers
for V regions of immunoglobulins (Kuettner et al., 1972;
Eichmann, 1975; Weigert and Potter, 1977). In nearly all
systems studied linkage has been observed between the idiotype
under investigation and the Igh locus, which determines allotypes present on C_H regions. This has been interpreted as
reflecting close linkage between genes controlling V_H and
C_H polypeptides. Since L chains frequently contribute to the
formation of idiotypic determinants (Hopper and Nisonoff,
1971), and genes controlling L and H chains are unlinked,
the linkage of idiotype to the Igh locus without reference
to the L chain might seem paradoxical. A possible explanation is that either of the pair of strains used in each such
genetic study was capable of providing L chains required for
the expression of the idiotype; i.e., that they had similar
L chain repertoires. Support for this view has come from
investigations involving strains of mice whose normal L
chains yield a tryptic peptide map of cysteine-containing
peptides from the V_K region that differ from those of other
strains; the 4 strains originally identified are AKR/J, C58/J,
PL/J and RF/J (Edelman and Gottlieb, 1970). The inheritance
of this genetic marker (called the I_B peptide marker) follows
classical Mendelian genetics and the genetic locus, designated Igk-Trp (Green, 1979) is closely linked to the locus
controlling a polymorphic alloantigen, Lyt-3,present on the
surface of thymocytes (Gottlieb, 1974; Gottlieb and Durda,
1977; Boyse et al., 1971; Itakura et al., 1972). Other

laboratories have demonstrated that the normal L chains (Gibson, 1976) or the L chains of purified antiphosphocholine antibodies of these 4 strains (Claflin, 1976) exhibit iso-lectric focusing patterns that differ from those of other strains, and both groups have demonstrated similar linkage of these properties to the Lyt-3 locus (Claflin et al., 1978; Gibson et al., 1978).

Our investigations on linkage of idiotype and allotype have made use of the major idiotype associated with anti-p-azophenylarsonate (anti-Ar)antibodies of A/J mice (Kuettner et al., 1972). The idiotype is also present on anti-Ar anti-bodies of C.AL-20 mice, a congenic strain with the allotype of the AL/N strain on a BALB/c background (Pawlak et al., 1973). Since BALB/c mice are idiotype-negative this de-monstrates close linkage of idiotype and heavy chain allo-type. A similar linkage was observed in backcross experi-ments, using the idiotype-negative BALB/c, CBA and C57BL/6 strains as mating partners with A/J (Laskin et al., 1977). However, when the PL or C58 strains, both of which are Lyt-3.1 positive and exhibit the I_B peptide marker, were used in breeding studies with A/J, it was found that the ability to produce the cross-reactive idiotype (CRI) required the pre-sence of genes controlling A/J L chains as well as A/J H chains (Laskin et al., 1977; Gottlieb et al., 1979). Offspring that were homozygous for Lyt-3.1, characteristic of strains PL or C58, failed to produce the idiotype despite the demon-strated presence of genes for the Ig-1^e (A/J) allotype. Mice that were Lyt-3.1, Lyt-3.2 heterozygotes and also positive for Ig-1^e produced anti-Ar antibodies bearing the CRI. These findings are consistent with the hypothesis that BALB/c, CBA and C57BL/6 mice can provide the L chains necessary for the expression of the CRI whereas PL and C58 cannot. It is not known whether the L chain differences among strains reflect the activity of structural or regulatory genes, but Swan and coworkers (1979) have shown that structural genes for mouse kappa chains are on the chromosome determining the L chain polymorphism (chromosome 6).

We have now carried out experiments to test this hypo-thesis directly. By appropriate breeding of the A/J and PL strains, mice were obtained that were homozygous for Lyt-3.1 and heterozygous for Ig-1^e; such mice failed to produce the CRI. These mice were mated to BALB/c or C57BL/6 mice, both of which are idiotype-negative strains. It was found that all Ig-1^e- positive offspring of the mating of such pairs of idiotype-negative mice were idiotype-positive. This is direct evidence for the production of the appropriate L chains by BALB/c or C57BL/6 mice. It also provides a rapid method for testing various strains of mice for their capacity to provide the requisite L chains. This can be done by mating mice which are doubly homozygous for Ig-1^e and Lyt-3.1 with mice of any given strain. If the latter mice can provide the required light chains all offspring should produce the idiotype. There is no requirement for testing the allotype or the Lyt phenotype of the offspring, except as an occasional control, since these phenotypes will be determined by the parental strains used.

Assay for the CRI in Parental Mice. Table 1 shows the results of idiotype analyses on anti-Ar antibodies produced by the individual mice used as parents in the breeding study. The parental mice were immunized by repeated inoculations in complete Freund's adjuvant of the p-azophenylarsonate derivative of keyhole limpet hemocyanin (KLH-Ar), by the same procedure used to immunize their offspring. The mice of Group D, Table 1, were obtained by backcrossing PL mice to F$_1$(PL x A/J) mice and selecting male offspring that were homozygous for Lyt-3.1, according to a cytotoxicity assay on thymus cells (Boyse et al., 1971), but heterozygous for Ig allotype (Ig-1^{a,e}) as determined by radioimmune assays (Bosma et al., 1975). It is evident that all of the mice were idiotype-negative, in accord with previous results.

The data in the lower portion of Table 1 show the results of idiotype analyses (Kuettner et al., 1972) of anti-Ar antibodies produced by offspring of the mating of mice of Group D, Table 1 (males; Lyt-3.1, Ig-1^{a,e}) with female mice of the PL, BALB/c or C57BL/6 strains. Offspring of the mating with PL, which would necessarily be homozygous for Lyt-3.1, produced anti-Ar antibodies which lacked the CRI. Those offspring of the matings with C57BL/6 or BALB/c (all Lyt-3.1, 3.2) which were negative for Ig-1^e likewise failed to produce anti-Ar antibodies with the CRI. However, the idiotype was present in all offspring of the latter matings which expressed Ig-1^e. The results indicate that C57BL/6 and BALB/c mice are capable of providing L chains required for the expression of the major CRI.

Measurements were carried out to ascertain whether the mice utilizing L chains of BALB/c or C57BL/6 origin to synthesize CRI produced anti-Ar antibodies with an idiotype

Table 1. Formation of anti-Ar antibodies possessing the CRI by offspring of parents that do not produce the idiotype.

Group Desig- nation	Strain	Sex	No. of Mice	Ig-1 allo- type	20	50	100	500	1,000
							--Assay for CRI-- ng anti-Ar antibody tested as inhibitor		
Parental Mice							% inhibition, mean (range)		
A	PL/J	F	2	a				0 (0)	5 (0-1)
B	BALB/cJ	F	2	a				6 (0-15)	10 (1-20)
C	C57BL/6J	F	2	b				0 (0-7)	2 (0-8)
D	Offspring of backcross*	M	2	e,a				0 (0)	0 (0)
Offspring of Matings									
A x D			5	e,a				2 (0-11)	12 (0-44)
A x D			2	a				0 (0)	0 (0)
B x D			4	e,a	51 (21-80)	66 (41-90)	83 (60-99)	97 (92-100)	
B x D			5	a				1 (0-4)	6 (0-13)
C x D			8	e,b	45 (4-73)	67 (20-88)	78 (34-95)	92 (52-100)	
C x D			3	a,b				0 (0)	12 (2-29)

*Offspring of backcross, PL/J x F_1(PL/J x A/J); selected for phenotypes Ig-1[e,a] and Lyt-3.1(+), 3.2(-).

content comparable to that of A/J antibodies. The results, obtained with specifically purified anti-Ar antibodies, are shown in Table 2. The data on maximum percentage of labeled, purified anti-Ar precipitable by anti-CRI were obtained by a double precipitation assay, using excess goat anti-rabbit Fc, adsorbed with mouse globulin, to precipitate complexes made with 10 ng of ^{125}I-labeled purified anti-Ar and increasing amounts of anti-id; the plateau values are reported. By this criterion and by that of weight of anti-Ar antibody required to cause 50% inhibition in the standard radioimmune assay for idiotype (Table 2), the antibodies from the backcross offspring have an idiotype content about half as great as that of the A/J mice. It is not certain whether this is statistically significant since individual mice vary considerably with respect to the idiotype content of their anti-Ar antibodies. If it proves to be a consistent finding, the difference may be attributable to gene dosage for the $Ig-1^e$ allotype, the L chain locus, or both, since the offspring tested were heterozygous at both loci (Table 2). It is evident that BALB/c or C57BL/6 are comparable to A/J mice with respect to their capacity to provide the requisite light chains.

Evidence for Microheterogeneity in Antibodies Expressing the Major CRI. Another aspect of the present studies deals with evidence indicative of microheterogeneity in the major CRI associated with anti-Ar antibodies of the A/J strain. This evidence is based on investigations with hybridomas secreting anti-Ar antibodies that were prepared with splenic lymphocytes from A/J mice immunized with KLH-Ar and the nonsecreting SP2/0-Ag14 line of Shulman et al. (1978). The method used for cell fusion was that of Köhler and Milstein (1976) as modified by Gefter et al. (1977). After expansion of clones in microtiter wells, individual clones were isolated in agarose by transferring 10 to 1,000 cells into 60 mm Petri dishes. Clones selected from the agarose were expanded in microtiter plates, grown in mass culture and finally in the ascites of F_1(A/J x BALB/c) mice. Hybridoma products (HP's) were selected for purification on the basis of their anti-Ar activity and the presence of the serum cross-reactive idiotype (CRI), as estimated by their inhibitory capacity in the standard radioimmune assay for the idiotype (Kuettner et al., 1972). About 25% of initial wells with anti-Ar activity exhibited the CRI. Each protein was specifically purified by affinity chromatography on Sepharose 4B conjugated with BGG-Ar or with Ar derivative of normal mouse IgG, followed

Table 2. Quantitative expression of the CRI in mice possessing L chains of A/J, BALB/c, or C57BL/6 Origin*

Source of Purified Antibody	Ig-1 Allotype	Lyt Phenotype	Maximum % of Labeled, Purified anti-Ar Precipitable by anti-CRI†	Assay for CRI ng anti-Ar Required for 50% Inhibition
A/J	e	3.2	50%	22
Offspring of (Balb/c x Backcross**)	e,a	3.1, 3.2	27%	41
Offspring of (C57BL/6 x Backcross**)	e,b	3.1, 3.2	26%	57

*Antibodies were specifically purified from serum by affinity chromatography on bovine IgG-Ar-Sepharose and elution with 0.2 M p-aminobenzenearsonate.

**Backcross - PL x F_1(PL x A/J): Offspring selected for mating were Lyt-3.2(-), Lyt-3.1(+), Ig-1^e(+).

†Using increasing amounts of rabbit antiidiotype and goat antirabbit Fc to precipitate the complexes.

by elution with 0.2 M or 0.5 M arsanilate, pH 7.5 to 8. In most instances, prior to affinity chromatography the protein was precipitated from ascites by the addition of ammonium sulfate to 50% saturation, followed by ultracentrifugation. All HP's used in these experiments were homogeneous by the criterion of electrophoresis in SDS polyacrylamide gels; samples were reduced with 2-mercaptoethanol just prior to loading into the gel (Laemmli, 1970). Samples were also homogeneous by the criterion of disc electrophoresis (Davis, 1964) or amino acid sequence analysis. Among the HP's the bands varied markedly with respect to their electrophoretic mobilities.

We investigated 14 hybridoma products (HP's) that were found capable of causing at least 50% inhibition of the reaction of labeled serum idiotype (A/J anti-Ar) with its rabbit antiidiotypic antibody. All were IgG-kappa; the IgG subclass is indicated in Table 3, which presents data on inhibition by specifically purified hybridoma products of the binding of 10 ng of ^{125}I-labeled specifically purified A/J anti-Ar antibodies by its rabbit antiidiotypic (anti-id) antibodies. Complexes of ^{125}I-labeled antibody and anti-id were precipitated with a slight excess of goat antirabbit Fc. The anti-id antiserum had previously been adsorbed twice with normal mouse globulin conjugated to Sepharose 4B. In addition, 20μl of normal A/J serum was present in each assay.

Two of the HP's (nos. 93G7 and 16.7) were comparable to serum antibody in their inhibitory capacity, as reflected by the weight of antibody needed to cause 50% inhibition in the assay. Both of these HP's were IgG$_1$. Three other HP's (nos. 13.4, 20.4 and 26.5) were almost as effective as inhibitors. Two of these are IgG$_3$, the other is IgG2b. With another group of 4 HP's (3 IgG2b and 1 IgG2a) considerably more unlabeled HP (180 to 460 ng) was required for 50% inhibition. Four other HP's (two of which are IgG$_1$) were relatively poor inhibitors; 1800 to 3200 ng were required for 50% inhibition. It should be emphasized that the majority of anti-Ar HP's (about 75% in these experiments) fail to cause 50% displacement, even when very high concentrations are tested.

There is a direct correlation between the effectiveness of an HP as an inhibitor, as estimated from the 50% inhibition point, and the degree of inhibition by a very large amount (2,000 ng). The best inhibitors give maximum values of 90-94% while the poorest yield a plateau at about 50% inhibition.

Table 3. Displacement of Labeled A/J anti-Ar From Its Rabbit Anti-idiotypic Antibodies by Unlabeled A/J anti-Ar Antibodies or Hybridoma Products with anti-Ar Activity*

Unlabeled Inhibitor	ng Required for 50% Inhibition	% Inhibition by 2 µg	Unlabeled Inhibitor	ng Required for 50% Inhibition	% Inhibition By 2 µg
Serum anti-Ar	11	97	HP# 20.4 (G2b)	14	86
			23.2 (G2b)	200	66
HP# 93G7 (G1)	12	90	17.5 (G2b)	460	63
16.7 (G1)	9	94	10.8 (G2a)	180	60
121D7 (G1)	300	71	22.4 (G2a)	3,200	49
123E6 (G1)	1,900	51	24.6 (G2a)	1,800	52
124E1 (G1)	2,900	47	13.4 (G3)	21	87
9.3 (G2b)	300	65	26.5 (G3)	17	85

*Each assay utilized 10 ng ^{125}I-labeled, specifically purified A/J anti-Ar antibodies and slightly less than an equivalent amount of antidiotype.

The hybridoma products were selected for specific purification and testing on the basis of their anti-Ar activity and their ability to cause inhibition in the standard radioimmune assay for CRI. About 75% of HP's with anti-Ar activity lacked the CRI.

Studies with Antiidiotypic Antiserum Prepared Against
an HP Carrying the Major Idiotype. Table 4 shows the results of measurements of inhibition of binding of HP 93G7
(IgG_1) to its autologous rabbit anti-id antibodies. (The
data discussed so far were all obtained with anti-id directed against A/J anti-Ar antibodies). The test system utilized
10 ng of ^{125}I-labeled, specifically purified HP 93G7,
sufficient rabbit anti-id to bind 69% of the labeled HP, and
a slight excess of goat antirabbit Fc to precipitate complexes of id and anti-id. Unlabeled inhibitors were pooled,
specifically purified A/J anti-Ar antibodies or the HP's
indicated in Table 4, each of which possessed an idiotype
related to the major serum CRI, as evidenced by its capacity
to cause 50% inhibition of binding in the conventional assay. Whereas 80 ng of unlabeled 93G7 caused 50% inhibition
of binding of labeled 93G7 to its autologous anti-id, 2,000
ng of each of the other HP's failed to cause 50% inhibition;
the values ranged from 14 to 39%, with nearly all proteins
yielding maximum inhibition of 20%-30%. Pooled A/J anti-Ar
antibodies inhibited the binding of labeled 93G7; however
1,600 ng were required for 50% inhibition. The requirement
for 80 ng of unlabeled 93G7 to cause 50% displacement of 10
ng of ^{125}I-labeled 93G7 indicates a relatively low affinity
of the anti-id, so that an excess of anti-id antibody was
required to bind the ligand.

These results are consistent with the view that HP
93G7 possesses one or more unique idiotypic determinants
that are not present on the other 13 HP's, although all 14
proteins share determinants with antibodies comprising the
serum CRI. In addition, HP 93G7 has one or more idiotypic
determinants which are present at very low concentration or
absent from pooled A/J anti-Ar antibodies, since the latter
caused a maximum of 55% inhibition with a 200/1 ratio of
unlabeled inhibitor to labeled ligand.

Table 4 also presents data obtained with labeled protein 93G7 as ligand but reacting with anti-id prepared
against serum anti-Ar. Here the data on inhibition are
strikingly different. Each of the HP's tested, as well as
A/J anti-Ar antibodies, was capable of causing 50% inhibition of binding; with 2,000 ng of unlabeled competitor, the
inhibition was virtually complete in most instances. Many
of the HP's, as well as A/J antibody, were about as effective
as unlabeled 93G7 in displacing the labeled 93G7. The data
may be readily explained on the basis that anti-id prepared

Table 4. Displacement of ^{125}I-Labeled HP 93G7 From Antiidiotypic Antibodies Directed Against HP 93G7 Or Against A/J anti-Ar Antibodies*

Unlabeled Inhibitor	Anti-Id prepared vs. HP 93G7	Anti-Id prepared vs. Serum anti-AR	Unlabeled Inhibitor	Anti-Id prepared vs. HP 93G7	Anti-Id prepared vs. Serum anti-Ar
	ng Required For 50% Inhibition	ng Required For 50% Inhibition		ng Required For 50% Inhibition	ng Required For 50% Inhibition
Serum anti-Ar	1,600	10			
HP 93G7 (G1)	80	12	HP 23.2 (G2b)	>2,000	30
16.7 (G1)	>2,000	13	20.4 (G2b)	>2,000	13
121D7 (G1)	>2,000	60	10.8 (G2a)	>2,000	50
123E6 (G1)	>2,000	600	22.4 (G2a)	>2,000	170
124E1 (G1)	>2,000	250	24.6 (G2a)	>2,000	75
9.3 (G2b)	>2,000	18	13.4 (G3)	>2,000	17
17.5 (G2b)	>2,000	28	26.5 (G3)	>2,000	25

*See footnote, Table 3; 10 ng of ^{125}I-labeled HP 93G7 was used as ligand in all experiments.

against serum antibody does not contain antibodies against
the unique idiotypic determinants of protein 93G7, but only
against shared determinants.

There is a good correlation, although not a perfect one,
between the inhibitory capacity of individual HP's in this
system and in the system involving labeled serum idiotype
as ligand and its autologous antiidiotype (Table 3). For
example, in both systems proteins 13.4, 16.7 and 20.4 are in
the group of strongest inhibitors, whereas proteins 24.6,
22.4 and 124E1 are relatively weak inhibitors.

Thus there is marked heterogeneity among those HP's
which cross-react idiotypically with A/J anti-Ar antibodies.
This is shown by the presence of unique idiotypic determinants on protein 93G7 and by the large differences in inhibitory capacity among HP's in the conventional assay (labeled serum id vs. its autologous anti-id, Table 3). If the HP's
are representative of serum antibodies one would have to conclude that the major idiotype in serum is actually a collection of closely related but nonidentical molecules. That the
HP's are related to one another is shown by their shared
capacity to displace labeled 93G7 from anti-id prepared
against serum antibodies. Also all the HP's have in common
the capacity to displace 50-90% of serum antibody from its
homologous antiidiotype; i.e., to react with most of the
molecules of anti-id directed against serum antibodies.

To account for these data we would postulate that the
major cross-reactive idiotype is encoded by a small number
of germ line genes and that these undergo somatic variation
to encode a large number of related antibodies whose structure is reflected by hybridoma products. The nature of
the variation may be elucidated by further serological
studies and, in greater detail, by the sequence analyses of
HP's being carried out by P. Estess and J.D. Capra. It seems
probable that individual molecules which comprise the major
CRI will prove to differ from a prototype sequence by a
small number of substitutions which vary with respect to
their position and with respect to the nature of the sub-
stitution at a given position in the sequence. This would
account for the fact that V regions of heavy chains isolated from serum antibody molecules bearing the idiotype
exhibit a single major sequence (Capra et al., 1977; Capra
and Nisonoff, 1979).

In addition to the heterogeneous group of molecules comprising the major CRI, hybridoma products reflect the presence of anti-Ar antibodies in A/J antisera which do not appreciably inhibit the binding of labeled serum anti-Ar to anti-id but which still react with a small proportion of the anti-id (Gill-Pazaris et al., 1979). Such HP's are detected initially by the capacity of anti-id to block the binding of the HP to BSA-Ar on a polyvinyl microtiter plate. Individual antisera vary markedly with respect to their content of these "minor" cross-reactive idiotypes. A set of data on the serological properties of 2 such HP's, obtained with the SP2/0-Ag14 cell line, is shown in Table 5. The HP's, nos. 19.9 and 21.1, were purified by affinity chromatography, then labeled with ^{125}I for the tests. More than 80% of each labeled HP could be bound by anti-id but the binding capacity per ml of the anti-id was 4 to 10 times lower than its binding capacity for labeled serum anti-Ar. The data in Table 5 confirm the wide variation in inhibitory capacity of individual anti-Ar sera, noted previously with other non-inhibitory HP's which react with the anti-id (Gill-Pazaris et al., 1979). However, all sera tested were able to cause 50% inhibition of binding of HP 19.9 and the majority caused 50% inhibition of binding of labeled HP 21.1 Comparisons of serological properties of individual HP's belonging to the group of "minor idiotypes" have indicated that they are quite heterogeneous although some are serologically related to one another (Gill-Pazaris et al., (1979).

Antiidiotypic antibodies have been prepared against several other HP's which cross-react with the major serum CRI. These reagents should permit us to obtain further information on the degree of serological microheterogeneity among these proteins.

Microheterogeneity has also been observed among major cross-reactive idiotypes associated with murine antibodies directed to other antigens. These include antibodies to the synthetic copolymer, glu-ala-tyr (Ju et al., 1979) in strain DBA/1 mice and antibodies to the hapten, 3-nitro-4-hydro-xyphenylacetyl (NP) in the C57BL strain (Imanishi-Kari et al., 1978). In each case microheterogeneity was demonstrated through studies of hybridoma products sharing idiotype with the major serum CRI. Heterogeneity of the major cross-reactive idiotypes may have a counterpart among BALB/c myeloma proteins which bind bacterial levans (Lieberman et al., 1975). Many of these myeloma proteins share idiotypic

Table 5. Displacement of Hybridoma Products Lacking the
CRI, but Reactive with Antiidiotype, From Antiidiotypic
Antibodies Prepared Against A/J anti-Ar Antibodies*

Unlabeled Inhibitor, A/J anti-Ar Serum From Mouse No.	^{125}I-Labeled Ligand	
	HP 21.1	HP 19.9
	ng Required for 50% Inhibition	
1709	170	5
1625	190	--
1606	320	8
1911	440	--
2012	600	40
1814	1,500	32
1902	2,500	17
2013	4,200	90
112	>10,000	14
1604	>10,000	--
1620	>10,000	6
1821	>10,000	9
Pooled A/J anti-Ar	600	40
HP 21.1	9	>2,000
HP 19.9	>2,000	10

Each assay utilized 10 ng of labeled ligand (HP 21.1 or
19.9) and sufficient antiidiotype to bind 46–52% of the
ligand. The two HP's were specifically purified on BGG-
Ar-Sepharose.

determinants but, in addition, possess unique individual idiotypic specificities. Studies of sequences at the protein and DNA level should elucidate the question as to whether similar mechanisms of generation of diversity are operative in the various systems.

Acknowledgements

The excellent technical assistance of Ms. Anne Kezer is acknowledged. This work was supported by NIH grants AI-12127 (to J.D.C.), CA-15808 (to P.D.G.), AI-12907 and AI-12895 (to A.N.), CA-14051 from the National Cancer Institute to MIT, and by grant PCM76-22411 from the National Science Foundation (to J.D.C.)

References

Bosma MJ, Marks R, Dewitt CL (1975).Quantitation of mouse immunoglobulin allotype by a modified solid-phase radioimmune assay. J Immunol 115:1381.
Boyse EA, Itakura K, Stockert E, Iratani CA, Miura M (1971). A third locus specifying alloantigens expressed on thymocytes and lymphocytes. Transpl Bull 11:351.
Capra JD, Nisonoff A (1979). Structural studies on induced antibodies with defined idiotypic specificities VII. The complete amino acid sequence of the heavy chain variable region of anti-p-azophenylarsonate antibodies from A/J mice bearing cross-reactive idiotype. J Immunol 123:279.
Capra JD, Tung AS, Nisonoff A (1977). Structural studies on induced antibodies with defined idiotypic specificities. V. The complete amino acid sequence of light chain variable regions of anti-p-azophenylarsonate antibodies from A/J mice bearing cross-reactive idiotype. J Immunol 119:933.
Claflin JL (1976). Genetic marker in the variable region of kappa chains of mouse anti-phosphorylcholine antibodies. Eur J Immunol 6:666.
Claflin JL, Taylor BA, Cherry M, Cubberly M (1978). Linkage in mice of genes controlling an immunoglobulin kappa chain marker and the surface alloantigen Ly-3 on T lymphocytes. Immunogenetics 6:379.
Davis BJ (1964). Disc electrophoresis II. Method and application to human serum proteins. Ann NY Acad Sci 121:404.
Edelman GM, Gottlieb PD (1970). A genetic marker in the variable region of light chains of mouse immunoglobulins.

Proc Natl Acad Sci, USA 67:;;92.

Eichmann K (1975). Genetic control of antibody specificity in the mouse. Immunogenetics 2:491.

Gefter ML, Margolies D, Scharff MD (1977). A simple method for polyethylene glycol-promoted hybridization of mouse myeloma cells. Somatic Cell Genet 3:231.

Gibson D (1976). Genetic polymorphism of mouse immunoglobulin light chains revealed by isoelectric focusing, J Exp Med 144:298.

Gibson D, Taylor BA, Cherry M (1978). Evidence for close linkage of a mouse light chain marker with the Ly-2,3 locus, J Immunol 121:1585.

Gill-Pazaris LA, Brown AR, Nisonoff A (1979). The nature of idiotypes associated with anti-p-azophenlyarsonate antibodies in A/J mice. Ann Immunol. (Inst. Pasteur) 130C:199.

Gottlieb, PD (1974). Genetic correlation of a mouse light chain variable region marker with a thymocyte surface antigen. J Exp Med 140:1432.

Gottlieb PD, Durda PJ (1977). The I_B-peptide marker and the Ly-3 surface alloantigen. Structural studies of a V-region polymorphism and a T-cell marker determined by linked genes. Cold Spring Harbor Symp Quant Biol 41:805.

Gottlieb PD, Wan H-CW, Brown AR, Nisonoff A (1979). Role of the light chain in studies of linkage of genes controlling idiotype and heavy chain allotype. Proc 12th Leukocyte Culture Conf. Academic Press, NY p. 317.

Green MC (1979). Genetic nomenclature for the immunoglobulin loci of the mouse. Immunogenetics 8:89.

Hopper JE, Nisonoff A (1971). Individual antigenic specificity of immunoglobulins. Adv Immunol 13:58.

Imanishi-Kari T, Reth M, Hammerling GJ, Rajewsky K (1978). Analysis of V gene expression in the immune response by cell fusion. Curr. Top. Microbiol. Immunol. 81:20.

Itakura K, Hutton JJ, Boyse EA, Old LJ (1972). Genetic linkage relationships of loci specificying differentiation of alloantigens in the mouse. Transplant Bull 13:239.

Ju S-T, Pierres M, Waltenbaugh C, Germain RN, Benacerraf B, Dorf ME (1979). Idiotypic analysis of monoclonal antibodies to poly ($glu^{60}-ala^{30}-tyr^{10}$). Proc Natl Acad Sci USA 76:2942.

Köhler G, Milstein C (1976). Derivation of specific antibody-producing tissue culture and tumor lines by cell fusion. Eur J Immunol 6:511.

Kuettner MG, Wang AL, Nisonoff A (1972). Quantitative investigations of idiotypic antibodies. Vl. Idiotypic speci-

ficity as a potential genetic marker for the variable
regions of mouse immunoglobulin polypeptide chains.
J Exp Med 135:579.

Laemmli UK (1970). Cleavage of structural proteins during
the assembly of the head of bacteriophage T4. Nature
227:680.

Laskin JA, Gray A, Nisonoff A, Klinman NR, Gottlieb PD (1977).
Segregation of a locus determining an immunoglobulin
genetic marker for the light chain variable region affects
inheritance of expression of an idiotype. Proc Natl
Acad Sci USA 74:4600.

Lieberman R, Potter M, Humphrey W, Mushinski EB, Vrana M
(1975). Multiple individual and cross-specific idiotypes
on 13 levan-binding myeloma proteins of BALB/c. J Exp
Med 142:106.

Pawlak L, Mushinski EB, Nisonoff A, Potter M (1973). Evidence for the linkage of the IgC_H locus to a gene control-
ing the idiotype specificity of anti-p-azophenylarsonate
antibodies in strain A mice. J Exp Med 137:22.

Shulman M, Wilde CD, Köhler G (1978). A better cell line
for making hybridomas secreting specific antibodies.
Nature 276:279.

Swan D, D'Eustachio P, Leinwand L, Seidman J, Keithley D,
Ruddle FH (1979). Chromosomal assignment of the mouse K
light chain genes. Proc Natl Sci USA 76:2735.

Weigert M, Potter M (1977). Antibody variable-region
genetics: Summary and abstracts of the Homogeneous Immunoglobulin Workshop Vll. Immunogenetics 4:401.

Gearhart: How can you map idiotype to the allotype when
the idiotype may be heterogenous in its
antigenicity?

Nisonoff: Idiotype is defined by an anti-idiotypic
antiserum. The idiotype I discussed is found
in A/J but not Balb/c mice. The phenotype is
the ability to react with the antiserum.
Genetic studies of this phenotype can
therefore be carried out.

Gearhart: Have you looked at the strain distribution of
the hybridomas?

Nisonoff: This has not yet been done. We have had the
sera only a short time.

Kabat: Maybe previous idiotype linkage studies
measure J and C, not V and C?

Nisonoff: That is not known. Yes, it might be a
regulatory gene turning on either V_H or J.

Kohler: The idiotype story is getting very
complicated. Can you help by defining
"idiotype"?

Nisonoff: The major or public idiotype is found in all
A/J mice. Private idiotypes were obtained
after suppressing the major idiotype.
Private idiotypes are very difficult to
identify in other mice. "Crossreacting
idiotype" has been used interchangeably with
"major idiotype".

Knight: Do the antigens corresponding to the unique
idiotypes crossreact with monoclonal antibody?

Nisonoff: It is not yet known.

McKearn: What proportion of minor idiotypes would you
find in animals challenged with arsenate?
What about animals not challenged with
arsenate?

Nisonoff: Not a high percentage, about 5-10% in immunized animals. Very little if any in immunized mice. Some of the minor idiotypes might
be quite widespread since they are heterogeneous and identified by cross-idiotypic
reactions which can be of low affinity.

Pages 249–261, Membranes, Receptors, and the Immune Response
© 1980 Alan R. Liss, Inc., 150 Fifth Avenue, New York, NY 10011

PRIMARY STRUCTURAL ANALYSIS OF MONOCLONAL ANTI-p-AZOPHENYL-ARSONATE ANTIBODIES

Pila Estess and J. Donald Capra

Department of Microbiology, The University of Texas Southwestern Medical School, Dallas, Texas 75235

Efforts in our laboratory over the past ten years have been devoted to the serological and structural dissection of an induced antibody system in an attempt to understand its molecular and genetic implications. All A/J mice, when immunized with the hapten p-azophenylarsonate (Ar) coupled to keyhole limpet hemocyanin, make a restricted anti-Ar response, 20-70% of which bears a cross-reactive idiotype (CRI) when analyzed with an appropriately absorbed rabbit antiserum (Kuettner et al. 1972). The CRI is linked to the immunoglobulin heavy chain locus (Pawlak et al. 1973), and has been one of the V-region markers used to demonstrate linkage of variable and constant regions of immunoglobulin heavy chains in mice. Recently, linkage of the CRI to the kappa chain locus has been demonstrated as well (Laskin et al. 1977; Brown et al. 1980).

All structural analyses done to date indicate that the serum anti-Ar response is extremely restricted. Thus, CRI-positive heavy chains isolated from conventional anti-Ar antibodies exhibit a homogeneous sequence including their hypervariable regions (Capra et al. 1975a; Friedenson et al. 1975; Capra and Nisonoff, 1979). CRI-negative heavy chains are homogeneous and identical to the CRI-positive chains with the exception of their hypervariable regions, which are quite heterogeneous. CRI-positive light chains appear to be drawn from at least three different V_k-subgroups, but also have homogeneous and identical hypervariable region sequences (Capra et al. 1975b; Capra et al. 1976; Capra et al. 1977). The CRI-negative light chains were too heterogeneous to sequence.

These results suggest that the CRI-positive anti-Ar response is under strict genetic control, that the immunoglobulin chains likely represent products of germ-line genes and that the cross-idiotypic specificity measured serologically is comprised entirely of amino acids in the hypervariable regions. In order to further explore the relationships between the CRI-positive and CRI-negative molecules and to verify the presumed homogeneity of the serum anti-Ar response, we undertook the generation of monoclonal anti-Ar antibodies by somatic cell fusion. Serologic analysis of the hybridoma antibodies presented in the paper by Lamoyi et al. (1980) indicates heterogeneity in their ability to react with a conventional anti-idiotypic reagent raised against serum anti-Ar, and suggests that each hybridoma · product possesses in addition to the cross-reactive idiotypic determinant(s), unique antigenic specificities (Brown et al. 1980; Lamoyi et al. 1980; Gill-Pazaris et al. 1979). We have previously reported on the amino-terminal amino acid sequences of two such monoclonal anti-Ar hybridomas (Estess et al. 1979) and here extend those findings to an additional six molecules.

RESULTS

Production and Characterization of Anti-Ar Producing Hybridomas.

The eight monoclonal anti-Ar antibodies subjected to amino terminal amino acid sequence analysis were generated in two separate fusion experiments. In the first experiment, 21/54 hybrids were positive for anti-Ar activity. Since the frequency of positive wells was high, hybridoma products (HPs) 93G7, 91A3, 92D5 and 94B10 were cloned by limiting dilution to insure their monoclonality. In the second experiment, only 39 out of 268 potentially positive hybrids exhibited anti-Ar activity. Since the Poisson distribution predicts that when no greater than 66% of the items under study are positive for a given parameter each positive represents the result of a single event and since the frequency of anti-Ar positive hybridomas in this experiment was only 15%, the cells were not cloned and four of the hybrids, HPs 121D7, 123E6, 124E1 and 123E4 were chosen for further study. Sequence analyses indicate that in terms of the anti-Ar producing population of cells, the hybrids are monoclonal. With respect to other parameters, the hybrid cells may be heterogeneous and each culture may contain cells derived from more than one fusion event. This should not interfere with studies performed on an isolated, specific product.

Supernatants from the eight cell lines, as well as purified anti-Ar antibody from (Balb/c X A/J)F_1 mice (CAF_1) ascites, were tested for their ability to inhibit the binding of radiolabeled, purified, CRI-positive antibodies from A/J mice to the rabbit anti-CRI reagent. As indicated in Table I, four of the hybridoma products effectively inhibit the binding of the ^{125}I-labeled CRI-positive antibodies by 50%, although marked quantitative differences in their ability to do so are evident. One hybridoma product, HP93G7, appears almost as effective as serum anti-Ar as an inhibitor of the CRI/anti-CRI reaction. The remaining four anti-Ar antibodies are unable to inhibit the reaction at all, even in very large amounts. By Ouchterlony analysis, all eight hybridoma products are of the IgG1 subclass.

Amino Terminal Amino Acid Sequence Analysis.

Eight monoclonal anti-Ar antibodies were selected for amino acid sequence analysis. Four of these molecules bear the A/J anti-Ar CRI as defined by their ability to inhibit by at least 50% the reaction between serum or ascites CRI-positive molecules and a rabbit anti-CRI reagent. The other four molecules are negative for the idiotype. Isolated heavy and light chains from each of the eight molecules were subjected to automated sequence analysis. Each PTH amino acid was subjected to three analytical procedures and unambiguous assignments could be made at every position. The results are shown in Figures 1 and 2, where the first framework segments are compared to the previously reported structures of anti-Ar heavy and light chains isolated from hyperimmunized A/J mice.

DISCUSSION

The amino-terminal framework sequences of eight individual anti-Ar antibodies obtained by somatic cell fusion of A/J spleen cells with a non-immunoglobulin secreting tumor cell line have been analyzed. The sixteen chains (eight heavy and eight light) of these hybridoma antibodies

TABLE I

DISPLACEMENT OF LABELED A/J ANTI-AR FROM ITS RABBIT ANTI-

IDIOTYPIC ANTIBODIES BY UNLABELED A/J ANTI-AR ANTIBODIES OR

HYBRIDOMA PRODUCTS WITH ANTI-AR ACTIVITY*

Unlabeled Inhibitor	Ng Required for 50% Inhibition	% Inhibition by 2 ug
Serum anti-Ar	11	97
HP# 93G7	12	90
121D7	300	71
123E6	1,900	51
124E1	2,900	47
91A3	**	4
123E4	**	2
94B10	**	0
92D5	**	4

*Each assay utilized 10 ng of ^{125}I-labeled, specifically purified A/J anti-Ar antibodies and slightly less than an equivalent amount of anti-idiotype.

**50% inhibition never achieved.

ANTI AR HYBRIDOMA HEAVY CHAINS

```
                                      10                      20                        30
CRI+ SERUM   GLU VAL GLN LEU GLN GLN SER GLY ALA GLU LEU VAL LYS ALA GLY SER SER VAL LYS MET SER CYS LYS ALA THR GLY TYR THR PHE SER

CRI+ HP
   93G7      _____ SER _____ THR _____
  121D7      _____
  124E1      _____ ARG THR _____ THR _____
  123E6      _____ THR _____ SER THR _____ SER SER _____

CRI- HP
   91A3      _____ GLY _____
  123E4      _____ ARG _____ GLU _____ SER _____ LYS _____
   94B10     ASP _____ GLU _____ PRO GLY _____ PRO SER GLN _____ LEU SER LEU THR _____ THR VAL _____ SER ILE THR
    9D5      ASP _____ GLU _____ PRO GLY _____ PRO SER GLN _____ LEU SER LEU THR _____ THR VAL _____ SER ILE THR
```

Figure 1 Comparison of the amino acid sequences of the CRI-positive and CRI-negative hybridoma heavy chain variable regions with the sequence of CRI-positive heavy chains found in serum. Identical residues are indicated by a line and only differences are noted.

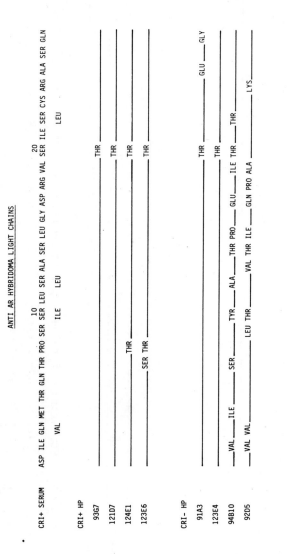

Figure 2 Comparison of the amino acid sequences of the CRI-positive and CRI-negative hybridoma light chains with the sequence of CRI-positive light chains found in serum. Identical residues are indicated by a line and only differences are noted. The major framework sequence of pooled antibody is listed on top with the minor sequence noted below for positions 3, 10, 12 and 22.

are compared to the previously sequenced heavy and light chains of anti-Ar antibodies isolated from hyperimmunized A/J mice (Capra et al. 1975a; Capra and Nisonoff 1979; Capra et al. 1975b; Capra et al. 1976; Capra et al. 1977; Capra et al. 1978). In the previous studies, the only detectable sequence differences between anti-Ar antibodies with and without the cross-reactive idiotype lay within the hypervariable regions of the heavy chains (CRI-negative light chains were too heterogeneous to sequence). Except in mice suppressed for the CRI, CRI-positive and CRI-negative heavy chains gave a homogeneous and identical framework sequence. In addition, the heavy and light chain hypervariable regions of CRI-positive antibodies were homogeneous while those of CRI-negative antibodies were very heterogeneous. The slight framework heterogeneity found in CRI-positive light chains was attributable to the presence of at least three different framework structures associated with identical hypervariable regions (Capra et al. 1975b; Capra et al. 1976; Capra et al. 1977). Since the only detectable structural difference between CRI-positive and CRI-negative anti-Ar antibodies lay within the hypervariable regions, and these two types of molecules were known to differ serologically with respect to a cross-reactive idiotype, it was of interest to us to further investigate the possible structural relationships between them.

CRI-positive anti-Ar hybridoma heavy chains are similar but not identical to CRI-positive anti-Ar heavy chains isolated from serum or ascites.

Four different CRI-positive anti-Ar hybridoma heavy chains have been sequenced and the first thirty residues are compared in Figure 1 to the CRI-positive heavy chain sequence previously reported (Capra et al. 1975a; Capra and Nisonoff, 1979). While antibodies isolated from hyper-immune A/J serum consistently gave a nearly homogeneous sequence (Capra et al. 1975a; Friedenson et al. 1975), clear differences from this sequence exist in the heavy chains of the hybridoma antibodies. With the exception of the Lys-Ser interchange at position thirteen in HP123E6, all of the CRI-positive heavy chain substitutions could have arisen from a single base change in the DNA encoding the major (serum) sequence.

CRI-negative anti-Ar heavy chains may either be very similar to CRI-positive heavy chains or be completely different.

The four CRI-negative heavy chains can be divided into two groups according to their amino-terminal framework sequences (see Figure 1). Two of the molecules, HP91A3 and HP123E4, are clearly as related to the serum heavy chain sequence as are the CRI-positive hybridoma heavy chains. That is, they belong to the immunoglobulin heavy chain variable region $(V_H)_{II}$-subgroup of mouse immunoglobulin heavy chains (Capra et al. 1975a). Again, however, definite differences from the serum sequence are noted in each of the chains. As with the CRI-positive chains, substitutions are found at several different positions, but appear to be more random with respect to the variant amino acid.

Variability in anti-Ar hybridoma light chains parallels that found in the heavy chains.

The sequences of both CRI-positive and CRI-negative anti-Ar hybridoma light chains are illustrated in Figure 2, along with the sequences found in serum A/J anti-Ar antibodies positive for the cross-reactive idiotype. Several striking features are apparent. First with respect to V_k-subgroup, the hybridoma molecules are more restricted than the CRI-positive molecules in A/J serum. Although only one heavy chain V-region subgroup is present in the serum CRI-positive molecules, it is found in association with at least three different light chain V-region subgroups (Capra et al. 1975b; Capra et al. 1976; Capra et al. 1977). Six of the eight hybridoma light chains (four with the CRI and two without) clearly belong to the same V_k-subgroup as the major population of serum anti-Ar light chains, while none belong to the two other subgroups. As in the monoclonal heavy chains, amino acid substitutions are found in the framework portions of all of the hybridoma light chains.

Implications of the Amino-Terminal Amino Acid Sequence Analysis of Anti-Ar Hybridoma Antibodies.

In light of the work that has been done on the arsonate system, these results have important implications with regard to our thinking on what constitutes an idiotypically homogeneous antibody population as well as on the general concept of idiotypic inheritance. It is clear that, in the absence of trivial explanations, the anti-Ar antibody population in the A/J mouse, while appearing homogeneous when serum or ascites are analyzed, is not. To some extent, the microheterogeneity found in the hybridoma chains is not inconsistent with the previously reported sequences. Thus, the substitutions at positions 7, 8 and 20 in the light chains and positions 16 and 25 in the heavy chains can be found in pools of anti-Ar antibodies derived from several animals (Capra et al. 1975a; Friedenson et al. 1975; Capra and Nisonoff, 1979; Capra et al. 1975b). It is interesting to note that the Ser at position 25 in the heavy chain of the CRI-positive hybridoma product HP123E6 was only seen in the CRI-negative serum pool (Capra et al. 1975a).

Thus, the A/J anti-Ar system which heretofore has appeared to be a restricted population by both the criteria of idiotypic cross-reactivity and amino acid sequence analysis may be, in fact, very heterogeneous. The extent of this "microheterogeneity" and its implications for the origins of antibody diversity are being explored by additional sequencing studies combined with serological analysis of the individual and cross-reacting idiotypic determinants on the monoclonal anti-Ar antibodies. These studies should lead to the precise chemical definition of both the cross-reactive idiotype and the individual antigenic specificities associated with these molecules.

SUMMARY

Amino terminal amino acid sequence analyses have been performed on the heavy and light chains of induced monoclonal antibodies with specificity for the hapten p-azophenylarsonate. Four of the eight antibodies react with conventional antisera to the previously described A/J anti-arsonate cross-reactive idiotype (CRI). Of the sixteen chains analyzed, all but one contain sequence differences in their first framework segment (residues 1-30) which distinguish them from the heavy and light chain sequences found in anti-arsonate antibodies isolated from A/J serum or ascites fluid. The presence of such framework differences appears to be independent of whether or not the hybridoma antibodies bear the CRI. In spite of the framework substitutions, all four of the CRI-positive hybridoma antibodies have V-region frameworks that are very similar

to each other and to the CRI-positive molecules found in A/J
serum. Two of the four CRI-negative molecules are also
structurally similar to the serum antibodies. Two others,
however, are strikingly different from any serum anti-
arsonate antibody thus far described and appear to reflect a
completely separate repertoire of anti-arsonate antibodies
in the A/J mouse. Serological analyses by Lamoyi et al.
(1980) with anti-idiotypic antisera generated against CRI-
positive hybridoma products suggest in addition that each
monoclonal antibody may possess individual antigenic specificities different from the determinant(s) detected with the
conventional rabbit anti-CRI. The consistent appearance
of framework substitutions in what has been thought to be a
homogeneous antibody population has important implications
for our understanding of the generation of antibody diversity
and for the precise chemical definition of an idiotype.

REFERENCES

Brown AR, Estess P, Lamoyi E, Gill-Pazaris L, Gottleib PD,
  Capra JD, Nisonoff A (1980) Studies of genetic control
  and microheterogeneity of an idiotype associated with
  anti-p-azophenylarsonate antibodies of A/J mice. In
  Cohen EP, Köhler H (eds): "Membranes, Receptors and the
  Immune Response," New York: Alan R. Liss.
Capra JD, Ju S-T, Nisonoff A (1978). Structural studies on
  induced antibodies with defined idiotypic specificities.
  VI. Amino terminal sequences of the heavy and light chain
  variable regions of anti-p-azophenylarsonate antibodies
  from A/J mice suppressed for a cross-reactive idiotype.
  J Immunol 121:953.
Capra JD, Klapper DG, Tung AS, Nisonoff A (1976). Identical
  hypervariable regions in light chains of differing V_K
  subgroups. Cold Spring Harbor Symposium on Quantitative
  Biology, Vol XLI, p 847.
Capra JD, Nisonoff A (1979). Structural studies on induced
  antibodies with defined idiotypic specificities. VII. The
  complete amino acid sequence of the heavy chain variable
  region of anti-p-azophenylarsonate antibodies from A/J mice
  bearing a cross-reactive idiotype. J Immunol 123:279.
Capra JD, Tung AS, Nisonoff A (1975a). Structural studies on
  induced antibodies with defined idiotypic specificities.
  I. The heavy chains of anti-p-azophenylarsonate antibodies from A/J mice bearing a cross-reactive idiotype.
  J Immunol 114:1548.

Capra JD, Tung AS, Nisonoff A (1975b). Structural studies on induced antibodies with defined idiotypic specificities. II. The light chains of anti-p-azophenylarsonate antibodies from A/J mice bearing a cross-reactive idiotype. J Immunol 115:414.

Capra JD, Tung AS, Nisonoff A (1977). Structural studies on induced antibodies with defined idiotypic specificities. V. The complete amino acid sequence of the light chain variable regions of anti-p-azophenylarsonate antibodies from A/J mice bearing a cross-reactive idiotype. J Immunol 119:993.

Estess P, Nisonoff A, Capra JD (1979). Structural studies on induced antibodies with defined idiotypic specificities. VIII. NH₂-terminal amino acid sequence analysis of the heavy and light chain variable regions of monoclonal anti-p-azophenylarsonate antibodies from A/J mice differing with respect to a cross-reactive idiotype. Mol Immunol, in press.

Friedenson B, Tung AS, Nisonoff A (1975). Constancy of amino terminal amino acid sequences of antibodies of defined specificity and shared idiotype from individual inbred mice. Proc Natl Acad Sci USA 72:3676.

Gill-Pazaris LA, Brown AR, Nisonoff A (1979). The nature of idiotypes associated with anti-p-azophenylarsonate antibodies in A/J mice. Annals d'Immunol Inst Pasteur, Paris 130C:199.

Kuettner MG, Wang, A-L, Nisonoff A (1972). Quantitative investigations of idiotypic antibodies. VI. Idiotypic specificity as a potential genetic marker for the variable regions of mouse immunoglobulin polypeptide chains. J Exp Med 135:579.

Lamoyi E, Estess P, Capra JD, Nisonoff A (1980). Heterogeneity of an intrastrain cross-reactive idiotype associated with anti-p-azophenylarsonate antibodies of A/J mice. Submitted for publication.

Laskin JA, Gray A, Nisonoff A, Klinman NR, Gottleib PD (1977). Segregation at a locus determining an immunoglobulin genetic marker for the light chain variable region affects inheritance of expression of an idiotype. Proc Natl Acad Sci USA 74:4600.

Pawlak L, Mushinski EB, Nisonoff A, Potter M (1973). Evidence for the linkage of the IgC_H locus to a gene controlling the idiotypic specificity of anti-p-azophenylarsonate antibodies in strain A mice. J Exp Med 137:22.

Coutinho: How are the Ia molecules assembled? Does
            I-A-alpha ever bind to I-E-beta?

Capra: A-alpha and A-beta have markedly different
            charges, so they may attract each other on a
            charge basis alone. E-alpha and E-beta,
            however, have a similar IEF and obviously need
            some other recognition system. One never finds
            an A-alpha on an E-beta.

Kabat: Are the 30 amino acid residues which are
            different between the E-alpha chains from
            different haplotypes present in one segment, or
            are they spread?

Capra: We do not know; so far we cannot correlate the
            peptide maps with the molecular weight
            difference.

Humphries: Could a disulfide bond in the reduced state
            exist with the disulfide bonded state? Could
            adding iodoacetamide shift the equilibrium? In
            other words, how valid are the iodoacetamide
            lysis experiments?

Capra: Iodoacetamide is used to prevent such
            interchanges.

Claflin: How can one align 25 tryptic peptides for the
            complete sequence?

Capra: We have chymotryptic peptides for overlaps.

Williams: As a word of warning . . . recall the KH-11
            mutation in which the expression of a non H-2
            gene is controlled by H-2. How reliable are
            congenic mice?

Capra: We have done some of our studies on different
            backgrounds as well as on B10 backgrounds and
            find no differences.

UNKN: With microheterogeneity not found, how can we
            be certain that we are looking at the correct
            end of the molecule?

Capra: We have looked throughout the molecule, not
            just at the N-terminus.

Quintans: I thought Katz found a difference in GL-theta response between recombinants and F_1 mice.

Capra: That is what I meant by the gene dosage effect. Not all mice have an expressed E-alpha chain. Mice without E-alpha chains do not form as many possible molecules as do the recombinant. We find about 50:50 cis:trans molecules. In a true F_1 with an expressed E-alpha, we would expect to find 25% of each.

Pages 263—277, Membranes, Receptors, and the Immune Response
© 1980 Alan R. Liss, Inc., 150 Fifth Avenue, New York, NY 10011

ANTI-ALLOTYPE ANTIBODY RESPONSE IN MICE: EXPRESSION of a
CROSS-REACTIVE IDIOTYPE AND ITS REGULATION BY AUTO-ANTI-
IDIOTYPIC ANTIBODIES IN MATERNALLY ALLOTYPE SUPPRESSED F_1
HYBRIDS.

Constantin BONA

C.N.R.S. and Pasteur Institute

28 rue du Docteur Roux, 75015 Paris, FRANCE.

ABSTRACT. Anti-IgG_{2a}^b allotype antibodies produced by
various responder strains of mice expressed a cross-reactive idiotype. This cross-reactive idiotype was evidenced with
BAB.14 and CXBI anti-idiotypic sera raised following immunization with affinity chromatography purified BALB/c anti-
CBPC 101 (IgG_{2a}^b) antibodies originating from a single BALB/c
mouse. F1 hybrids of BALB/c X C.B20 parents, which have
been maternally suppressed for IgG_{2a}^b allotype as a result
of immunization with CBPC 101, produced anti-allotype antibodies lacking cross-reactive idiotype. Furthermore, these
mice produced auto-antibodies directed at the IdX of anti-
IgG_{2a}^b allotypic antibodies.

1. INTRODUCTION

There is increased evidence that the cooperation between T
and B lymphocytes or macrophages in the humoral or cell
mediated immune response is genetic (Rosenthal 1978,
Doherty et al. 1976) and isotype allotype and idiotype
restricted. Thus, the level of immunoglobulin (Ig) classes
of antibodies in response to antigen may be regulated by T
cells which are specific for an Ig class (Elson et al.1979,
Black et al. 1979, Kishimoto et al. 1979).Janeway et al.
(1977) have presented some suggestive evidence that one
of synergizing T cells that the observed in adoptive
transfer system is Ig specific. In this experiment primed
T cells from agammaglobulinic mice failed to show synergy.
Herzenberg et al.(1976) clearly demonstrated that T cells
specific for allotype helped hapten primed allotype bearing
B cells to produce antibody of IgG_{2a} class. Furthermore,
T suppressor cells generated during allotype suppression

in mice exert their regulatory effect on allotype specific
T helper cells. Finally, it was shown in various systems
that idiotype bearing T helper cells collaborate in the
immune response only with idiotype positive and not with
idiotype negative bearing B cells (Ward et al. 1977,
Hetzelberger et al. 1979). These data indicate that the antigenic determinants of Ig molecules of lymphocyte receptors
play an important role in the regulation of the immune response since they restrict the collaboration between T and
B lymphocytes and they might serve as sites of regulatory
effects of anti-isotypes, anti-allotype and anti-idiotype
antibodies.

Because of such findings we considered that it is important to study the regulation of anti-allotype response.
We have studied the response to allotypic determinants of
$\underline{b}$ allele of IgG_{2a}. We have shown that this response is under
the genetic control and that only the mice of $H_2\ \underline{d}$, $\underline{b}$, $\underline{q}$,
$\underline{r}$, $\underline{s}$ and $\underline{p}$ haplotype are responders(Bona et al. in press).

In this communication we present the results concerning the expression of a cross-reactive idiotype (IdX) on
anti-allotype antibody of responder mice strains and the
regulation of IdX^+ component of anti-allotype. antibody response by auto-anti-IdX antibodies.

2. EXPRESSION OF CROSS-REACTIVE IDIOTYPE ON ANTI-
(IgG_{2a}^b) ALLOTYPE ANTIBODIES.

A. Anti-idiotypic sera specific for anti-allotype antibodies
Mice of $\underline{d}$, $\underline{b}$, $\underline{r}$, $\underline{p}$, $\underline{q}$ and s H_2 haplotype following immunization with CBPC 101 myeloma protein developed a vigorous
anti-IgG_{2a}^b allotype response. CBPC 101 myeloma is a IgG_{2a}^b
protein originating from C.B20 mice which are of H_2^d type
and possess b allelic form IgG_H region gene. BALB/c mice
(H_2^d) subsequent immunization with CBPC 101 myeloma protein
developed a high titer ($\geqslant$ 18(log.2)) of anti-IgG_{2a}^b allotype
antibodies. Their sera agglutinated as well SRBC coated
with either CBPC 101 myeloma protein and Ig of C57BL/6.
BAB.14 and CXBI mice were immunized with affinity chromatography purified anti-CBPC 101 antibodies coupled with KLH
according to a described previously technique (Bona et al.
1979). The anti-CBPC 101 antibodies used for immunization
originated from a single BALB/c mouse. BAB.14 and CXBI mice
developed antibodies which agglutinated SRBC-coated with
BALB/c anti-CBPC 101 antibody. These sera had little or no
activity against SRBC coupled with UPC 10 (IgG_{2a}^a) MOPC 195
(IgG_{2b}^a) MOPC 31 (IgG_1^a) and UPC 61 (IgA^a) myeloma proteins
(table 1). Furthermore, the agglutinating ability of these

sera was not altered by addition of high amounts of BALB/c
Ig (table 2). These results indicated that after immunization of BAB.14 or CXBI mice with purified BALB/c anti-CBPC
101 antibody originating from a single BALB/c mouse, we
obtained antisera containing anti-Id antibodies directed
against Id determinants of anti-allotype antibodies. These
anti-Id antibodies excellently bound 3H-BALB/c anti-CBPC 101
purified antibodies in RIA (Fig. 1).

Fig.1. Binding of ^{3}H–BALB/c anti-CBPC101 antibody to anti-
Id antibodies.

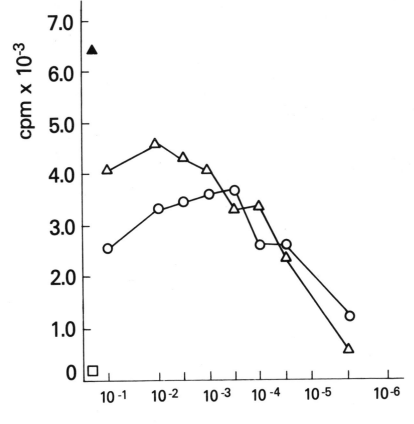

DILUTION OF SERUM

Plates coated with: ● BALB/c serum (1:10), ⬤ C57B1/6 Ig
◑ BAB.14 anti-Id serum, △ CXBI anti-Id serum

Table 1: Hemagglutination of BALB/c anti-CBPC101 antibody-coated SRBC by BAB.14 and CXBI anti-Id sera

Sera from/No	SRBC coated with:				
	BALB/c anti-CBPC101	UPC10	MOPC195	MOPC/31	UPC61
BAB14 mice immunized with BALB/c anti-CBPC101					
1	24*	1	2	1	1
2	24	2	4	3	3
3	24	1	1	2	3
4	24	0	1	4	2
CXBImice immunized with BALB/c anti-CBPC 101					
1	24	4	3	2	3
2	24	3	4	3	4
3	24	2	2	3	2
Rabbit anti-mouse κ - chain	12	7	12	12	12

*HA titer

Table 2: Failure of BALB/c Ig to inhibit hemagglutination

Inhibitors	HI titer ($\log_2$)	
	BAB.14 anti-Id serum	CXBI anti-Id serum
BALB/c anti-CBPC101 antibody (1.0mg/ml)	8	7
BALB/c Ig (5mg/ml)	0	0
BALB/c Ig (10mg/ml)	0	0
BALB/c Ig (20mg/ml)	0	2

SRBC coated with BALB/c anti-CPBC101 were used as indicators.

B. Expression of cross-reactive idiotype on anti(IgG_{2a}^b) allotype antibodies in all mice of BALB/c strain.

The ability of anti-(IgG_{2a}^b) allotype antibodies from 9 individuals BALB/c mice to inhibit agglutination of BALB/c anti-CBPC 101 coated-SRBC by BAB.14 and CXBI anti-Id sera was tested. In parallel of HI, the ability of these sera to inhibit the binding of anti-Id antibodies to 3H-BALB/c anti-CBPC 101 also was tested. The sera from 9 individuals BALB/c mice inhibited the interaction between anti-Id sera and BALB/c anti-CBPC-101 antibody used to raise anti-Id sera. These findings indicate that cross-reactive idiotype is uniformely expressed on BALB/c anti-allotype antibody. However, it should be noted that the individual BALB/c anti-sera were capable of inhibiting CXBI anti-Id capacity at higher dilutions than of BAB.14 anti-Id serum. There are two possible explanations for this observation:
a) that BAB.14 and CXBI anti-Id sera, each recognizes a group of cross-reactive idiotypes (IdX) expressed on anti-allotype antibody and that the sera from individual BALB/c mice tested contained more IdX recognized by CXBI anti-Id serum.
b) That the titer of BAB.14 anti-Id serum is higher than that of CXBI anti-Id serum and thus more IdX bearing anti-allotype antibodies are required for inhibition.
In fact in HA assay we found that BAB.14 anti-Id serum had a HA titer ($log._2$) of $8X10^6$ whereas RICXBI $2X10^6$($log._2$).

C. Expression of cross-reactive idiotype on anti(IgG_{2a}^b) allotype antibody from responder strain of mice.

Anti(IgG_{2a}^b) allotype antisera from each strain of responder mice appear to contain IdX bearing antibodies (i.e BALB/c, BALB.B, B.C8, CXBG, CXBJ, RIII, CAL.20, DBA/2 P/J and 129/sw strains of mice). This was demonstrated by the ability of these sera to inhibit the interaction between anti-Id sera and BALB/c anti-CBPC 101 antibodies used to raise anti-Id sera. It should be noted that mice strain bearing H_2^b haplotype have a relatively lower level of IdX than mice of d, r and p MHC types (Table 3). The expression of an IdX by anti-immunoglobulin antibodies is in agreement with the observation of Kunkel et al. (1974) who showed that monoclonal human IgM proteins specific for IgG, classified into two major groups (Wa and Po) share an IdX and that the light chain of these proteins demonstrated a stricking restriction of V_L region subgroup (Capra et al. 1972). It should be mentioned that Roland

Table 3: IdX on anti-allotype (IgG$_{2a}^b$) antibodies produced in various strains of mice.

Strain	H2	allotype	HA titer (log2) with SRBC-CBPC101	HI titer (log2) SRBC-BALB/c anti-CBPC101		Inhibition of RIA*	
				BAB.14 anti Id serum	CXBI anti Id serum	BAB.14 Id serum	CXBI-anti Id serum
BALB/c	d	a	12	8	8	1000	1000
BALB.B	b	a	7	3	2.6	10	0
B.C8	b	a	11.5	6	3.5	5	3
CXBG	b	a	9.5	6	8	30	650
CXBJ	b	a	12	6	5	3	100
DBA/2	d	c	12	8	8	1000	1000
CAL.20	d	d	11.3	8	8	1000	60
RIII	r	g	12	8	8	650	1000
P/J	p	h	12	8	8	650	200
129/SW	bc	a	12	6	7	100	30

*Expressed as 1/dilution of serum for 50% inhibition.

et al.(1979) have shown that rabbit anti-b4 allotype antibodies also expressed a common idiotype. Within responder
strains the ability to produce anti-allotype antibody was
equally distributed in mice of $\underline{a}$, $\underline{d}$, $\underline{c}$,g and h IgC_H types.
This sharing of IdX among antibodies of a variety of IgC_H
types has already been reported in other antigenic systems
such as phosphocholine (Cancro et al. 1978; Riesen, 1979)
galactan (Mushinski et al. 1977) and GAT (Ju et al. 1978).
Anti-αm (1) cryoglobulins in several members of a family
expressed a cross-reactive idiotype. Inheritence of this
idiotype was not related with HLA nor to Gm allotype among
the members of this family.

3. OCCURRENCE OF ANTI(ANTI-ALLOTYPE)-ANTIBODIES IN
MATERNALLY ALLOTYPE-SUPPRESSED (BALB/c x C.B20)F_1HYBRIDS.

Allotype suppression was obtained in F_1 hybrids prepared
by mating C.B20 males with BALB/c females which had been
immunized with CBPC 101. Low titers of anti-allotype antibodies were detected in the sera of these F_1 hybrids until
approximately 4 wk of age. At 3 mo of age, 22 of 24
suppressed F_1 hybrids failed to express detectable IgG_2a^b
allotypic determinants, as judged by HI assay. These 22
mice were immunized with CBPC 101 myeloma protein. Of these,
20 developed a low titer of anti-allotype antibodies
(titer log_2 2-6) as determined by HA assay with CBPC 101
or C57BL/6 Ig-coated SRBC. In contradistinction to anti-
allotype antibodies produced in BALB/c mice and mice of
other responsive types, which express IdX, the anti-allotype
antibodies produced by suppressed F_1 hybrids were IdX$^-$.
Thus, sera from these mice did not inhibit agglutination of
BALB/c anti-CBPC 101 antibody-coated SRBC by BAB.14 or
CXBI anti-Id sera (Table 4). Surprisingly, when sera from
these immunized suppressed mice were used in inhibition of
RIA, we observed an increase in the binding of ^{3}H-BALB/c
anti-CBPC 101 antibodies to plates coated with BAB.14
anti-Id serum.

This observation suggested to us that F_1 antisera
lacking IdX$^+$ anti-allotype antibodies might contain anti-
IdX antibodies. Therefore, we tested that ability of these
sera, when coated on microtiter plates, to bind ^{3}H-BALB/c
anti-CBPC 101 antibodies. We found that sera from each
mouse bound ^{3}H-BALB/c anti-CBPC 101 antibodies. This
binding appears to be due to the presence of anti-Id antibodies and not to the presence of IgG_2a^b immunoglobulin

molecules, since these sera contain anti-IgG_{2a}^b antibodies (Table 5).

Table 4: Absence of IdX on anti(IgG_{2a}^b) allotype antibodies produced by maternally allotype-suppressed (BALB/c x C.B210)F_1 mice immunized with CBPC101 myeloma protein

F_1 no.	HA titer ($\log_2$)			HI titer ($\log_2$)	
	CBPC101	C57BL/6 Ig	UPC10	BAB14 anti-Id	CXB1 anti-Id
1	0	0	0	0	0
2	5	5	0	0	0
3	5	5	0	0	0
4	5	5	0	0	0
5	2	2	0	0	0
7	5	5	0	0	0
8	3	3	0	0	0
9	3	4	0	0	0
10	6	6	0	0	0
11	4	4	0	0	0
12	6	5	0	0	0
13	4	4	0	0	0
15	4	5	0	0	0
16	5	5	0	0	0
17	4	5	0	0	0
18	2	1	0	0	0
19	5	4	0	0	0
20	5	0	0	0	0
21	5	4	0	0	0
22	3	5	0	0	0
23	4	5	0	0	0
24	1	1	0	0	0

Table 5: Binding of 3H-BALB/c anti-CBPC101 antibodies to BAB.14 anti-idiotypic serum and to spontaneous auto-anti-idiotypic antibodies produced by maternally allotype suppressed (BALB/c x C.B20)F₁ hybrids immunized with CBPC 101 myeloma protein.

origin of serum:	No of mice	Binding of 3H-BALB/c anti-CBPC101* antibody to microplates coated with various sera
BAB14 anti-Id serum (diluted 5x10⁻⁴)	pool	2,560**
BAB 14 normal serum (diluted 5x10⁻⁴)	pool	103
BALB/c normal serum (diluted 1:10)	pool	87
serum from non immunized maternally suppressed F₁ hybrids (diluted 1:2)	10	350***, 283, 275, 252, 258 211, 183, 122, 118, 98

dilution of sera:

origin of serum:	No of mice	1:2			1:8		
serum from maternally suppressed F₁ hybrids immunized with myeloma proteins	19	2,510	2,150	1,835	1,132	1,637	935
		1,675	1,501	1,487	756	736	831
		1,408	1,395	1,291	830	812	805
		1,187	1,185	1,184	799	795	786
		1,073	1,052	856	603	601	592
		833	720	710	556	570	534
			650			490	

* 15.000cpm of 3H-BALB/c anti-CBPC101 was added for each well

** cpm   *** each represents an individual mouse tested

These results suggest that the absence of IdX^+ anti-allotype antibodies in suppressed F_1 mice can be related with the appearence of auto-anti-Id antibodies. The initial event in production of auto-anti-idiotypic antibodies may be a result of priming of F_1 anti-Id antibody forming cells with maternal transferred anti-allotype antibodies. Upon challenge of these F_1 mice with CBPC 101, these primed cells may be boosted by one of two possibilities:

a) residual maternal anti-CBPC 101 antibodies undetectable by HIA assay may complex with injected CBPC 101 and this complex may stimulate.

b) IdX^+F cells stimulated by injection of CBPC 101 may synthesize enogh IdX bearing molecules to boost the production of anti-Id antibodies.

These results as well as another reported in autologous or syngeneic systems for the immune response to various antigens (Kluskens et al. 1974, Cosenza 1976, Bona et al. 1978, Bankert et al. 1976, Tasiaux et al. 1978, Brown et al. 1979, Morgan et al. 1979, Goidl et al. 1979) clearly illustrate that the occurrence of auto-anti-idiotypic antibodies has an important role in the functional network regulatory mechanisms of the immune response (Jerne 1974, 1976; Cazenave 1977, Urbain et al. 1979; Bona 1979; Bona and Hiernaux in press).

4. DISCUSSION AND CONCLUSIONS

The main observation of this study is the similarity of anti-$IgG_2{}_a^b$ anti-allotype antibodies which express an IdX among the responder strains. This observation suggests that the ability to produce anti-allotype antibody or in a larger extent anti-Ig antibody is a highly conserved function. This function is encoded by a single V gene or a closely related family of V region genes. In particular experimental conditions such as the immunization of maternally allotype suppressed mice these IdX bearing anti-allotype antibodies elicited the spontaneous production of anti-Id auto-antibodies. The occurrence of such auto-anti-idiotypic antibodies suppressed the differentiation and proliferation of clones able to produce IdX^+ bearing anti-allotype antibody. This suppression permits the stimulation of a minor clone by CBPC 101 myeloma protein which was able to produce a small amount of anti-allotype antibodies which lack IdX. Therefore, the expression of clones which produce anti-allotype antibodies and in a

larger extent anti-Ig antibodies, phenomenon which could
seriously disturb the mechanisms of the immune defence, is
under the control of other clones which produce anti-Id
antibodies which suppressed the dominant anti-allotype
response.

One may ask why the capacity to produce anti-allotype
antibodies should be of sufficient significance so that this
ability would exhibit this degree of conservation. One
obvious possibility is that the V_H genes which encode the
combining site may also code for T cell receptor which
regulate the expression of B cells able to synthesize
various clones of Ig. Alternatively, the concentration of
immunoglobulins represents an important component of
homeostasis of macromolecules which requires its maintai-
nance in narrow limits   implaying a high degree of
conservation of genes which regulate the synthesis of Ig.
Our data taken collectively show the complexity of the
mechanisms of the control of production of anti-Ig antibodies which is governed by a single or closed related family
of V region gene conserved during evolution of a species.
The expression of this gene is under the control of genes
of MHC locus. In addition the differentiation and proliferation of clones able to produce anti-allotype antibody
can be suppressed by auto-anti-Id antibodies which
spontaneously occur in maternally allotype suppressed
F_1 hybrids in which the production of anti-allotype antibody was actively induced. This fine control and rigorous
control of production of anti-Ig antibodies could be
related to the important role of Ig recognition of production of class, allotype and idiotype of antibodies.

Bankert R.B. and Pressman D. (1976). Receptor-blocking
    factor present in immune serum resembling auto-anti-
    idiotype antibody. J. Immunol. 117: 457.
Black S.J. and Herzenberg L.A. (1979) B cell influence
    on the induction of allotype suppressor T cells. J. Exp.
    Med. 150:174.
Bona C., Lieberman R·., Chien C.C., Mond J., House S.,
    Green I., and Paul W.E. (1979) Immune response to levan
    I kinetics and ontogeny of anti-levan and anti-inulin
    antibody response and of expression of cross-reactive
    idiotype. J. Immunol. 120: 1436.

Bona C., Hooghe R., Cazenave P.-A., Le Guern C., and Paul W.E. (1979). Cellular basis of regulation of expression of idiotype II. Immunity to anti-MOPC 460 idiotype antibodies increases the level of anti-trinitrophenyl antibodies bearing 460 idiotypes. J. Exp. Med. 149:815.

Bona C., Mongini P., Stein K.A. and Paul W.E. Anti-allotype antibodies I. Production of anti-IgG$_2$$_a^b$ allotype antibodies is controlled by an H$_2$ linked Ir gene and single V gene (submitted).

Bona C. Regulation of the growth of myeloma tumor cells and non neoplastic B cell clones by anti-idiotypic antibodies in Porter M (eds) Progress in myeloma. Elsevier North Holland Amsterdam and New York (in press).

Bona C. and Hiernaux J. Immune response: idiotype-anti-idiotype network. Critical Review in Immunology (in preparation).

Brown J.C. and Rodkey I.S. (1979) Autoregulation of an antibody response via network-induced auto-anti-idiotype. J. Exp. Med. 150: 67.

Cancro M.P., Sigel N.H. and Klinman N.R. (1978) Differential expression of an equivalent clonotype among BALB/c and C57BL/6 mice. J. Exp. Med. 147:1.

Capra J.D., Kehoe J.M., Williams R.C., Feizi T. and Kunkel H.G. (1972) Light chain sequences of human IgM cold agglutinins. Proc.Natl. Acad.Sci. (USA) 69:40.

Cazenave P.-A.(1977). Idiotypic anti-idiotypic regulation of antibody synthesis in rabbits. Proc.Natl. Acad. Sci. (USA) 74: 5122.

Cosenza H. (1976) Detection of anti-idiotype reactive cells in the response to phosphorylcholine. Eur.J. Immunol. 6:114.

Doherty P.C., Blanden R.V., and Zinkernagel R.M.(1976). Specificity of virus-immune effector T cells for H-2K or H-2D compatible interactions: implications for H-antigen diversity. Tranpl. Rev. 29:90.

Elson C.O., Heck, J.A. and Strober W. (1979) T-cell regulation of murine Igl synthesis. J. Exp. Med. 149:632.

Goidl E.A., Schrater A.F., Siskind G.W., and Thorbecke G.J. (1979). Production of auto-anti-idiotypic antibody during the normal immune response to TNP-Ficoll. II. Hapten-reversible inhibition of anti-TNP plaque forming cells by immune serum as an assay for auto-anti-idiotypic antibody. J. Exp. Med. 150:154.

Herzenberg L.A., Okumura K., Cantor H., Sato V.L., Shen F.W, Boyse E.A., and Herzenberg L.A. (1976). T cell regulation of antibody responses: demonstration of allotype-specific helper T cells and their specific removal by suppressor T cells. J. Exp. Med. 144:33.

Hetzelberger D. and Eichmann K. (1978) Recognition of idiotypes in lymphocyte interactions I. Idiotypic reactivity in the cooperation between T and B lymphocytes. Eur. J. Immunol. 8:846.

Janeway C.A., Murgita R.A., Weinbaum F.I., Asofsky R. and Wigzell H. (1977). Evidence for an immunoglobulin dependent antigen specific helper T cell. Proc. Natl. Acad. Sci. (USA) 74:4582.

Jerne N.K. (1974) Towards a network theory of the immune system. Ann. Immunol. (Inst. Pasteur) 125C: 373.

Jerne N.K. (1976). The immune system: a web of V domains. Harvey Lectures: series 70. Academic Press, New York, San Francisco, London p.93.

Ju S.T., Benacerraf B. and Dorf M.E. (1978). Idiotypic analysis of antibodies to poly (Glu^{60}, Ala^{10} Tyr^{10}): interstrain and interspecies idiotypic cross reactions. Proc. Natl. Acad. Sci. (USA) 75:6192.

Kluskens L. and Köhler H. (1974) Regulation of immune response by autogenous antibody against receptor. Proc. Natl. Acad. Sci. (Usa) 71: 5083.

Kunkel H.G., Winchester R.J., Joslin F.G. and Capra J.D. (1974) Similarities in the light chains of anti-γ-globulins showing cross idiotypic specificities. J. Exp. Med. 139: 128.

Morgan A.C., Rossen R.D. and Twomey J.J. (1979) Naturally occurring circulating immune complexes: normal human serum contains idiotype-anti-idiotype complexes dissociable by certain IgG antiglobulins. J. Immunol. 122: 1672.

Mushinski E.B. and Potter M. (1977) Idiotypes on galactan binding myeloma proteins and anti-galactan antibodies in mice. J. Immunol. 119:1888.

Riesen W.F. (1979). Idiotypic cross-reactivity of human and murine phosphorylcholine-binding immunoglobulins. Eur.J. Immunol. 9:421.

Roland J. and Cazenave P.-A. (1979) Mise en evidence d'idiotypes anti-b4 apparentés chez les lapins de phénotype a3$^+$ immunisés contre l'allotype b4. C.R. Acad. Sci. Paris 288:571.

Rosenthal A.S. (1978) determinant selection and macrophage function in genetic control of the immune response. Immunol. Rev. 40:136.

Tasiaux N., Leuwenbroon R., Bruyns C. and Urbain J. (1979) Possible occurrence and meaning of lymphocytes bearing auto-anti-idiotypic receptors during the immune response. Eur.J. Immunol. 8:464.

Urbain J., Collignon J., Franssen J.D., Mariamé B., Léo O., Urbain-Vansanten G., Van de Valle P., Wikler M., and Wuilmart C. (1979). Idiotypic networks and self recognition in the immune system. Ann. Immunol. (Inst.Pasteur) 130C:281.

Ward K., Cantor H., and Boyse E.A. (1977). Clonally restricted interactions among T and B cell subclasses in: Sercaz E.A., Herzenberg L.A., and Fox C.F. eds) ICN-UCLA Symposia on Molecular and Cellular Biology Immune system: genetic and regulation. Academic Press New York, San Francisco, London, Vol.VI p.397.

Acknowledgments: The skilful secretarial assistance of Mrs Nina Canto is greatly appreciated.

UNKN: Can you obtain allotype-suppressed mice in combinations other than the CB-20 x Balb/c cross?

Bona: Yes. Herzenberg studied genetic requirements of allotype suppression in SJL x Balb/c.

UNKN: Is suppression long-lasting?

Bona: I have not checked two months after suppression, because we must clear maternal allotype from the serum. Suppression is broken after six months, however.

Kohler: Similar crossreactivity with T15 has been found with Balb/c and A mice by isoelectric focusing.

Kohler: Did you detect small amounts of anti-idiotype sera in allotype-suppressed mice?

Bona: Twenty of twenty-two animals had anti-idiotype antibody.

Kohler: Could this not be a technical problem due to complexes of idiotype and anti-idiotype?

Bona: Complexes create problems when trying to detect small amounts of anti-idiotype in RIA 150. Many people found this auto-antiidiotype. In this case we tried to precipitate and I think that there are a lot of pitfalls to be sure with gradient IgG_{2a}.

Pages 279—293, Membranes, Receptors, and the Immune Response

INDICATIONS FOR AN INTERNAL REGULATION IN THE IMMUNE SYSTEM

A. Coutinho and
L.Forni, C.Martinez-A, R.R.Bernabé, E.-L.Larsson,
M.Reth, A.A. Augustin, P.-A.Cazenave,

Basel Institute for Immunology
487 Grenzacherstrasse, CH-4005 Basel 5,Switzerland

1.   The Definition of the problems
     The prevalent concepts of the immune system still
suffer from the historical origin of immunology as a by-
product of microbiology. Although few would deny the idea
that anti-microbial defense is a main purpose of the immune
system, there are wide disagreements on the strategies
used by the system to accomplish that function. Classical
views consider the immune system essentially resting,
awaiting for foreing antigen (Cohn et al., 1974) or mitogen
(Coutinho and Möller, 1975). The system is "blank" before
the introduction of environmental stimuli. The alternative
concept pays a fundamental importance to the activity
developed within the system itself (Jerne, 1974), and
assumes that the ability to respond to non-self antigens is
acquired and developed by ongoing responses to self (Vaz and
Varela, 1978).
     The choice between these opposing concepts is fundament-
al for any further theoretical considerations on the origin
of antibody diversity and on the functional basis for the
self-nonself discrimination. While the network ideas of
Jerne, as they were formulated, can in fact account for
practically all observations available at present, this is
exactly the problem with the concept, namely that it explains
formally contradictory observations. Because of its lack of
precision it cannot distinguish the fundamental pathways of
idiotype anti-idiotype interactions, from those which
are only apparent in artificial experimental situations.
This is actually the concern of Jerne, when asking the

question whether the network is fundamental for the economy of the system, or whether one can show that idiotypes are important in some situations but they are a mere sophistication without which the immune system could function nearly as well. The whole question is difficult to approach because of the very nature of network concepts, namely the influence of the postulated internal regulation at all levels of the immune ontogeny, steady states and responses. In other words, analytical approaches, are, by the fact of being analytic, limiting of a network concept and assumptions. In essence, network concepts require a theoretical and experimental approach which escapes that ascribed to natural sciences (analysis-synthesis), and which is basically a philosophical one (synthesis-synthesis). Considering the difficulties in developing pictures of the immune system as a network, we might recall the remarks of A. Toynbee about societies which are "complete networks of relationships between individuals", and the components of which are, primarily, the existing relationships rather than the individuals themselves. As he says, "a group, as opposed to a society , may be collected, dispersed, photographed or destroyed".

Many independent observations have recently accumulated to indicate the overall validity of network ideas. They have not given the answers to these questions, but they have deeply shaken the foundations of the classical views of an immune system turned to the outside only. We, as many others, have accumulated small pieces of experimental evidence which can hardly, if at all, be accounted for by classical concepts. In our search for the general rules presiding to the actual physiology of the normal immune system, however, we still see these as the Holy Grail. We will discuss here a few of these findings and some of the colours the grail could have.

2. Some of the main questions

Somatic diversification of antibody genes is now established (Möller Ed., 1977). Whatever the molecular mechanism for the generation of somatic variants, these are necessarily rare, and consequently, the relative importance of their contribution to the antibody repertoire is directly related to the efficiency of the mechanisms that positively select for variants. The very large numbers of antibody-forming cell precursors generated and wasted in a normal steady state (Osmonde, 1979), would allow for the

occurrence of these variants. Actually, this is the most
obvious reason why this high turnover of cells should
constitute a major property of the B lymphocyte and antibody
system. On the other hand, even if one accepts that the
available repertoire is primarily made up of germinal specificities, one still has to accept that not all of these are
expressed with the same frequencies throughout the life time
of the individual. In fact, good evidence has been produced
to indicate profound alterations in the actual repertoire of
individuals along development (Cancro and Klinman, 1979).
"Germ-line" points of view would use the high turnover of
cells to select available repertoire from the germ line
pool rather than for the somatic generation of new variants.
Consequently, independently of the somatic or germinal
origin of the majority of the repertoire, it is clear that
there must exist mechanisms which select for the actual
repertoire expressed by the individual at any time point.
Since those changes in the available, expressed repertoires
occur in the absence of "foreign antigen", this selection
must use tools which are available internally. These,
however, are not necessarily components of the immune system,
nor do they have to be recognized as antigens. It is likely,
on the other hand, that the selection of the available
repertoire is done at the level of precursor cells, before
acquisition of immunocompetence, since the overwhelming
majority of antigen-reactive cells (which constitute the
available repertoire) are resting, noncycling lymphocytes.
Furthermore, many experiments indicate that this selection
is, at least partially, based on the idiotypic specificity
of the precursor cells (Cosenza and Köhler, 1972, Eichmann
and Rajewsky, 1975, Cazenave, 1977, Urbain et al., 1977).
It is even more striking to find that in a "primed" steady
state induced by the injection of antigen, the frequency of
antibody specificities expressed by immunocompetent cells
is regulated by idiotypic, rather than by combining site,
specificities (Eichmann et al., 1977). From these observations we conclude that a normal immune system is constitutive-
ly capable of generating a very large number of precursor
cells and that the process of stimulation of these cells
must include a mechanism for selecting on idiotypic basis,
out of all potential clones, those which differentiate into
immunocompetence. These questions on the driving forces of
precursor cell expansion and on the selective pressures

they are submitted to, have not been the major concern in
both classical and network views of the immune system. In
fact, the suggestion that the internal, network recognition
could be used as a mechanism for selecting immunocompetent
cells from the precursor pool, is not included in the original formulations of the concept, and it has been proposed
later by Adam and Weiler (1976). The original network
concepts are concerned with a mature immune system and its
regulation. Obviously, also here, the problems involved in
this approach, and the attraction of its clear elegance
require thoughtful experiments and conclusions. We know,
for example, that T helper cells exist in normal individuals
that can specifically react with self idiotypes (Janeway et
al., 1975; Julius et al.,1977; Woodland and Cantor, 1979;
Eichmann et al. 1979). It is still not clear, however, how
these observations can be accommodated with the problem of
self-nonself discrimination by T cells, and what is the
importance of helper T cells in the overall regulation of an
immune network. While recent experiments would strongly
suggest an important functional role for auto-anti-idiotypic
T cells, it is also true that T-cell deprived mice (nude)
appear normal as to the basic features of the B cell-anti-
body system.

3.   Indications in favour of a role for idiotype-anti-
idiotype interactions in the process of expansion and
selection of precursor cells.

In search of specific reagents for mitogen receptors on
B lymhocytes, we tried the same experimental approach previously used for other non-immunological receptors (Sege and
Peterson, 1978). In short, we assessed the ability of anti-
idiotypic antibodies against a dextran-binding antibody combining site to recognize polyclonally distributed mitogen
receptors for dextran α 1-3 -a thymus-independent antigen
and mitogen (Blomberg et al. 1972). We found that these
anti-idiotypic antibodies could bind to a dextran-specific
surface structure on a large fraction of all B lymphocytes
(10-15%) in the spleen of adult mice, from a number of
inbred strains, regardless of the genetic determination for
expression of that idiotype on antibody molecules, previously
determined in the same strains (Coutinho et al. 1978). This
surface structure was functionally defined as a mitogen
receptor since these purified anti-idiotypic antibodies
could trigger roughly the same numbers of B lymphocytes into
clonal expansion and maturation to immunoglobulin secretion

(Coutinho et al., 1978). These findings were extended to
several other idiotypic systems, in which the specific
antigen was also a direct B cell mitogen, such as dextran α
1-6 and levan. We soon found, however, that the same could
apply to anti-idiotypic antibodies against other myeloma
proteins with binding specificity for antigens that are not
B cell mitogens, such as the haptens TNP and NIP. The
availability of monoclonal reagents with the same anti-
idiotypic specificities (Buttin et al., 1978; Reth et al.,
1979) which were found to have these polyclonal properties,
made it even more unlikely the possibility that we were
dealing with experimental artifacts. We had, consequently,
to revise our original simplistic interpretation of the
finding that highly specific reagents for determinants on
variable regions of antibody molecules recognize a large
fraction of all mature B lymphocytes. With the testing of
more anti-idiotype reagents, and the finding of positive and
negative antisera, we were led to conclude preliminarily,
that antibodies to "public" or "major" idiotypes had this
property, while antibodies against "private, "individual" or
"minor" idiotypes did not. In support of this conclusion,
we had found that while antibodies to a levan-binding idiotype (EPC-109) which is expressed on antibody molecules from
every mouse with a BALB/c immunoglobulin haplotype were
polyclonal mitogens, similar antisera to a "private" levan-
binding idiotype (ABPC-48) did not have these properties
(Forni, Coutinho, Lieberman and Cazenave, to be published).

With further experiments, however, this picture did not
hold any longer. As the introduction of monoclonal anti-
idiotypic reagents and better detection methods apported
further precision and complexity to the current definitions
of "public" versus "private" idiotypes, the testing of such
reagents in our systems had the same consequences. Thus,
while we find monoclonal antibodies which react with a
minority of anti-NIP heteroclytic antibodies to be strongly
positive in our assays, another monoclonal anti-idiotype
which recognizes the large majority of all anti-NIP antibodies
produced by the same strains is completely negative, as to
binding to B cells other than those which express the
corresponding idiotypes on antibody receptors. In essence,
antibodies to "public" and "major" idiotypes can be totally
negative, while antibodies to "minor", although "public"
idiotopes can be strongly positive (Coutinho, Forni, Cazena-

*ve, Reth and Rajewsky, to be published). Furthermore, also
antibodies to rabbit idiotypes, which have been described
(Oudin and Michel, 1963), and are currently considered as
typical "private" idiotypes, appear to recognize surface
determinants on a large fraction all peripheral B cells
(Forni, Kelus and Coutinho, to be published).*

*These considerations bring us to the discussion of the
specificity of anti-idiotypic reagents and their cross-
reactivity, in terms of what we can conclude from our findings. It appears now clear that a "major" idiotype is in
fact a mixture of several distinct antibody species which
share one or several idiotopes (Berek et al., 1979; Gill-
Pazaris et al., 1979; Reth et al., 1978). It follows that a
pool of different antibodies in conventional anti-idiotypic
reagents recognize a family of idiotypically related molecules. Our findings indicate that there are structures on
the B cell surface which are certainly not immunoglobulins
but share with them antigenic determinants recognized by
conventional pools of anti-idiotypic antibodies . It is
clearly impossible to ascribe to any particular antibody
this cross-reactivity, which, on the other hand, must exist
between those mitogen receptors and the immunizing myeloma
protein. With monoclonal anti-idiotypic reagents, these
considerations proceed to a higher level of resolution,
since we are now dealing with antibodies to determinants,
or idiotopes. It is clear, however, that these reagents
are still antibodies and, consequently, they might recognize
many different, cross-reactive antigenic determinants, on
immunoglobulin molecules or not. Depending upon which*

** The non-immunoglobulin nature of the membrane molecules
detected by anti-idiotypes on μ^+ cells in adult spleen
is supported by the observation that all B cell blasts
induced in cultures by a given anti-idiotype, bear membrane
determinants cross-reactive with that particular idiotype.
In contrast, only a minority (around 1%) of all plasma
cells induced in these cultures, which are direct descend-
ants of those blasts, contain immunoglobulin molecules
bearing these idiotypic determinants. It follows that,
keeping to the postulates of clonal selection theory, the
surface structure recognized by the anti-idiotypic antibodies cannot be immunoglobulin.*

particular idiotope is recognized on the antibody molecule
and upon the fine specificity of the recognizing monoclonal
anti-idiotype, we might find various reagents as positive
or negative in our assays. In fact, while we have found so
far two different monoclonal anti-idiotypes to be positive,
we have also failed to detect with monoclonal anti-idiotypic
antibodies, cross-reactivities that could clearly be found
with the corresponding conventional antisera, (e.g. anti-
J558 and anti-TEPC 15 antibodies). It is clear from these
elaborations that the study of the physiological significance
and genetics of these idiotype-cross-reactive B cell receptors,
and their relationship with antibody idiotypes has to be
done with monoclonal reagents since, using conventional
antisera, the anti-idiotypes which react with such receptors
might be different from those which react with the particular
antibodies we are detecting in our experiments. It should
be pointed out, however, that all the genetics and functional studies on idiotypes have so far been done using conventional reagents, previously considered by many to provide
clonal markers for individual antibody molecules.

In spite of all the reservations as to the basic rules
and the detailed significance of our findings, we consider
it very stimulating and intriguing the observation that the
same anti-idiotypic antibodies which react with large
mature B cell subsets in the adult spleen, also react
specifically with cell populations containing B cell precursors, namely foetal liver an adult bone marrow. As described before (Forni et al., 1979), individual anti-idiotype
reagents may stain specifically as many as 5% of all nuclea-
ted cells in the marrow, what represents roughly 20% of all
lymphoid cells in this organ. The majority of these cells,
and all those stained by the anti-idiotypes in the foetal
liver, did not express membrane bound or intracytoplasmic
immunoglobulins.

If these cells could be shown to be precursors for B
lymphocytes, as the μ^+, δ^- phenotype of the spleen cells
stained in the same conditions would suggest, it would be
important to establish the functional consequences of the
interactions between anti-idiotypic antibodies with these
cells. Experiments were performed in which immunoglobulin-
negative cells purified from bone marrow or obtained from
foetal livers, were incubated with a number of anti-idiotypic reagents. We observed basically three effects of

*these reagents: 1) an increase in the spontaneous proliferat-
ion detected in these cultures, with the consequent recovery
of higher numbers of cells, 2) an increase in the number
of small lymphocytes, expressing membrane-bound IgM that
could be recovered from these cultures, 3) an increase in
the numbers of IgM PFC developed in anti-idiotype treated
cultures upon stimulation by lipopolysaccharide at later
culture periods. These results demonstrate that B cell
precursors are targets for anti-idiotype recognition and
that interaction with anti-idiotypic antibodies may result
in enhanced proliferation and induction of differentiation
amongst those precursors. If we postulate the availability
of anti-idiotypic antibodies at threshold concentrations
(these effects are observed with a few nanograms of antibody)
at the sites for B cell generation, these could in fact
constitute the driving force for the expansion of B cell
precursors. The postulate appears reasonable, since such
antibodies can be envisaged to be passively transferred
from the mother, or even produced in situ by embryonic
cells which differentiate to this type of effector function.
   In such a framework, it is possible to design a number
of models describing the mechanisms how anti-idiotypic
interactions could select for precursors on the basis of
antibody idiotypes, simultaneously with providing the basis
for continuous expansion. In particular, it is relatively
easy to elaborate models based on the cross-reactivity of
two functionally distinct receptors where variants would be
selected for, a primary requirement for concepts of somatic
generation of antibody diversity. Some results supporting
these possibilities have now been obtained. Thus, the
stimulation of bone marrow precursors with monoclonal anti-
idiotypes against TNP or NIP-binding proteins, results in a
relative increase in the number of IgM clones selected for
immunocompetence in these cultures with specificity for TNP
or NIP respectively. In contrast, the same cell populations
do not contain a proportionally higher number of clones
secreting the idiotype against which the stimulatory
reagent was directed. These results will have to be analyzed
in further detail, but they already provide good indications
that the hypothesised mechanisms may in fact be operative
in the generation of antibody diversity. The available
anti-idiotypes which could provide the driving forces and
the pressures selecting cells into the immunocompetent pool*

are, in the adult, components of the steady state, originating
from the internal activity in the system and "feeding back"
at its origin. It is to be expected, therefore, that
alterations in this steady state, induced by antigen (Eichmann
et al. 1977) or by idiotypic or anti-idiotypic immunizations
(Cazenave, 1977; Urbain et al., 1977) will be reflected
also in the relative frequencies of precursors which are
being selected. In fact, preliminary experiments designed
to directly test for these assumptions have demonstrated
population changes induced by anti-idiotypic immunization,
amongst immunoglobulin-idiotype negative precursors in the
marrow which expresses the non-reactive structure (Bernabé,
Forni, Cazenave and Coutinho, to be published).
4. The regulation of the mature immune system by its own
elements.

A number of other findings that we have recently obtained
relate directly to this point. One demonstration of internal
regulation has been obtained in experiments steming from the
analysis of the antibody-mediated enhancement and suppression
of antigen-dependent immune responses. We have found that
some, but not all, IgM antibodies when injected in nanogram
amounts into untreated recipients can induce the appearance
of plasma cells secreting antibodies of the same specificity
(Forni, Coutinho and Köhler, to be published). This finding
is compatible with the idea that all the antigens (or corresponding functional substitutes) exist within the immune
system (Jerne, 1974) and it cannot be accommodated with
classical views of an immune system turned to the outside
only. We still do not know whether this effect of passively
administered antibodies is due to their idiotypic or to
their combining site properties, an important point to be
established in order to clarify the mechanism of induction
of such an antigen-independent responses. On the other
hand, we already know that these responses are T cell dependent, bringing into the discussion, once again, the role of
auto-reactive helper cells in the establishment and mainten-
ance of the normal steady states. This situation could in
fact be similar to the previous demonstrations of idiotype-
specific helper cells which function in an antigen-independent fashion. We, as others (Julius et al., 1977; Eichmann
et al., 1979; Augustin and Julius, to be published), could
raise and enrich for T helper cells which specifically
recognize an autologous antibody idiotype (Augustin, Marti-

nez, Forni, Bernabé and Coutinho, to be published). Upon interaction with syngeneic B lymphocytes, and in the absence of antigen, such helper T cells induce idiotype-bearing antibodies. We have found in addition, that those cellular interactions also result in the activation of a large number of B cells which do not express that idiotype on antibody molecules, and that idiotype-specific helper T cells can as well induce B cells originating from strains in which no antibodies can be detected with that idiotype. It appears, therefore, that we are in the same situation as discussed above for the cross-reactivity of antibody idiotypes with other B cell surface structures, as it is seen, in the latter case, by helper T cells. Since, on the other hand, a sizable fraction of the helper activity mediated by normal T cells to B lymphocytes reacting with heterologous red cells appears to have an anti-idiotypic specificity (Bernabé et al., 1979), these findings suggest higher levels of complexity in such an internal regulation, which is not limited to the idiotype-anti-idiotype interactions occurring with antibody molecules and T cell receptors. Finally, while our results reinforce the reservations that must be taken in the interpretation of the genetic determination of T cell receptors on the basis of reactivities with anti-idiotypic reagents, a large body of evidence is now available demonstrating that such reagents do in fact recognize specific structures on T cell surfaces (Binz and Wigzell, 1977; Rajewsky and Eichmann, 1977). These remarks are important in the speculations concerning the T cell system. T cell activation has been reported upon interaction with anti-idiotypic antibodies (Eichmann and Rajewsky, 1975; Cosenza et al., 1977; Binz et al., 1979). Although some of these experiments (Binz et al, 1979) appear to contradict basic rules of T cell activation (Larsson and Coutinho, 1979a) and we have indications that antibodies to polyclonally distributed T cell receptors may also result in triggering (Larsson and Coutinho, 1979b), it is clear that T cell function may be influenced by anti-idiotypic antibodies. It follows that the completeness of the antibody repertoire would necessarily result in the possibility of stimulating all immunocompetent T cells, as T cell idiotypes would not escape that completeness of recognition. The consequences of these elaborations in the functional development and control of specific T cell clones at the periphery remain to be further developed.

Adam G, Weiler E (1976). Lymphocyte population dynamics during ontogenetic generation of diversity. In Cunningham AJ (ed): "The generation of antibody diversity. A new look New York - London: Acad. Press, p.1.

Berek C, Schreier MH, Sidman CL, Jaton JC, Kocher HP, Cosenza H (1979) Phosphorylcholine-binding hybridoma proteins of normal and idiotypically-suppressed Balb/c mice. I. Characterization and idiotypic analysis. Eur J Immunol in press.

Bernabé RR, Martinez-Alonso C, Coutinho A (1979). The specificity of non-specific T cell replacing factor. Eur J Immunol 9:546.

Binz H, Wigzell H (1977) Antigen binding, idiotypic T-lymphocyte receptors. Contemporary Topics Immunobiol 7:113.

Blomberg B, Geckeler WR, Weigert M (1972). Genetics of the antibody response to dextran in mice. Science 177:178.

Buttin G, LeGuern G, Phalente L, Lin ECC, Medrano L, Cazenave PA. (1978) Production of hybrid cell lines secreting monoclonal anti-idiotypic antibodies by cell fusion on membrane filters, Curr Topics Microbiol Immunol 81:27.

Cancro M., Klinman NR (1979) The genetic control of antibody diversification. In Cooper M, Mosier DE, Scher I, Vitetta ES (Eds) "B lymphocytes in the immune response" Elsevier-North Holland, p. 172.

Cazenave PA (1977) Idiotypic-anti-idiotypic regulations of antibody synthesis in rabbit. Proc Natl Acad Sci USA 74:5122

Cohn M, Blomberg B, Geckeler G., Raschke W, Riblet R, Weigert M (1974) First order considerations in analyzing the generation of diversity. In Sercarz EE, Williamson AR, Fox, CR "The immune system, genes, receptors, signals" New York: Acad Press p 89.

Cosenza H, Koehler H (1972) Specific suppression of the antibody response by antibodies to receptors. Proc Natl Acad Sci USA 69:2701.

Cosenza H, Augustin AA, Julius MH (1977). Induction and characterization of "autologous" anti-idiotypic antibodies. Eur J Immunol 7:273.

Coutinho A, Möller G. (1975) Thymus-independent B cell induction and paralysis. Adv Immunol 21:114.

Coutinho A, Forni L, Blomberg B. (1978) Shared antigenic determinants by mitogen receptors and antibodies to the same thymus-independent antigen. J exp Med 148:862.

Eichmann K, Rajewsky K. (1975) Induction of T and B cell immunity by anti-idiotypic antibodies. Eur J Immunol 5:661.

Eichmann K, Coutinho A, Melchers F (1977) Absolute frequencies of lipopolysaccharide-reactive B cells producing A5A idiotype in unprimed streptococcal A-carbohydrate-primed, anti-A5A idiotype-sensitized and anti-5A-idiotype suppressed A/J mice. J exp Med 146:1436.

Eichmann K, Falk I, Rajewsky K (1979) Recognition of idiotypes in lymphocyte interactions. II.Antigen-independent cooperation between T and B lymphocytes that posses similar and complementary idiotype. Eur J Immunol 8:853.

Forni L, Cazenave PA, Cosenza H, Forsbeck K, Coutinho A (1979) Expression of V-region-like determinants on Ig-negative precursors in murine fetal liver and bone marrow. Nature (London) 280:241.

Gill-Pazaris LA, Brown AR, Nisonoff A. (1979) The nature of idiotypes associated with anti-p-azophenylarsonate in A/J mice. Ann Immunol (Inst Pasteur) 130C:199.

Janeway CAJr, Sakato N, Eisen HN (1975) Recognition of immunoglobulin idiotypes by thymus-derived lymphocytes. Proc Natl Acad Sci USA 72:2357.

Jerne NK (1974) Towards a network theory of the immune system. Ann Immunol (Inst Pasteur) 125C:373.

Julius MH, Augustin AA, Cosenza H (1977) Recognition of a naturally occurring idiotype by autologous T cells. Nature (London) 265:271.

Larsson EL, Coutinho A (1979a) On the role of mitogenic lectins in T cell triggering. Nature (London) 280:239.

Larsson EL, Coutinho A (1979b) Mechanism of T cell activation I. A screening of "step-one" ligands. Eur J Immunol in press.

Möller G (Ed) "Molecular Aspects of V Genes" Transplant. Reviews 36

Osmonde DG (1979) Generation of B lymphocytes in the bone marrow. In Cooper MD, Mosier DE, Scher I, Vitetta ES (Eds) "B lymphocytes in the immune response" Elsevier-North Holland, p 63.

Oudin J, Michel M (1963) Une nouvelle forme d'allotypie des globulines gamma du sérum de lapin, apparemment liée à la fonction et à la spécificité anticorps. CR Acad Sci (Paris) 257:805.

Rajewsky K, Eichmann K (1977) Antigen receptors of T helper cells Contemporary Topics Immunobiol 7:69.

Reth M. Hämmerling GJ, Rajewsky K (1978) Analysis of the repertoire of anti-NP antibodies in C57BL/6 mice by cell fusion. I. Characterization of antibody families in the primary and hyperimmune response. Eur J Immunol 8:393.

Reth M, Imanishi-Kari T, Rajewsky K (1979) Analysis of the repertoire of anti-NP antibodies in C57BL/6 mice by cell fusion. II. Characterization of idiotopes by monoclonal anti-idiotope antibodies. Eur J Immunol in press.

Sege K, Peterson PA (1978) Use of anti-idiotypic antibodies as cell-surface receptor probes. Proc Natl Acad Sci USA 75:2443.

Urbain J, Wikler M, Franssen JD, Collignon C (1977) Idiotypic regulation of the immune system by the induction of antibodies against anti-idiotypic antibodies. Proc Natl Acad Sci USA 74:5126.

Vaz NM, Varela FJ (1978) Self and nonsense: an organism-centered approach to immunology. Med Hypotheses 4:231.

Woodland R, Cantor H (1979) Idiotype-specific T helper cells are required to induce idiotype-positive B memory cells to secrete antibodies. Eur J Immunol 8:600.

Quintans: Could anti-idiotype selection be simply
             anti-idiotype suppression?

Coutinho: Yes. If the two receptors crossreact, cells
             are driven to proliferate and diversify Ig.
             If there is no crossreaction the precursors
             would proceed straight to immunocompetence.

Quintans: Do IgM antibodies select T cells which prime
             B cells?

Coutinho: Yes.

Quintans: How long does it take for these to appear?

Coutinho: Specific plaques appear in 5 days. This
             implies that auto-reactive helper cells are
             preexistent.

Lutz: Have you noticed the phenomenon with any
             other class besides IgM?

Coutinho: No. The phenomenon is specific for IgM
             antibodies. One monoclonal antibody,
             injected in mice (and even in vitro) induces
             an enormous response of all specificities.
             This response is T-independent, and
             consequently the phenomenon is distinct from
             what I just described. Not all IgM
             antibodies work; some clones do not respond
             at all.

Lutz: Does it work only in vitro?

Coutinho: It works only in vivo.

Bona: Does this work in CeH/HeJ mice?

Coutinho: It works on C3H/HeJ mice, and on all other
             strains.

Bona: Could you have LPS contamination in the
             reagents from bacterial growth?

Coutinho: We get the preparations in low concentrations.
             They are then diluted one millionfold to show
             optimal activities in culture. If it were
             LPS contamination, we would need to have in
             the order of 50g LPS/ml in the original
             preparation.

Bona: Problem: 10 picograms of LPS in cultures just by leaving the bottle out, shipment, etcetera. Could bacteria have grown in the medium?

Coutinho: These are not borderline results. They were as good or better than the LPS-induced PFC response, three orders of magnitude higher than the backgrounds.

Pages 295–311, Membranes, Receptors, and the Immune Response
© 1980 Alan R. Liss, Inc., 150 Fifth Avenue, New York, NY 10011

IMMUNOLOGICAL MEMORY: CELL SELECTION

David W. Talmage

Department of Microbiology and the Webb-Waring
Lung Institute, University of Colorado Health
Sciences Center, Denver, Colorado 80262

Few would quarrel today with the statement that the
major process in immunological memory is cell selection,
i.e. the selective multiplication of that small fraction of
lymphocytes that happen to have immunoglobulin receptors
with affinity for antigen.

Much has happened in the past 23 years to fill in the
details of the molecular events that make cell selection
possible. However, the basic concept developed simultaneously at the Hall Institute in Melbourne and here at the
University of Chicago in the year 1956. That this should
happen independently in two distant places can only mean
that the time was ripe for this development and that the
concept of cell selection was based logically on preceding
knowledge and ideas.

It would seem appropriate on this occasion to recount
the story of cell selection in order that we might speculate
on the process of scientific advance and pay tribute to those
forebears who made the discoveries and formulated the
concepts on which cell selection was based.

The concept of immunological memory has been around a
long time and was based on the common observation that those
who survived an attack of smallpox rarely suffered a second
attack. The deliberate inoculation of a susceptible person
with pustular material from a relatively mild case of smallpox (known as variolation) was practiced in the Near East
for several centruies before it was introduced into
Western Europe in 1718 by Lady Mary Montague, wife of the

British Ambassador in Constantinople.

Almost eighty years later Edward Jenner, who studied
medicine under John Hunter and was practicing in his home
town, Berkeley in Gloucestershire, took note of a common
local belief that dairy maids who had caught cowpox could not
catch smallpox. In perhaps the most successful and far
reaching single clinical experiment of all time (Figure 1)
Jenner took matter from the hand of Sarah Nelmes, a local
dairy maid and injected it into the arm of James Phipps, a
healthy eight year old boy. Six weeks later he introduced
smallpox matter into the boy's arm without ill effect.

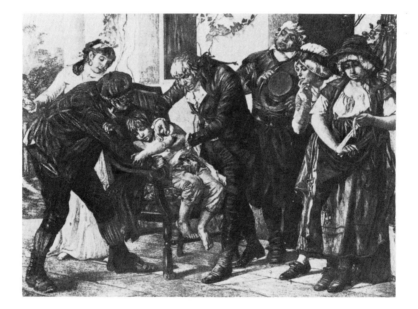

Figure 1. Edward Jenner gave the first vaccination for
smallpox to James Phipps in England in 1796. (Reprinted
from Rosen 1971.)

Although he may not have understood all of the
immunological implications of his work, Jenner had
demonstrated that the specificity of immunity was not
absolute. It was not necessary to inject the disease

producing organism to develop immunity. A related less
virulent organism would work equally well. Surprisingly, it
was eighty years before Pasteur generalized this concept to
other diseases: chicken cholera, anthrax, swine erisepelas
and rabies.

Although Pasteur understood the practical implications
of vaccination he did not have a clear idea of how the
immune system worked. Nor did anyone else at that time.
The findings of Metchnikoff with cells and von Behring and
Kitosato with antitoxins set off an early controversy between
adherents of cellular and humoral immunity.

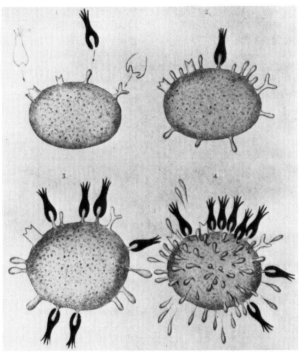

Figure 2. Ehrlich's conception of the multiplication and
shedding of natural cellular receptors after their
combination with antigen. From Ehrlich (1900).

It was at this point that Ehrlich (1900) introduced his
side chain theory. As shown in Figure 2, Ehrlich had a
clear concept of the interaction between antigen and antibody molecules and the relationship between cells, cell

receptors and humoral antibodies. It was a logical
synthesis of the cellular and humoral theories. It should
have been the beginning of cellular immunology, but science
was not yet ready. Two things interfered with the general
acceptance of Ehrlich's ideas. One was his arrogant
insistence that he was right in all details and the other
was his belief that the side-chains were physiologically
important to the acquisition of nutrients by the cells. When
Landsteiner (1915) showed that antibodies could be made to
newly synthesized chemicals the side chain theory and the
study of cells was dropped and forgotten for more than 30
years. See Landsteiner (1945).

It is surprising that Landsteiner was not able to make
the necessary modifications of Ehrlich's theory to adapt it
to his own findings because he came very close to it in his
discussion of Malkoff's findings (Table 1). Malkoff (1900)
reached the conclusion that a normal serum contains as many
specific agglutinins as there are sorts of cells that are
agglutinated by the serum. Because of the large number of
different substances which could be specifically agglutinated,
and because each of them amounted to several micrograms per
milliliter of serum, Landsteiner (1945) rejected this
hypothesis. He was able to purify the agglutinins by
absorption and elution from red cells and to show that the
purified agglutinins acted most strongly on the red cells
used for absorption, but also agglutinated other sorts of
blood. He concluded that "if one assumes that normal serum
contains a sufficient number of agglutinins, each reacting
with a certain proportion of all bloods, a given sort of
blood will absorb from a serum all those agglutinins for
which it has affinity and there will remain after absorption
some that react with freshly added blood of other species...
One may conjecture that there exists a much greater variety
of globulin molecules in a serum than would appear from
physicochemical examination, some of which by virtue of
accidental affinity to certain substrates are picked out as
antibodies".

The preceding conclusion of Landsteiner attributed the
specificity of natural antibodies to unique combinations of
natural globulins. An extension of this concept to
include immune antibodies might have seemed likely, because
of the similarity of Landsteiner's own results with
synthetic haptenes to those of Malkoff with natural
agglutinins (see Tables 1 and 2). However, Landsteiner

rejected this concept as an explanation of the specificity of immune antibodies, apparently because of a firm conviction that immune antibodies were different from natural antibodies.

Table 1. Malkoff's results (1900)

Blood	Unab-sorbed serum	Goat serum absorbed with				
		Pigeon blood	Rabbit blood	Human blood	Pigeon and rabbit blood	Pigeon and human blood
Pigeon blood	+	0	+	+	0	0
Rabbit blood	+	+	0	+	0	+
Human blood	+	+	+	0	+	0

Table 2. Results obtained by Landsteiner and van der Scheer. Since the test antigens contained the same proteins, unrelated to the horse serum used for immunization, the protein component could not be responsible for the differential reactions. (1936)

Immune sera for m-aminobenzene sulfonic acid after absorption with	Azoproteins made from chicken serum and			
	o-Amino-benzene sulfonic acid	m-Amino-benzene sulfónic acid	m-Amino-benzene arsenic acid	m-Amino-benzoic acid
o-Aminobenzene sulfonic acid*	0	++±	±	+
o-Aminobenzene sulfonic acid†	0	+++±	±	+
m-Aminobenzene arsenic acid*	+±	˙+++	0	+
m-Aminobenzene arsenic acid†	++	++++	0	++±
m-Aminobenzoic acid*	+±	+++	±	0
m-Aminobenzoic acid†	++	++++	±	±
Unabsorbed immune serum*	++	+++±	+	++±
Unabsorbed immune serum†	+++	++++	++	++±

* After standing 1 hour at room temperature.
† After standing overnight in the icebox.

But it was Landsteiner and Chase who started the trend back to cellular studies in immunology. Landsteiner had proposed that contact sensitivity to simple chemicals was a typical immune response to a complex of the chemical and some body protein. This idea had been attacked by Strauss and Coca (1937) who performed the experiment depicted in Figure 3. They produced an isolated cuff of skin on the arm of a monkey and applied poison ivy extract to this cuff. After a few days they found that the skin of the cuff was sensitive to the extract but the rest of the body was not.

Although Strauss and Coca's results have never been adequately explained, Landsteiner was obviously skeptical of their interpretation. He set out on a series of experiments with contact sensitivity to determine if it could be due to humoral antibodies. This culminated in the report with Chase (1942) demonstrating the most unique feature of delayed hypersensitivity, its ability to be transferred only with cells.

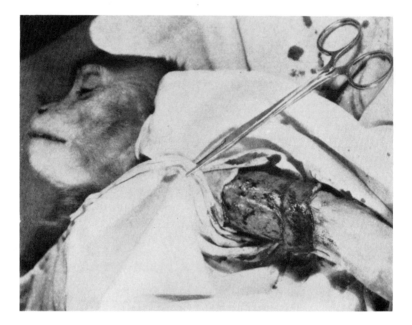

Figure 3. The mutual isolation of two areas of skin by surgical operation on the left arm of the rhesus monkey. From Strauss and Coca (1937).

Within the next few years after the Landsteiner and Chase experiment, Coons (1942) had introduced immuno-fluorescence, Fagraeus (1948) had shown that antibodies were made in plasma cells and Dixon (1951) had pioneered the use of radioactive labels in immunology. I had the privilege of working with Dixon in a roof top laboratory in St. Louis and remember our concern with the fate of antigen and its relation to the subsequent appearance of antibody.

It was at this time that Burnet and Fenner's (1949) book on Antibody Production appeared. These authors strongly attacked the current antigen template theory of antibody formation and the isolation of immunology from the mainstream of biology. They considered antibody formation analogous to adaptive enzyme synthesis in bacteria and introduced the term protein synthesizing unit (ribosomes were unknown at that time).

Burnet and Fenner's book had an obvious influence on Dixon's group as illustrated by our proposed explanation of the radiosensitive and radioresistant phases of antibody formation (Figure 4) (1952).

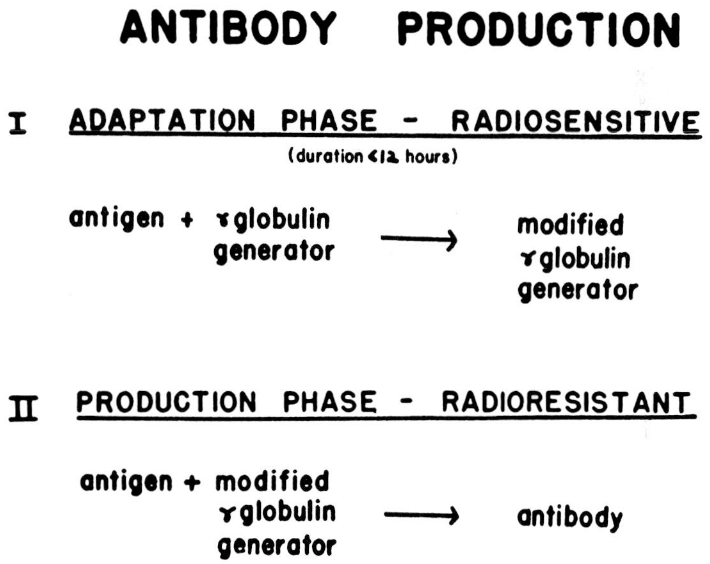

ANTIBODY PRODUCTION

I **ADAPTATION PHASE - RADIOSENSITIVE**

(duration < 12 hours)

antigen + γglobulin
generator

$\longrightarrow$

modified
γglobulin
generator

II **PRODUCTION PHASE - RADIORESISTANT**

antigen + modified
γglobulin
generator

$\longrightarrow$

antibody

Figure 4. A modification of Burnet and Fenner's globulin synthesizing unit was adopted as an explanation of the radiosensitive and radioresistant phases of antibody production in an article published by Dixon, Talmage and Maurer (1952).

The same year, 1952, I left Dixon's group and came to the University of Chicago. I was fortunate to make here a close collaboration with Tolly and Lucy Taliaferro who had independently made observations on the radiosensitive and radioresistant phases of the hemolysin response in rabbits (1952). Tolly (Figure 5) had started out as a zoologist at Hopkins and become interested in the host response to parasitic infection. He and Lucy together with numerous students and collaborators had made detailed studies of the cellular responses to trypanosome and malarial infections. They had introduced the term lymphocyte-macrophage system to indicate the cells most involved in immunity. Tolly was convinced that lymphocytes were stem cells which could differentiate into other cells such as monocytes, macrophages and plasma cells. The marked radiosensitivity of both lymphocytes and the immune response was a strong argument for the importance of lymphocytes to the immune response. I was privileged to absorb all of this cellular theory during weekly lunches in Tolly's office.

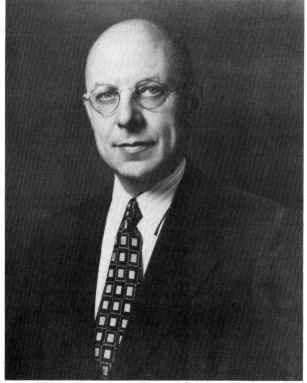

Figure 5. William Hay Taliaferro (1895-1973).

The Taliaferros had switched from studying parasites to measuring the hemolytic antibody response in rabbits to injections of sheep red cells. They had developed an accurate sensitive and quantitative assay which could be performed on a small sample of blood. This permitted them to make frequent serial bleedings on the same animal. Using this method they determined the precise length of the induction period, the logarithmic rise in antibody (1951) (Figure 6) and the log normal distribution of peak antibody titers (1954) (Figure 7). All of these seemed to fit in with Burnet and Fenner's concept of a natural protein synthesizing unit.

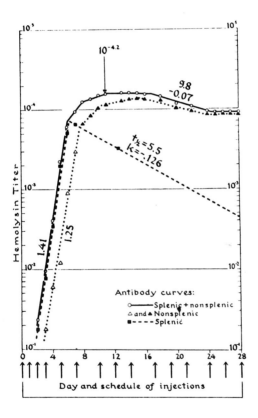

Figure 6. Mean daily hemolysin curve for 14 repeatedly injected intact rabbits and the hypothetical separation of this curve into splenic and nonsplenic antibody. From Taliaferro and Taliaferro 1951.

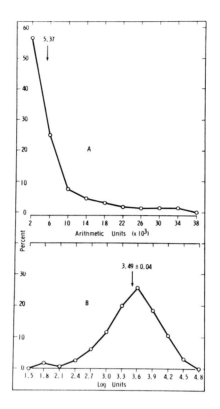

Figure 7. Frequency polygons and means of peak hemolysin titer in 164 nonirradiated rabbits after one intravenous injection of 10 sheep red cells per kg when graphed arithmetically (A) and logarithmically (B). (From Taliaferro and Taliaferro 1954 and 1964.)

Some of those who supported the antigen template theory of antibody production had suggested that anamnestic antibody responses were due to the release of preformed antibody. Tolly and I determined to test this hypothesis in a critical experiment (Taliaferro and Talmage 1955) (Figure 8). A rabbit preimmunized with bovine serum albumin (BSA) was given a second injection of BSA and over the next five days ten injections of 0.2 mc of ^{35}S labeled yeast hydrolysate. At the end of this time the spleen cells of the rabbit were synthesizing highly labeled antibody as indicated by radioactivity counts in the antigen antibody precipitates. The spleen cells of this animal were removed, washed and

injected into an unlabeled recipient. Within 2 days the
serum of the recipient rabbit contained measurable amounts
of antibody. The fact that this antibody was not labeled
indicated that antibody formed during the anamnestic response
was newly synthesized. Since only living cells could
transfer antibody synthesis in this way, the cells themselves
must contain antibody synthesizing units.

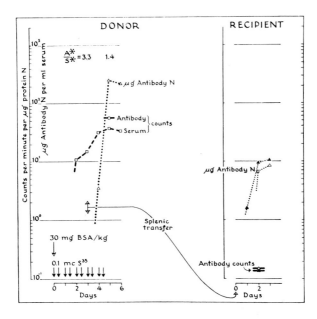

Figure 8. A comparison of the antibody formed and its
specific radioactivity in labeled donor 14 and its two
unlabeled recipients 14A and 14B. In addition, the relation
of the specific radioactivity of antibody and serum proteins
(A*/S*) are shown in the donor. From Taliaferro and
Talmage (1955).

The results of this experiment were also incompatible
with Jerne's Natural Selection Theory (1955) which came out
the same year. Jerne had postulated a large set of
natural globulins which had been diversified in some random
fashion. The function of antigen was to combine with the
globulin with which it made a chance fit, transport it into
an antibody forming cell which would then make identical
copies of the globulin presented to it.

It seemed unlikely if not impossible that protein molecules could be replicated. But it was a simple matter to substitute randomly diversified cells for randomly diversified globulin molecules and develop a cell selection theory of antibody formation. This I did in an article for the Annual Review of Medicine (Talmage 1957) in 1956 with considerable encouragement from William Taliaferro.

The following year Burnet published his first paper amplifying the cell selection concept and giving it a catchy name, Clonal Selection Theory (1957). I still prefer the name, cell selection, because it emphasizes the fact that a cell, not a clone, is the unit of selection. The word "clonal" derives from an analogy to mutant clones of bacteria. Since antibody diversity is not thought to depend on somatic mutation, the term clonal no longer seems appropriate.

When the concept of cell selection was originally advanced, the main argument used against it was that the amount of DNA present in a cell was inadequate to account for the antibody responses to the innumerable antigens in nature. As already mentioned, Burnet's solution to this problem was somatic mutation, which if present could account for an almost infinite variety of antibodies. In 1959 I suggested another solution that depended on Jenner's original observation that the specificity of immunity is not absolute.

I had been trying to separate labeled antibodies by absorbing and eluting them from an insoluble column as illustrated in Figure 9 (Talmage 1954). I was impressed with the fact that antibodies came with many avidities, some very high that were difficult to elute, others very low in avidity that were difficult to distinguish from normal globulin. Thus, antibodies appeared to be just an extreme case of the spectrum of avidities present in normal globulin (Figure 10) (Talmage 1959). Since each antigenic determinant would have a different spectrum of avidities the combination of globulins which were selected as antibodies would be different for each antigenic determinant.

Since that time the finding that immunoglobulins are made up of two chains containing variable and constant regions has greatly simplified this explanation. A more recent discovery is that the genes for the variable and constant regions are separated in the chromosome by gaps and that these are removed during cell differentiation and gene expression (Figure 11) (Talmage 1979; Weigert, Gatmaitan, Loh, Schilling, Hood 1978; Brock, Herama, Lenhard-Schuller, Tonegawa 1978; Honjo, Kataoka 1978). Thus, it is possible to say 23 years after first proposing a cell selection theory, that the genetic mechanism of cell diversity on which it depends have been well established. But the molecular mechanisms of selective cell activation and replication are poorly understood. How does combination of antigen with specific receptors on the surface of a lymphocyte lead to both an increase in antibody production and immunological memory? I believe that only after we understand and can control this cell selection will we be able to apply fully the tremendous advances in immunology to numerous human diseases such as cancer, diabetes and organ transplantation.

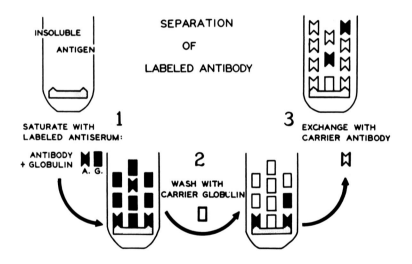

Figure 9. A diagrammatic representation of the separation of labeled antibody by exchange with unlabeled carrier antibody. From Talmage, Baker and Akeson (1954).

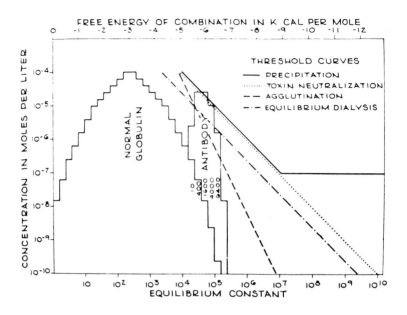

Figure 10. The relationship between antibody concentrations, the energy of combination of antigen and antibody, and the threshold required for detection. The threshold calculations are based on the Goldberg theory and the following assumptions: Agglutination involves a suspension of 10^8 particles per milliliter, each particle containing 6 x 10^5 sites; precipitation and toxin neutralization involve antigen molecules with a valence of 6 and antibody molecules with a valence of 2, and an optimal ratio of antigen to antibody; equilibrium dialysis requires the binding of at least 20 percent of the haptene in the antiserum compartment. From Talmage (1959).

DNA in Undifferentiated Cell

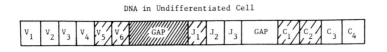

DNA in Differentiated Cell

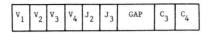

RNA as Transcribed

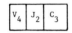

RNA as Translated

$$V_4 \quad J_2 \quad C_3$$

Figure 11. The immunoglobulin (Ig) chain is formed from a much greater number of genes than it ultimately contains by the steps shown in the diagram. Some details have not been explicitly demonstrated experimentally, in particular those dealing with excision of J genes. The dark cross-hatched areas are always excised in the next step; the light cross-hatched areas are the additional genes which were excised in the particular cell illustrated. The variability in the excision of V and J genes in the differentiation step accounts for the diversity in lymphocyte specificity. (Modified from Talmage 1979.)

References

Brock C, Herama M, Lenhard-Schuller R, Tonegawa S (1978). A complete immunoglobulin gene is created by somatic recombination. Cell 15:1.

Burnet FM (1957). A modification of Jerne's theory of antibody production using the concept of clonal selection. Aust J Science 20:67.

Burnet FM, Fenner F (1949). "Production of Antibodies." Melbourne: MacMillen.

Coons AH, Creech HJ, Jones RN, Berliner E (1942). Demonstration of pneumococcal antigen in tissues by use of fluorescent antibody. J Immunol 45:159.

Dixon FJ, Bukantz SC, Dammin GJ, Talmage DW (1951). Fate of I^{131} labelled bovine gamma globulin in rabbits. Fed Proc 10:553.

Dixon FJ, Talmage DW, Maurer PH (1952). Radiosensitive and radioresistant phases in the antibody response. J Immunol 68:693.

Ehrlich P (1900). On immunity with special reference to cell life. Proc Roy Soc London B 66:424.

Jerne NK (1955). The natural-selection theory of antibody formation. Proc Natl Acad Sci US 41:849.

Fagraeus A(1948). The plasma cellular reaction and its relation to the formation of antibodies in vitro. J Immunol 58:1.

Honjo T, Kataoka T (1978). Organization of immunoglobulin heavy chain genes and allelic deletion model. Proc Natl Acad Sci US 75:2140.

Landsteiner K (1945). "The Specificity of Serological Reactions." Cambridge, Mass: Univ. Press, p. 6.

Landsteiner K, Chase MW (1942). Experiments on the transfer of cutaneous sensitivity to simple compounds. Proc Soc Exptl Biol Med 49:688.

Landsteiner K, van der Scheer J (1936). On cross reactions of immune sera to azo proteins. J Exptl Med 63:325.

Malkoff GM (1900). Beitrag zur frage der agglutination der rathen Blutkorperchen. Deut med Wochschr 26:229.

Rosen G (1971). Jenner, Edward. In the World Book Encyclopedia 11:73, Chicago: Field Enterprises Educ. Corp.

Straus HW, Coca AF (1937). Studies in experimental hypersensitiveness in the Rhesus monkey. III. On the manner of development of the hypersensitiveness in contact dermatitis. J Immunol 33:215.

Taliaferro WH, Taliaferro LG (1951). The role of the spleen in hemolysin production in rabbits receiving multiple antigen injections. J Infect Diseases 89:143.

Taliaferro WH, Taliaferro LG (1954). Effect of X-rays on hemolysin formation following various immunization and irradiation procedures. J Infect Diseases 95:117.

Taliaferro WH, Taliaferro LG, Janssen EF (1952). The localization of X-ray injury to the initial phases of antibody response. J Infect Diseases 91:105.

Taliaferro WH, Taliaferro LG, Jaroslow BN (1964). "Radiation and Immune Mechanisms." New York & London: Academic.

Taliaferro WH, Talmge DW (1955). Absence of amino acid incorporation into antibody during the induction period. J Infect Diseases 97:88.

Talmage DW (1957). Allergy and immunology. Ann Rev Med

8:239.

Talmage DW (1959). Immunological specificity. Science 129:1643.

Talmage DW (1979). Recognition and memory in the cells of the immune system. American Scientist 67:173.

Talmage DW, Baker HR, Akeson W (1954). The separation and analysis of labelled antibodies. J Infect Diseases 94: 199.

Weigert M, Gatmaitan L, Loh E, Schilling J, Hood L (1978). Rearrangement of genetic information may produce immunoglobulin diversity. Nature 276:785.

Session V.
T and B Cell
Idiotypes

Pages 315–323, Membranes, Receptors, and the Immune Response
© 1980 Alan R. Liss, Inc., 150 Fifth Avenue, New York, NY 10011

MOUSE T CELL CLONES HAVING DEFINED IMMUNOLOGICAL FUNCTIONS.

F. W. Fitch, A. L. Glasebrook, and M. Sarmiento

The Department of Pathology and the Committee
on Immunology, The University of Chicago,
Chicago, Illinois 60637, U.S.A.

Several different approaches, some of them considered elsewhere in this volume, have been used to characterize properties of antigen receptors on T lymphocytes. Immuno- logical properties of such receptors have been inferred using anti-idiotypic antibodies obtained by immunization with antibodies (Binz et al. 1974) or with T lymphocytes (Binz and Wigzell 1975, Krammer and Eichmann 1977). Recep- tors extracted from T cells (Binz et al. 1978) or shed either spontaneously (Binz and Wigzell 1976) or after binding to insoluble antigens (Krawinkel et al. 1977) have been partially characterized using allotype specific or anti-idiotypic antisera. Interpretation of results obtained using these approaches is complicated by the heterogeneity of receptors and of antibodies used to characterize them. Antibody preparations used in reported studies almost certainly contained a mixture of antibody molecules differing in molecular class and in reactivity for antigens even though conditions were chosen to limit the range of response and absorptions were used to remove unwanted reactivities. In all cases, the T lymphocytes being studied have consisted of a heterogeneous mixture of sub-populations of cells.

It should be possible to overcome the problem of heterogeneity of antibody molecules using the hybridoma technology developed by Kohler and Milstein (1975). This methodology is being used both to provide homogeneous material for use as immunogen and to obtain monoclonal antibodies reactive with different idiotypic determi- nants. Hybridoma antibodies should answer definitively questions regarding the role of different immunoglobulin classes and the importance of particular idiotypes in the activation and suppression of specific immune responses. However, the heterogeneous nature of lymphocyte populations and the limited number of cells of any given reactivity still will hamper studies involved with the isolation and characterization of T lymphocyte receptors.

A promising approach for overcoming some of these problems of T cell heterogeneity is the development of clones of normal T lymphocytes having defined immunological functions (Fathman and Hengertner 1978, Nabholz et al. 1978, Baker et al. 1979, Glasebrook and Fitch 1979). We have been able to develop cloned lines of mouse T lymphocytes which have either amplifier or cytolytic activity. These clones, which will be described in detail elsewhere, have been derived by restimulating cells from a primary mixed leukocyte culture (MLC) (Cerottini et al. 1974) with the original stimulating alloantigen and then cloning at limit dilution in the presence of alloantigen and supernatant fluid from a secondary MLC (Ryser et al. 1978). Culture wells containing proliferating cells were screened for cytolytic activity using a ^{51}Cr-release assay (Brunner et al. 1968). Both non-cytolytic and cytolytic cells were found. Cells from selected wells were cloned again at limit dilution and then characterized further. So far, clones have been obtained from cultures prepared with C57BL/6 or A/J spleen cells reacting against irradiated DBA/2 spleen cells.

The reactivity patterns of 4 representative cytolytic clones is shown in Table 1. Two of the clones appear to be specific for antigens of the major histocompatibility complex; clone L3 is cytolytic toward target cells bearing H-2D^d antigens, while B18 is cytolytic for target cells bearing H-2K^d or H-2I^d antigens. Other clones exhibit more complex patterns of cytolytic activity. For example, C25, in addition to lysing target cells bearing H-2K^d or H-2I^d antigens, is also cytolytic for H-2^k tumor target cells but not for concanavalin A (Con A)-induced blast cells bearing H-2^k antigens. Clone G20 is cytolytic for a wide variety of target cells including rat Con A-induced blasts. A comparable spectrum of reactivity has been observed with several monoclonal rat antibodies directed against rat Ag-B alloantigens (McKearn et al. 1979).

Table 1
SPECIFICITY OF CYTOLYTIC CLONES[a]

Target cell	H-2 K I S D	Cytolytic Clones L3(B6)	B18(B6)	C25(A)	G20(B6)
P-815 tumor	d - - d	+	+	+	+
B10.D2*	d d d d	+	+	+	+
B10.A*	k k d d	+	-	-	+
AKR-A tumor	k - - k	-	-	+	+
B10.BR*	k k k k	-	-	-	+
B10.AL*	k k k d	+	-	-	N.D.[b]
B10.OH*	d d d k	-	+	+	N.D.
EL-4 tumor	b - - b	-	-	-	N.D.
RBL-5 tumor	b - - b	N.D.	N.D.	N.D.	+
Lewis rat*		-	-	+	+
BN rat*		-	-	-	+

a. Cytolytic activity was measured using a ^{51}Cr-release assay employing the indicated tumor or Con A-induced blast (*) target cells.   b. N.D. = Not done.

Other clones of cells were not cytolytic when tested with target cells bearing the stimulating alloantigen. These cells also lacked cytolytic activity when incubated with target cells in the presence of Con A using conditions shown previously to enable "non-specific" lysis by cytolytic T lymphocytes (Tartof and Fitch 1977). The nature of alloantigens stimulating proliferation of these cells was evaluated in MLC prepared with various stimulating cells. The results observed with 4 representative clones are shown in summary form in Table 2.

Proliferation of these cloned non-cytolytic cells was stimulated by spleen cells bearing the Mls determinants of the original stimulating strain regardless of the MHC haplotype. No stimulation was produced by cells bearing the MHC antigens of the original stimulating strain if they were syngeneic with the responding non-cytolytic clones at the M locus. We did not identify non-cytolytic clones which proliferate in response to MHC antigens. This may be due to the particular culture conditions which we employ. Other investigators, using these same conditions, found that the addition of I-region differences to

K-region differences did not increase the cytolytic response to H-2K antigens in MLC (Engers and MacDonald 1975).

Table 2
Specificity of MLR Responses Exhibited by
Non-cytolytic T Cell Clones[a]

Stim. Cells	Haplotype H-2	Mls	Non-cytolytic Clones (origin[b]) L2(B6)	Fal3(B6)	Fal5(B6)	Cl4(A)
DBA/2	d	a	46500	45000	33600	54500
BALB/c	d	b	3000	340	1800	78600
B10.D2	d	b	770	340	220	25000
AKR/J	k	a	47100	72400	10900	78900
CBA/J	k	d	72300	35200	38900	79000
C3H/HeJ	k	c	4400	420	1200	1100
B10.BR	k	b	1400	210	1000	8500
A/J	a	c	4400	1000	4700	1200
C57BL/6	b	b	1400	1200	1700	970

a. Non-cytolytic cloned T cells (10^4) were cultured with 10^6 irradiated spleen cells of different H-2 and Mls haplotypes in micro-well cultures for 2 to 4 days. Cultures were pulsed with 1 uCi ^{3}H-thymidine for 4 hours and then collected onto filter paper strips for counting. Peak values for ^{3}H-thymidine incorporation are expressed as mean d.p.m. for triplicate cultures.
b. B6= C57BL/6, H-2^b, Mls^b; A= A/J, H-2^a, Mls^c

All cytolytic and non-cytolytic clones bear Thy-1.2 antigens. The cytolytic lines tested so far bear Lyt-2.2 antigen; some but not all non-cytolytic lines bear Lyt-1.2 antigen. The antisera used for determining the Lyt phenotype of these cells were provided by Dr. Harvey Cantor.

Culture conditions necessary for proliferation were different for the cytolytic and non-cytolytic clones (Table 3). Non-cytolytic clones proliferated when cultured with stimulating alloantigen alone while cytolytic clones required the addition of supernatant fluid from secondary murine MLC or Con A-stimulated rat spleen cells for growth. Although irradiated spleen cells in addition to supernatant fluid were required for proliferation of cytolytic clones, syngeneic cells functioned as well as allogeneic cells, suggesting that the spleen cells provided a "medium-conditioning" effect.

Table 3
Incorporation of ^{3}H-Thymidine by
Non-cytolytic and Cytolytic T Cell Clones
Cultured Under Various Conditions[a]

T Cell Clone	Factor	Medium	C57BL/6	DBA/2
Non-cytolytic clone (L2)	Medium	200	1100	7500
	MLC SF	1100	1600*	8700
	LCA SF	560	10200	17200
Cytolytic clone (L3)	Medium	110	1000	1300
	MLC SF	920	3200*	13000
	LCA SF	700	30900	53300

a. The incorporation of ^{3}H-thymidine by non-cytolytic (L2) and cytolytic (L3) cloned T cells cultured with medium alone, or with irradiated syngeneic (C57BL/6) or allogeneic (DBA/2) spleen cells was measured in the presence of medium alone, supernatant fluid from secondary MLC (MLC SF) or supernatant fluid from Con A-stimulated Lewis rat spleen cells (LCA SF). Values are mean d.p.m. averaged from results of 12 different experiments except for values indicated by * which are the means of 2 different experiments.

Although cytolytic activity was not observed when either type of cloned cell was cultured with stimulating alloantigen, culture of both types of clones together with alloantigen resulted in generation of high levels of cytolytic activity (Table 4). Amplification of the expression of cytolytic activity did not require direct cellular interaction between the non-cytolytic and cytolytic clones. When non-cytolytic clones were cultured with alloantigen in the lower part of a Marbrook chamber, cytolytic clones in the upper chamber proliferated with an associated increase in cytolytic activity.

In order to study cell surface polypeptides of cloned cytolytic and non-cytolytic (amplifier) T cells, the cells were labeled with ^{125}I using the lactoperoxidase-glucose

Table 4
Cytolytic Activity Generated in Marbrook Chambers[a]

Culture Number	Cells in Lower chamber	Upper chamber	Lytic Units / Chamber
1	L2+L3+DBA/2		185
		None	0
2	L3+DBA/2		3
		DBA/2	0
3	L3+DBA/2		135
		L2+DBA/2	0
4	L2+DBA/2		0
		L3+DBA/2	65

a. Cultures were established in Marbrook chambers prepared with membrane filters having 0.2 micron pore size. Cytolytic activity was measured in both upper and lower chambers after 5 days of culture.

oxidase technique (Hubbard and Cohn 1972), and Nonidet P-40 (NP-40) extracts were analyzed on SDS-polyacrylamide gels (Sarmiento et al. 1980). Figure 1 shows an autoradiograph of the radioiodinated cell surface polypeptides obtained from cytolytic clones L3 and B18, non-cytolytic (amplifier) clones Fal3 and Fa 15, and C57BL/6 anti-DBA/2 MLC cells. The clones exhibit band patterns which are distinct from those of MLC cells. These differences are most evident in the high molecular weight region - 159,000 to 205,000 daltons.

The cytolytic clones L3 and B18 appear to have similar polypeptide profiles. The profiles of non-cytolytic clones Fal3 and Fal5, however, are different from each other and from those of the cytolytic clones. The cell surface polypeptide profile represented by L3 and B18 is characteristic of all cytolytic clones isolated from C57BL/6 mice (Sarmiento et al. 1980). Non-cytolytic clones, however, appear to exhibit broad variability in their cell surface polypeptides. The cloned T cells have profiles that are distinct from those of more heterogeneous populations such as MLC cells.

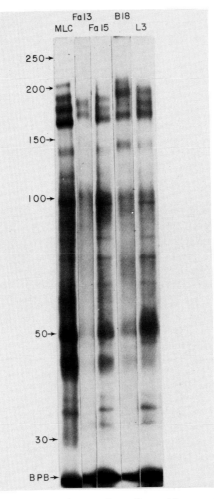

Figure 1. Autoradiograph of cell surface iodinated polypeptides obtained from C57BL/6 cytolytic clones L3 and B18, non-cytolytic (amplifier) clones Fa13 and Fa15, and unidirectional secondary C57BL/6 anti-DBA/2 MLC cells as analyzed on a 24 cm, 8 1/2% polyacrylamide slab gel crosslinked with DATD. Molecular weight scale indicated was determined by electrophoresis of known standards. BPB= position of bromphenol blue dye front.

Thus, we have been able to develop clones of cytolytic and non-cytolytic mouse T lymphocytes which bear Thy-1 antigens. The non-cytolytic clones, some of which bear Lyt-1 antigen, proliferate in response to alloantigens specified by the M locus and secrete a soluble factor that enables cytolytic clones to proliferate. Cytolytic clones, which bear Lyt-2 antigen, proliferate when exposed to supernatant factors obtained from activated lymphocytes. "Feeder cells" are required for both types of cells to proliferate. The availability of cloned murine T lymphocytes having different immunological functions should facilitate the characterization of antigen receptors on these cells.

References

Baker PE, Gillis S, Smith KA (1979). Monoclonal cytolytic T-cell lines. J Exp Med 149:273.

Binz H, Lindenmann J, Wigzell H (1974). Cell bound receptors for alloantigens on normal lymphocytes. I. Characterization of receptor-carrying cells by the use of antibodies to alloantibodies. J Exp Med 139:877.

Binz H, Wigzell H (1975). Shared idiotypic determinants on B and T lymphocytes reactive against the same antigenic determinants. I. Demonstration of similar or identical idiotypes on IgG molecules and T cell receptors with specificity for the same alloantigens. J Exp Med 142:197.

Binz H, Wigzell H (1976). Shared idiotypic determinants on B and T lymphocytes reactive against the same antigenic determinant. V. Biochemical and serological characteristics of naturally occuring, soluble antigen-binding T-lymphocyte-derived molecules. Scand J Immunol 5:559.

Binz H, Fischknecht H, Mercolli C, Wigzell H (1978). Partial characterization of cell surface idiotypes on alloantigen-activated T Lymphocytes. Scand J Immunol 7:481.

Brunner KT, Mauel J, Cerottini J-C, Chapuis B (1968). Quantitative assay of the lytic action of immune lymphoid cells on ^{51}Cr labeled allogeneic target cells in vitro. Inhibition by isoantibody and by drugs. Immunology 14:181.

Cerottini J-C, Engers HD, MacDonald HR, Brunner KT (1974). Generation of cytotoxic T lymphocytes in vitro. I. Response of normal and immune spleen cells in mixed leukocyte culture. J Exp Med 140:703.

Fathman CG, Hengartner H (1978). Clones of alloreactive T cells. Nature 272:617.

Glasebrook AL, Fitch FW (1979). T cell lines which cooperate in the generation of specific cytolytic activity. Nature 278:171.

Hubbard AL, Cohn ZA (1972). The enzymatic iodination of the red cell membrane. J Cell Biol 55:390.

Kohler G, Milstein C (1975). Continuous cultures of fused cells secreting antibodies of predefined specificities. Nature 265:495.

Krammer PH, Eichmann K (1977). T cell receptor idiotypes are controlled by genes in the heavy chain linkage group and the major histocompatibility complex. Nature 270:733.

Krawinkel U, Cramer M, Berek C, Hammerling G, Black SJ, Rajewsky K, Eichmann K (1976). On the structure of the T-cell receptor for antigen. Cold Spring Harbor Symp Quant Biol 41:285.

McKearn TJ, Fitch FW, Smilek DE, Sarmiento M, Stuart FP (1979). Properties of rat anti-MHC antibodies produced by cloned rat-mouse hybridomas. Immunol Rev 47 (In press).

Nabholz M, Engers HD, Collavo D, North M (1978). Clonal T-cell lines with specific cytolytic activity. Curr Topics Microbiol Immunol 81:176.

Ryser J-C, Cerottini J-C, Brunner KT (1978). Generation of cytolytic T lymphocytes in vitro. IX. Induction of secondary CTL responses in primary long-term MLC by supernatants from secondary MLC. J Immunol 120:370.

Sarmiento M, Glasebrook AL, Fitch FW (1980). Cell surface polypeptides of murine T cell clones expressing either cytolytic or amplifier activities. Proc Nat Acad Sci (In press).

Tartof D, Fitch FW (1977). Immunologically specific cytolytic activity induced in long-term mixed leukocyte culture cells by Concanavalin A. J Immunol 118:35.

Pages 325—344, Membranes, Receptors, and the Immune Response
© 1980 Alan R. Liss, Inc., 150 Fifth Avenue, New York, NY 10011

ANTIGEN-BINDING MYELOMA CELLS:
MONOCLONAL MODELS OF B CELL DIFFERENTIATION

R.G. Lynch, J.W. Rohrer, H.M. Gebel, B.F. Odermatt,
R.G. Hoover, G.L. Milburn, and R. Mordhorst
Department of Pathology, and Division of Biology
and Biomedical Sciences, Wash. Univ. Sch. Med.
660 So. Euclid Avenue, St. Louis, MO 63110

INTRODUCTION

Antibody-secreting cells are the differentiated progeny of non-secreting lymphocytic precursors that produce small quantities of antibody that is incorporated into the surface membrane. The surface membrane-localized immunoglobulin functions as: i) an antigen-specific receptor, and ii) a clone-specific receptor for anti-idiotypic immunoregulatory signals.

Although a great deal has been learned about some of the determinants that influence the differentiation of pre-secretory lymphocytes to antibody-secreting cells, certain limitations have been imposed on this analysis because: i) most antigen-induced B cell responses are clonally hetero-geneous, and ii) most studies have employed immune cell samples, such as spleen cells, in which the specifically responding B cells account for only a small fraction of the total sample analyzed. Because purified, clonally homo-geneous antibody-producing cells have not been available for study, many fundamental questions about the regulation of B cells have remained unanswered. An analogous impasse existed in the study of antibody molecules until the discovery that myeloma proteins were, in fact, monoclonal antibodies (Eisen et al., 1967).

Since myeloma proteins had proven to be such powerful tools for the study of antibodies we conducted studies to explore whether myeloma cells might provide useful models for the study of antibody-producing cells. Most of our studies have employed MOPC-315 which is: i) a mineral oil-induced plasmacytoma of BALB/c mice (Eisen et al., 1968); ii) a monoclonal B cell neoplasm that differentiates during in vivo growth in a fashion that mimics normal B cell differentiation (Rohrer et al., 1977); and iii) an IgA-producing tumor in which the surface membrane-associated immunoglobulin can function as a physiologically relevant receptor for TNP-antigens (Rohrer and Lynch, 1977, 1978) and anti-idiotypic effectors (Rohrer et al., 1979).

We recently reviewed most of our studies on the immunoregulation of MOPC-315 (Lynch et al., 1979) and the material to be discussed presently will limit its focus to three major points: i) MOPC-315 growth and differentiation can be regulated by host immune responses directed to the idiotypic antigens present on the surface membrane of the myeloma cells; ii) MOPC-315 growth and differentiation can be regulated by host immune responses directed to antigenic structures located on carriers that present TNP to the TNP-receptors on the surface of the myeloma cells; and iii) mice with established MOPC-315 tumors develop large numbers of circulating T lymphocytes that bear TNP receptors and M315 idiotypic antigens. Although a great deal of effort will be required before the cellular and molecular mechanisms of myeloma cell regulation are completely understood, it seems reasonable from the results thus far to anticipate that hapten-specific myeloma cells will provide unique, relevant and productive models with which to analyze the mechanisms of B cell regulation.

MOPC-315 CELLS ARE RESPONSIVE TO ANTI-IDIOTYPIC IMMUNOREGULATORY SIGNALS

BALB/c mice immunized with M315, the purified immunoglobulin produced by MOPC-315 cells, develop: 1) Idiotype-specific (a-Id^{315}) antibodies (Sirisinha and Eisen, 1971); ii) Idiotype-specific blockade of M315 secretion by MOPC-315 cells (Rohrer et al., 1979); and iii) Idiotype-specific transplantation resistance to challenge with myeloma cells (Lynch et al., 1972). Likewise, BALB/c mice immunized with M460 (another TNP-binding IgA produced by MOPC-460 cells) develop antibodies (Sirisinha and Eisen, 1971), transplantation resistance (Lynch et al., 1972) and secretory blockade (Rohrer et al., 1979) which are all specific for the idiotypic antigens expressed on M460. There is no cross-reactivity between anti-Id^{315} and anti-Id^{460} effectors.

A substantial body of evidence indicates that each of the effects induced by immunization with isologous myeloma protein reflects the activity of a separate lymphoid cell population.

Characteristics and Functional Significance of Anti-Idiotypic Antibodies

Anti-Id^{315} antibodies are the products of an oligoclonal B cell response (Odermatt et al., 1978). The majority of these antibodies are directed to antigenic determinants located in or near the TNP-binding sites of M315 (Lynch et al., 1972; Odermatt et al., 1978), and a minority of the antibodies appear to be directed to framework determinants. Greater than 90% of BALB/c anti-Id^{315} antibodies belong to the non-complement-fixing IgG$_1$ subclass (Frikke et al., 1977). Anti-Id^{315} antibodies bind in vivo (Rohrer et al., 1979) and in vitro (Milburn and Lynch, unpublished data) to surface membrane M315 on MOPC-315 cells and mediate a reversible clearance of M315 from the cell surface. In vitro, affinity-purified anti-Id^{315} antibodies (even when they are continuously present for up to three weeks) do not affect M315 secretion by MOPC-315 cells, are not cytotoxic, and do not influence the growth of MOPC-315 cells (Milburn and Lynch, unpublished data). Id^{315}-specific myeloma transplantation resistance is not passively transferred with serum from Id^{315}-immunized donors if the serum is given at the time of MOPC-315 cell challenge (Frikke et al., 1977). Collectively, these findings indicate that when the M315 idiotypes on the surface of MOPC-315 cells are engaged by BALB/c anti-Id^{315} antibodies, the only obvious effect is a reversible clearance of M315 from the cell surface membrane.

Idiotype-Specific Blockade of M315 Secretion

In contrast, when the M315 idiotypes on the surface of MOPC-315 cells are engaged by Id^{315}-specific products produced by T cells in Id^{315}-immunized mice the outcome is a reversible blockade of M315 secretion (Rohrer et al., 1979). That the secretory blockade is mediated by Id^{315}-specific T cell products rather than anti-Id^{315} antibodies is based on the following observations: i) Secretory blockade can be adoptively transferred to normal BALB/c mice with spleen cells from Id^{315}-immune donors and the transfer is abrogated by depletion of T cells with anti-θ serum plus complement (Rohrer et al., 1979); ii) M315 secretory blockade is mediated across the 0.1 μ pores of peritoneal diffusion chambers that contain MOPC-315 cells (Rohrer et al., 1979); iii) Secretory blockade in adoptively immunized hosts occurs in the absence of anti-Id^{315} antibody (Rohrer et al., 1979); and iv) Affinity-purified BALB/c anti-Id^{315} antibodies do not influence M315 secretion by MOPC-315 cells in vitro (Milburn and Lynch, unpublished data).

When MOPC-315 cells are blocked from secreting M315 in vivo they do not differ from control cells in their rates of growth or differentiation from lymphocytoid to plasmacytoid myeloma cells (Rohrer et al., 1978). Secretory blockade is reversed in vitro after exposure of the blocked myeloma cells to pronase. If blocked MOPC-315 cells continued to synthesize M315 at a normal rate it would be expected that the cells would accumulate large amounts of immunoglobulin that might result in the formation of Russell bodies or other cytoplasmic inclusions, or a decrease in cell growth and viability. Our failure to detect any of these changes in blocked MOPC-315 cells suggests that secretory blockade is accompanied by a down-regulation of M315 synthesis or an increase in its intracellular degradation. In contrast to TNP-antigen specific regulation of MOPC-315 by T cells (vide infra) secretory blockade appears to be: i) macrophage-independent, and ii) effected at the level of the actual secretory myeloma cells. If T cell-mediated idiotype-specific secretory blockade is an expression in myeloma cells of a component of the response repertoire of normal B cells then some forms of B cell tolerance and clonal suppression might be mediated at the level of the immunoglobulin-secreting cell.

Immunoglobulin Idiotypes Can Function as Transplantation Antigens

The third prominent effect induced in BALB/c mice by immunization with purified M315 is a resistance to transplantation with myeloma cells that express the M315 idiotypes (Lynch et al., 1972). The degree of transplantation resistance is modest when mice are challenged subcutaneously but is considerable when the challenge is systemic (Daley et al., 1978a). Idiotype-specific tumor immunity has been reported for a number of BALB/c myelomas (Meinke et al., 1974); Eisen et al., 1975) and for IgM-producing murine lymphomas (Sugai et al., 1975; Haughton et al., 1978).

Our original finding that a myeloma protein could function as a transplantation antigen (Lynch et al., 1972) was somewhat of a paradox. Even though Hannestad et al. (1972) showed that murine myeloma cells had surface membrane immunoglobulin and suggested that its presence at the cell surface created a potential target for immune effectors, it nonetheless was surprising that the secreted myeloma protein did not rapidly neutralize the cellular and/or humoral effectors that mediated the idiotype-specific tumor immunity. Early attempts to identify the mechanism of idiotype-specific tumor immunity were uniformly unsuccessful. Since the specificity of the induced antibodies and the transplantation resistance were identical, studies were carried out to determine if there was any relationship between serum anti-idiotypic antibodies and myeloma graft resistance. Frikke et al. (1977) failed to observe a constant relationship between the quantity of anti-Id^{315} antibody induced and the degree of resistance to MOPC-315 challenge. Furthermore, tumor immunity could not be related to a qualitative feature of the anti-Id^{315} antibody response and protection from MOPC-315 challenge. In the studies of Frikke et al. (1977) passive transfer of anti-Id^{315} sera did not protect recipients from MOPC-315 challenge. Moreover, neither sera nor spleen cells from M315-immunized mice were cytotoxic for MOPC-315 cells in vitro (Freedman et al., 1976).

The early failure to incriminate either Id^{315}-specific antibodies or cells in the mechanism of protection from MOPC-315 cells, reflected in part at least, the failure to consider that immunoregulation, rather than conventional tumor immunity, might play a fundamental role. Although the mechanism of idiotype-specific tumor immunity is still not totally established two findings suggest an immunoregulatory mechanism: i) tumor immunity is rapidly abrogated by post-immunization thymectomy (Daley et al., 1978b); and ii) MOPC-315 cells are responsive to some host immunoregulatory signals (vide infra).

Potential Relevance of Idiotype-Specific Regulation of MOPC-315 to the Regulation of Normal B Cells

The immunological consequences of immunization of BALB/c mice with the BALB/c immunoglobulin M315 are listed in Table 1. It is clear that host T cells and B cells can be induced to produce effectors which specifically recognize idiotypic antigens on M315. Although each of these effectors are

TABLE 1

IMMUNOLOGICAL CONSEQUENCES OF IMMUNIZATION OF BALB/c MICE WITH THE PURIFIED IgAϕ_2

ANTI-TNP ANTIBODY PRODUCED BY MOPC-315

	EFFECT	MECHANISM
1)	Id^{315}-specific tumor immunity (PNAS $\underline{69}$:1540, 1972)	Complex, involves T cells and B cells, rapidly abrogated by post-immunization thymectomy
2)	Id^{315}-specific "modulation" of surface immunoglobulin on myeloma cells	Anti-Id^{315} antibodies from an oligo-clonal B cell response, that is predominantly IgG$_1$
3)	Id^{315}-specific blockade of immuno-globulin secretion by MOPC-315 cells (JI $\underline{122}$:2011, 1979)	Id^{315}-specific T cells (products) that appear to act directly upon secretory MOPC-315 cells

targeted to the same region of the same surface membrane molecule (M315) a multiplicity of independent effects are observed, viz., suppression of clonal expansion, modulation of surface membrane immunoglobulin, and inhibition of immunoglobulin secretion. If one ignored for the moment that MOPC-315 is a malignant neoplasm and considered it only as a clone of anti-TNP B cells, the three different idiotype-specific effects provide three separate mechanisms that could result in the failure of a TNP-antigen to induce serum anti-TNP antibodies or anti-TNP plaque-forming cells. Although demonstration of a regulatory effect in a myeloma cell does not establish that the effect has a counterpart in normal B cells, observations made with myeloma cells may tell us how, where and when to examine normal B cells for effects that have previously escaped detection.

MOPC-315 CELLS ARE ANTIGEN SENSITIVE

MOPC-315 cells enclosed in peritoneal diffusion chambers differentiate during in vivo growth (Rohrer et al., 1977). Morphologically and functionally MOPC-315 differentiation mimics antigen-induced differentiation of normal B cells (Williamson et al., 1976). These similarities prompted us to assess whether MOPC-315 cells would respond to TNP-antigens. The experimental protocol utilized is summarized as follows: i) The immunization procedure of Chan and Henry (1976) was used to induce helper or suppressor T cells specific for sheep red blood cells; ii) TNP-derivitized sheep red blood cells were mixed with MOPC-315 cells and implanted in peritoneal diffusion chambers into the sheep red cell-primed mice; and iii) MOPC-315 cells were recovered sequentially and assayed for growth, TNP-binding cells, and anti-TNP secretory cells.

We observed that MOPC-315 growth and differentiation were enhanced when the myeloma cells were implanted with TNP-SRBC into mice in whom SRBC-specific helper T cells had previously been induced, and were suppressed in mice with SRBC-specific suppressor T cells (Rohrer and Lynch, 1977). Both the help and suppression of MOPC-315 were carrier-specific. Regulatory effects were observed when MOPC-315 cells were mixed with TNP-SRBC and implanted into mice having SRBC-specific regulatory T cells, or were mixed with TNP-RRBC and implanted into mice having RRBC-specific regulatory T cells. The criss-cross experiment did not result in MOPC-315 regulation, i.e., TNP-RRBC did not work in SRBC-primed mice and TNP-SRBC did not work in RRBC-primed mice. It is emphasized that the effects observed were alterations in the pattern of MOPC-315 cell growth and differentiation that occurs in normal hosts. It is clear that MOPC-315 cells survive, proliferate and differentiate when implanted into normal recipients. The effects of carrier-specific help and suppression are to modify the growth and differentiation that are already occurring.

As was observed by Mitchison (1971) in his classic studies of the carrier-effect we also found that carrier-specific regulation of myeloma cells required that the hapten be presented to the B cell by the same carrier that had induced the regulatory T cells (Rohrer and Lynch, 1977). Whereas regulatory effects were observed when TNP-SRBC were mixed with MOPC-315 cells in SRBC-primed mice, regulatory effects did not occur in SRBC-primed mice when TNP was presented on mouse erythrocytes (TNP-MRBC) with non-haptenated SRBC also present in the diffusion chamber. These findings implied that MOPC-315 regulation required an intimate association between carrier-specific effector, carrier, hapten, and hapten-binding sites on the MOPC-315 cell surface.

In subsequent studies we observed (Rohrer and Lynch, 1978) that carrier-specific regulation of MOPC-315 could be adoptively transferred to normal mice with nylon-wool column-purified T cells from carrier-primed donors, and that the adoptive transfer was abrogated by treatment of the donor cells with heterologous anti-Θ serum plus complement. The helper and suppressor T cells that regulate MOPC-315 appear to be distinct T cell populations. Using an adoptive transfer protocol we have observed that carrier-primed T cells given 1100 r γ-irradiation in vitro prior to transfer to normal mice still transferred help but no longer transferred suppression. In fact, irradiation of cells from suppressor donors eliminated the suppressor activity and resulted in the transfer of some help. These findings indicate that induction of carrier-specific T helper activity with 4×10^8 SRBC actually is accompanied by the induction of both helper and suppressor T cells, but the net regulatory activity that results is help. Conversely, immunization with 4×10^6 SRBC induces both helper and suppressor T cells but in this case suppression is dominant. The effects observed following γ-irradiation of the carrier-primed T cells results from the sensitivity of suppressor T cells and the insensitivity of helper T cells to irradiation. In other studies we have observed that the regulatory T cells and their precursors show the same patterns of sensitivity and resistance to hydrocortisone as has been found for T cells that regulate non-neoplastic antibody-producing cells. Collectively, these studies indicate that myeloma cell regulation is mediated by the normal immunoregulatory apparatus of the host.

Although purified T cells from carrier-primed donors are necessary and sufficient for adoptive transfer of MOPC-315 regulation to normal hosts, there is an additional requirement for macrophages to be present inside the diffusion chamber with the MOPC-315 cells and the TNP carrier (Rohrer and Lynch, 1978). When the macrophages that contaminate MOPC-315 ascites are depleted, diffusion chamber-enclosed MOPC-315 cells survive and behave as in normal hosts, but carrier-specific regulation does not occur. In preliminary studies we have observed a requirement for histocompatibility between the regulatory T cells and macrophages. Since the regulatory effects occur across the 0.1 μ pore diffusion chamber membrane it seems likely that a carrier-specific T cell product plays a major role. The T cell product could be a soluble factor or T cell vesicles that can penetrate the diffusion chamber pores. The requirement for histocompatibility between T cells and macrophages favors the view that macrophages do more than simply digest the TNP-antigen, and implies that the macrophage, or macrophage product, interacts with the T cell product.

One of the effects mediated by carrier-specific regulatory T cells is regulation of M315 secretion by MOPC-315 cells. As was discussed earlier M315 secretion is also regulated by Id^{315}-specific T cells (Rohrer et al., 1979). Since each of the effectors that regulate M315 secretion appear to involve an interaction with MOPC-315 cells via the variable regions of surface membrane M315 we carried out studies to examine the effect of simultaneous presentation of multiple immunoregulatory signals (Lynch et al., 1979). MOPC-315 cells that were presented with both a carrier-specific helper T cell signal and an Id^{315}-specific suppressor T cell signal showed an increased frequency of M315 secretory cells, but the cells were blocked from releasing M315 until they were treated with pronase. Therefore, the carrier-specific T cell signal did not influence Id^{315}-specific T cell signal (and vice versa) even though both signals engaged

MOPC-315 cells via the surface membrane M315 variable regions. In contrast, the carrier-specific suppressor T cell signal totally prevented expression of the Id^{315}-specific suppressor T cell-mediated secretory blockade. We have interpreted the results of these experments to mean that carrier-specific regulatory T cells affect M315 secretion by regulating the rate of progression of pre-secretory cells to the secretory stage, whereas Id^{315}-specific secretory blockade is effected at the level of the actual secretory cell.

The multiplicity and diversity of effects that may follow engagement of the variable regions of surface membrane M315 either through their idiotypic antigens or their TNP binding sites suggests that engagement per se does not dictate the character of the effect or even that a measurable effect will occur (TNP-SRBC alone has no overt effect). These observations suggest that the quality and intensity of the regulatory effect observed in the MOPC-315 cell is determined by: i) the effector that is captured, and ii) the suscepti- bility of the target cell to that effector at that point in the differentiation of the target cell. If this model is correct then the idiotypes and antigen-binding sites on cell surface immunoglobulin may simply function as exquisitely specific focusing devices.

M315 IDIOTYPES AND TNP RECEPTORS ON CIRCULATING LYMPHOID CELLS IN MICE WITH MOPC-315 TUMORS

In a symposium dealing with membrane receptors and immune responses it seems appropriate to briefly review our studies which have demonstrated that the TNP-binding sites and idiotypic antigens of M315 also appear on the surface of circulating lymphoid cells in mice with large MOPC-315 tumors (Gebel et al., 1979). The M315-bearing lymphoid cells are T lymphocytes, and they account for approximatey one-third of the circulating and splenic lymphocytes in mice with MOPC-315. On the basis of studies carried out in CBF_1 mice, it is clear that the T cells are derived from the host and not from the tumor. The T cell surface contains M315 constant regions ($\alpha\gamma2$) as well as M315 variable regions which suggests that the entire M315 molecule is present on the surface. The T cell surface M315 is produced by MOPC-315 cells and is passively acquired by the T cells. Preliminary studies suggest that the T lymphocytes express surface recep- tors for Fc-IgA. In normal BALB/c mice only 2-4% of T cells express surface receptors for Fc-IgA (Strober et al., 1978). Although the mechanism responsible for the increased number of Fc-IgA T cells in mice with MOPC-315 is unknown, their frequency is related to the level of M315 in the serum. It is of interest in this regard that Yodoi and Ishizaka (1979) have found increased numbers of Fc-IgE lymphocytes in rats with elevated serum levels of IgE, and Yodoi et al. (1979) have demonstrated that purified rat IgE induces rat lymphocytes in vitro to express surface membrane receptors specific for Fc-IgE. Since myeloma protein is commonly found on the surface of lymphocytes in murine and human myeloma, it may be that myeloma is accompanied by increased numbers of lymphocytes which express receptors for the isotope of the myeloma heavy chain.

There are several implications of the occurrence of TNP-receptors and M315 idiotypes on the surfaces of T lymphocytes in mice with MOPC-315:

i) Since it has been suggested (Moretta et al., 1977) that Fc receptor-bearing T cells are regulatory T cells, myeloma-bearing mice may be a rich source of regulatory T cells which can be purified on the basis of their passively acquired hapten binding sites.

ii) It provides an opportunity to experimentally determine whether passive acquisition of TNP-receptors and idiotypic antigens will render the T cells responsive to TNP-antigens and/or anti-Id^{315} antibodies.

iii) A natural consequence of the occurrence of M315 on the surface of regulatory T cells as well as MOPC-315 cells is that either anti-Id^{315} antibody, or TNP antigen could cross-link the regulatory cell and the antibody-producing cell. Studies presently underway are examining each of these issues.

CONCLUDING REMARKS

The studies reviewed here have demonstrated that MOPC-315 myeloma cells are responsive to antigen-specific and idiotype-specific immunoregulatory signals induced in the host. Perhaps it should not be surprising that the myeloma-bearing host can influence the growth and differentiation of

malignant antibody-producing cells since there already exists
in the mouse an elaborate immunoregulatory apparatus that
constantly orchestrates the expansion, contraction and
differentiation of normal B cell clones (Gershon, 1974).
Furthermore, regulation of neoplastic cells by the tumor-
bearing host is not a new concept. For example, neoplasms
that arise in endocrine target tissues (e.g., endometrium,
prostate, breast) often exhibit a pattern of hormonal
responsiveness that is characteristic of the original tissue
(Martin et al., 1979). Analogous effects have been observed
with hematopoietic neoplasms (Lotem and Sachs, 1978).
Although our studies have only employed MOPC-315 and
MOPC-460, it is clear that other B cell neoplasms are also
responsive to immunoregulatory signals (Meinke et al., 1974;
Eisen et al., 1975; Sugai et al., 1974; Haughton et al.,
1978; Manning and Jutila, 1974; Bosma and Bosma, 1977; and
Beatty et al., 1976). Furthermore, in preliminary studies
K. Schroer and P. Baker (personal communication) have made
the exciting observation that mice in whom low-zone tolerance
to pneumococcal polysaccharide SIII had been induced, were
resistant to challenge with a somatic cell hybrid clone that
produced anti-SIII antibody. Since low-zone tolerance to
SIII appears to be mediated by suppressor T cells that act
directly on B cells that produce anti-SIII antibodies
(Markham et al., 1978) it is likely that the failure of the
hybridoma to become established in low-zone tolerant mice is
one more example of specific host immunoregulation of neoplastic B cells. Finally, Fu et al. (1974) have observed
that human chronic lymphocytic leukemia cells can differentiate in vivo to plasma cells and the rate of differentiation
can be accelerated in vitro by helper T cells (Fu et al.,
1978).

We have proposed (Lynch et al., 1979) that hapten-
specific myelomas are appropriate B cell models and provide
powerful tools for the analysis of the cellular and molecular
mechanisms involved in B cell regulation. In the instance
of MOPC-315 the cells: i) are monoclonal, ii) produce an
easily purified anti-TNP antibody whose structure and binding
properties have been thoroughly characterized, iii) are
regulatable by antigen-specific and idiotype-specific
effectors, iv) differentiate during in vivo growth, v) are
readily adapted to in vitro growth, vi) have stem cells
which can be quantitated by in vivo and in vitro colony
forming assays, and vii) can be individually visualized to
determine their extent of immunoglobulin expression.

These features provide a system in which it may be possible to: i) determine the relative contributions of idiotype-specific and antigen-specific effectors to B cell regulation (Woodland and Cantor, 1978), ii) determine the developmental level of the B cell at which a given effector operates, iii) examine the molecular events that occur in the B cell coincident with and subsequent to the reception of an immunoregulatory signal, and iv) develop further understanding of immunologic circuits (Eardley et al., 1978) and networks (Jerne, 1974).

REFERENCES

Beatty PG, Kim BS, Rowley DA, Coppleson LW (1976). Antibody against the antigen receptor of a plasmacytoma prolongs survival of mice bearing the tumor. J Immunol 116:1391.

Bosma MJ, Bosma GC (1977). Prevention of IgG_{2A} production as a result of allotype-specific interaction between T and B cells. J Exp Med 145:743.

Chan EL, Henry C (1976). Coexistence of helper and suppressor activities in carrier-primed spleen cells. J Immunol 117:1132.

Daley MJ, Bridges S, Lynch RG (1978a). MOPC-315 spleen colonization: A sensitive quantitative in vivo assay for idiotype-specific immune suppression of MOPC-315. J Immunol Methods 24:47.

Daley MJ, Gebel HM, Lynch RG (1978b). Idiotype-specific transplantation resistance to MOPC-315: Abrogation by post-immunization thymectomy. J Immunol 120:1620.

Eardley DD, Haugenberger J, McVay J, Boudreau L, Shen FW, Gershon RK, Cantor H (1978). Immunoregulatory circuits among T-cell sets. I. T-helper cells induce other T-cell sets to exert feedback inhibition. J Exp Med 147:1106.

Eisen HN, Little JR, Osterland CK, Simms ES (1967). A myeloma protein with antibody activity. Cold Spring Harbor Symposia on Quantitative Biology 32:75.

Eisen HN, Simms ES, Potter M (1968). Mouse myeloma proteins with anti-hapten antibody activity. The protein produced by plasma cell tumor MOPC-315. Biochemistry 7:4126.

Eisen HN, Sakato N, Hall SJ (1975). Myeloma proteins as tumor-specific antigens. Transplant Proc 7:209.

Freedman P, Autry JR, Tokuda S, Williams RC (1976). Tumor immunity induced by pre-immunization with BALB/c mouse myeloma protein. J Natl Cancer Inst 56:735.

Frikke MJ, Bridges SH, Lynch RG (1977). Myeloma-specific antibodies: Studies of their properties and relationship to tumor immunity. J Immunol 118:2206.

Fu SM, Winchester RJ, Feizi T, Walzer PD, Kunkel HJ (1974). Idiotypic specificity of surface immunoglobulin and the maturation of leukemic bone-marrow derived lymphocytes. Proc Natl Acad Sci USA 71:4487.

Fu SM, Chiorazzi N, Kunkel HJ, Halper JP, Harris SR (1978). Induction of in vitro differentiation and immunoglobulin synthesis of human B leukemic lymphocytes. J Exp Med 148:1570.

Gebel HM, Hoover RG, Lynch RG (1979). Lymphocyte surface membrane immunoglobulin in myeloma. I. M315-bearing T lymphocytes in mice with MOPC-315. J Immunol 123:1110.

Gershon RK (1974). T cell control of antibody production. In Cooper M, Warner N (eds.): "Contemporary Topics in Immunobiology," New York: Plenum Press, 3:1.

Hannestad K, Kao MS, Eisen HN (1972). Cell-bound myeloma proteins on the surface of myeloma cells: Potential targets for the immune system. Proc Natl Acad Sci 69:2295.

Haughton G, Lanier LL, Babcock GF, Lynes MA (1978). Antigen-induced murine B cell lymphomas. II. Exploitation of the surface idiotype as tumor specific antigen. J Immunol 121:2358.

Jerne NK (1974). Towards a network theory of the immune system. Ann Immunol Inst Past 125c:373.

Lotem J, Sachs L (1978). In vivo induction of normal differentiation in myeloid leukemia cells. Proc Natl Acad Sci USA 75:3781.

Lynch RG, Graff R, Sirisinha S, Simms ES, Eisen HN (1972). Myeloma proteins as tumor-specific transplantation antigens. Proc Natl Acad Sci 69:1540.

Lynch RG, Rohrer JW, Odermatt B, Gebel HM, Autry JR, Hoover RG (1979). Immunoregulation of murine myeloma cell growth and differentiation: A monoclonal model of B cell differentiation. Immunol Rev (in press).

Markham RB, Stashak PW, Prescott B, Amsbaugh DF, Baker PJ (1978). Generation of low dose paralysis in the absence of the ability to secrete antibody. J Immunol 120:986.

Manning DD, Jutila JW (1974). Prevention of myeloma growth in BALB/c mice by injection of anti-immunoglobulin antisera. J Immunol 113:78.

Martin PM, Rolland PH, Gammerre M, Serment H, Toga, M (1979). Estradiol and progesterone receptors, histopathological examinations and clinical responses under progestin therapy. Int J Cancer 23:321.

Meinke GC, McConahey PJ, Spiegelberg HL (1974). Suppression of plasmacytoma growth in mice by immunization with myeloma proteins. Fed Proc 33:792.

Mitchison NA (1971). Carrier effects on the secondary immune response. II. Cellular cooperation. Eur J Immunol 1:18.

Moretta L, Webb SR, Grossi CE, Lydard PM, Cooper MD (1977). Functional analysis of two human T cell subpopulations: receptors for IgM or IgG. J Exp Med 146:184.

Odermatt BF, Perlmutter R, Lynch RG (1978). Molecular. heterogeneity and fine specificity of BALB/c antibodies elicited by isologous myeloma protein. Eur J Immunol 8:858.

Rohrer JW, Lynch RG (1977). Specific, immunologic regulation of differentiation of immunoglobulin expression in MOPC-315 cells during in vivo growth in diffusion chambers. J Immunol 119:2045.

Rohrer JW, Lynch RG (1978). Antigen-specific regulation of myeloma cell differentiation in vivo by carrier-specific T cell factors and macrophages. J Immunol 120:1066.

Rohrer JW, Vasa K, Lynch RG (1977). Myeloma cell immuno-globulin expression during in vivo growth in diffusion chambers: Evidence for repetitive cycles of differentiation. J Immunol 119:861.

Rohrer JW, Odermatt BO, Lynch RG (1978). Idiotype-specific suppression of MOPC-315 IgA secretion in vivo: Reversible blockade of secretory myeloma cells by soluble mediators. J Immunol 121:1799.

Rohrer JW, Odermatt B, Lynch RG (1979). Immunoregulation of murine myeloma: Isologous immunization with M315 induces idiotype-specific T cells that suppress IgA secretion by MOPC-315 cells in vivo. J Immunol 122:2011.

Sirisinha S, Eisen HN (1971). Autoimmune antibodies to the ligand binding sites of myeloma proteins. Proc Natl Acad Sci 68:3130.

Strober W, Hague NE, Lum LG, Henkart PA (1978). IgA-Fc receptors on mouse lymphoid cells. J Immunol 121:2440.

Sugai S, Palmer DW, Talal N, Witz IP (1974). Protective and cellular immune responses to idiotypic determinants on cells from a spontaneous lymphoma of NZB/NZW_{F1} mice. J Exp Med 140:1547.

Williamson AR, Zitron IM, McMichael AJ (1976). Clones of B lymphocytes: Their natural selection and expansion. Fed Proc 35:2195.

Woodland R, Cantor H (1978). Idiotype-specific T cells are required to induce idiotype-positive B memory cells to secrete antibody. Eur J Immunol 8:600.

Yodoi J, Ishizaka K (1979). Lymphocytes bearing Fc receptors for IgE. I. Presence of human and rat T lymphocytes
with Fc_ε receptors. J Immunol 122:2577.
Yodoi J, Ishizaka T, Ishizaka K (1979). Lymphocytes bearing
Fc receptors for IgE. II. Induction of Fc_ε-receptor
bearing rat lymphocytes by IgE. J Immunol 123:455.

ACKNOWLEDGEMENT

The studies reviewed here were supported by US Public
Health Service research and training grants from the National
Institutes of Health and a grant to the Department of
Pathology from the following companies: Brown & Williamson
Tobacco Corporation; Larus and Brother Company, Inc.; Liggett
& Myers, Incorporated; Lorillard, a Division of Loews
Theatres, Incorporated; Philip Morris, Incorporated; R.J.
Reynolds Tobacco Company; United States Tobacco Company; and
Tobacco Associates, Inc.

We gratefully acknowledge the excellent technical
contributions of Elizabeth Pertile and Shirley Carroll and
the skilled secretarial efforts of Diane Smerdon in the
preparation of this manuscript.

Capra: In my work with M. Cooper and S. Lawton, we
           looked at 3 patients with IgA myelomas and
           asked, "What is the origin of the antibody-
           forming cell?" We sequenced the N terminus of
           the heavy and light chains and produced an
           anti-idiotype. The anti-idiotype was absorbed
           with normal human serum and other myelomas
           matched for heavy and light chain sub-groups.
           We found large numbers of circulating B cells
           with idiotype in the bone marrow expressing the
           idiotype. Since the pre-B cell is defined as
           having cIgM and not sIg, we concluded that the
           myeloma process begins at the pre-B cell level.

Lynch: Your findings are very interesting and obviously
           add to the increasing evidence that human
           myeloma also is not simply a neoplasm of auto-
           nomous malignant plasma cells but instead each
           myeloma may consist of malignant B cells that
           are structurally and functionally heterogeneous.
           I should emphasize that in mice with MOPC-315
           there are two distinctly separate groups of
           lymphoid cells that express M315. One group
           consists of lymphocytoid myeloma cells, all of
           which have cytoplasmic M315 and some of which
           also express surface membrane M315. The surface
           membrane negative myeloma cells show a spectrum
           of intensity of cytoplasmic staining with
           fluorescein-conjugated anti-IgA and could be
           designated as pre-B myeloma cells. These cells
           may be the murine counterparts of the pre-B
           myeloma cells found in humans by Drs. Capra,
           Cooper and Lawton. The other group of lymphoid
           cells that expresses M315 are post-thymic
           lymphocytes that passively acquire M315 from
           the serum. As I pointed out, these cells are
           of host origin and are not members of the
           myeloma clone.

Coutinho: In mice bearing a MOPC-315 tumor, do you see
           PFCs of host origin of the same idiotype?

Lynch: We have not investigated this question.

Coutinho: Do secreting cells undergo division or are they
           terminally differentiated? I think it's not
           the latter, because when myeloma cells are
           grown in vitro, greater than 50% are secreting

cells and yet, we get a cloning efficiency of up to 100%.

Lynch: We don't have the answer to that question yet. Noel Warner has found that murine myelomas differ considerably from one another in: i) their stem cell frequency; ii) whether the stem cells are small or large; and iii) whether the stem cells co-sediment with secretory myeloma cells (Immunological Reviews, Volume 48, in press). Your question is an important one but I think we have to be careful not to infer too much about the in vivo situation from in vitro studies of long-passaged myeloma lines. For example, we have MOPC-315 lines with cloning efficiencies of 40-50% in soft agar, yet it takes greater than 10^6 cells to establish a tumor in normal or irradiated mice. It is also important to make a distinction between proliferating cells and clonogenic cells. I have no doubt that myeloma cells secreting antibody can divide, but I don't know whether they are able to form clones.

Cramer: Is there evidence that T cells express idiotypes, but not via the F_cR? i.e., as a consequence of passive absorption similar to human myelomas?

Lynch: We haven't seen that. All of the T cells which bear the M315 idiotype appear to passively acquire the entire M315 molecule. When the M315-bearing T cells are cultured in vitro all of them shed M315 and do not re-express it.

Bona: What is the specificity of idiotype-specific T cells? Do they react only with the V region?

Lynch: It is clear that the T cells that mediate secretory blockade are idiotype-specific but we do not yet have information on what portions of F_v^{315} are "seen" by the T cells. Jorgensen and Hannestad (Eur. J. Immunol. 7: 426, 1977) observed that Balb/c mice immunized with M315 developed Id^{315}-specific T cells, all of which were directed toward determinants located in V_L^{315}. This is provocative because we have found (Eur. J. Immunol. 8: 558, 1978) that

Id^{315}-specific B cells see binding-site
and framework determinants that are only
expressed when H^{315} and L^{315}, or Fd^{315}
and L^{315} are paired. A major difference
between the Id^{315}-specific T cells studied
by Jorgensen and those in our studies is
that their T cell is a "Mitchesonian" helper
T cell that mediates a carrier effect while
our T cell is a suppressor T cell that
appears to operate directly on secretory B
cells and does not require an adherent
accessory cell for its action.

Bhoopalam: Does the nature of the antigen have an effect
on the type of F$_c$R seen on T cells? For
example, if you give a mouse M104E or J558,
which both recognize the same antigen, do
you see T cells with F$_c$R for IgA?

Lynch: Those studies are presently in progress but
our bias is that the isotype of the myeloma
determines the specificity of the Fc receptor
on the T cell. In this regard, recent
studies from Ishizaka's laboratory may be
relevant. They have found that rats chron-
ically infected with the metazoan parasite
Nippostrongylus braziliensis develop elevated
levels of serum IgE and increased numbers of
lymphocytes with surface receptors for
Fc-IgE. The Fc-IgE receptor can be induced
in vitro by exposing normal rat spleen cells
to purified rat IgE. The induction is not
inhibited by inhibitors of DNA synthesis but
is blocked by inhibitors of RNA or protein
synthesis.

Silverstein: What is the nature of the accessory cell?
Is it a macrophage?

Lynch: The cell is probably a macrophage that
normally is present in the myeloma ascites
fluid. We do know that it is an adherent
cell. If we use MOPC-315 ascites cells
recovered from mice that were treated with
carrageenan the myeloma cells are not
responsive to antigen-specific regulatory signals but still respond to idiotype-
specific regulatory effectors.

Silverstein: Have you done an experiment with carrier-
              primed mice (say, with rabbit erythrocytes)
              and include TNP-SRBC in the diffusion
              chamber and RRBC on the outside?
Lynch: No, all we have done in that regard has been
              to add them both to the diffusion chamber.

Silverstein: Do the macrophages have F_cR or $C'R$?
Lynch: We have not looked.

Howard: Can you speculate on the mechanism that T
              cell helper effects permeate the diffusion
              chamber membrane? Why don't you put T cells
              into the diffusion chamber? Could it be
              antibody, e.g. anti-SRBC?
Lynch: We believe that the T cell helper effects
              are mediated by either soluble T cell
              products or T cell membrane fragments which
              could be derived from T cells on the outside
              of the chamber. It is certainly possible
              that intact T helper cells might gain access
              to the inside of the diffusion chamber, and
              we have not ruled out that possibility, but
              the rapidity of the effects on MOPC-315
              RFC's and PFC's suggest to us that soluble
              factors are probably involved. We do not
              put T cells in the diffusion chambers because
              we get the effects without having to do that.
              We do not know what role, if any, anti-SRBC
              antibody might play in the regulatory effects
              that occur in the myeloma cell. In our adop-
              tive transfer studies, help and suppression
              were transferred with nylon wool-purified T
              cells. Since recipients of T cells were
              implanted with diffusion chambers that
              contained TNP-SRBC in addition to MOPC-
              315 cells, it could be argued that the recip-
              ients developed anti-SRBC antibodies in
              response to TNP-SRBC that escaped from the
              chamber. Even though this might occur, the
              important observation is that the donor T
              cells determined the quality of the effect
              (i.e., help or suppression) regardless of
              anti-SRBC antibodies.

Pages 345–358, Membranes, Receptors, and the Immune Response
© 1980 Alan R. Liss, Inc., 150 Fifth Avenue, New York, NY 10011

ANTIGEN-SPECIFIC RECEPTOR MOLECULES ISOLATED FROM
MURINE T LYMPHOCYTES[x]

Matthias Cramer, Ulrich Krawinkel[xx] and
Rudolf Mierau
Institute for Genetics, University of Cologne
Weyertal 121, D-5000 Cologne 41, F.R.G.

Abstract. Hapten-specific receptor material can be isolated from sensitized murine T and B lymphocytes by the use
of hapten-coupled nylon discs. The structural element shared
between T and B cell receptors is the variable region of
immunoglobulin heavy chains (V_H), while known constant immunoglobulin domains appear not to be part of the T cell receptor molecule. The rules governing V_H expression (i.e. NP^b-
idiotype expression) in the B and the T cell compartments
are, however, different. Allotype-linked V_H (idiotype) expression on T cell molecules was used in genetic reconstitution experiments to prove that the material under study is an endogenous T cell product. With the data available it seems reasonable to view the T cell molecules as representing surface
receptors for antigen although this point needs further investigation.

INTRODUCTION

T lymphocytes as immunocompetent cells are able to react
specifically to antigenic stimuli. The analyses of the key
element(s) involved in these antigen recognition processes,
namely of the T cell receptor(s) for antigen, are generally
performed by one or a combination of the four experimental
approaches listed below:

x) Supported by the Deutsche Forschungsgemeinschaft through
   Sonderforschungsbereich 74
xx) Present address: MRC Laboratory of Molecular Biology,
    Hills Road, Cambridge, CB2 2QH, U.K.

1) <u>Functional</u> studies of T-cell mediated immune responses
   (for review see Rajewsky and Eichmann 1977, Binz and Wigzell 1977, Lindahl and Rajewsky 1979).
2) <u>Serological</u> studies on the T-cell surface (for review see
   Cazenave et al. 1977, Krammer and Eichmann 1978).
3) Analysis of spontaneously arising or induced <u>thymomas</u>
   (e.g.Moseley et al. 1979, Finn et al. 1979), of continuously
   growing <u>T cell lines</u> (for review see Haas and von Boehmer
   1978) and of <u>T cell hybridomas</u> (e.g. Taniguchi et al. 1979).
4) <u>Isolation</u> and subsequent characterization of T cell receptor material (for review see Rajewsky and Eichmann 1977,
   Binz and Wigzell 1977, Lindahl and Rajewsky 1979, Cramer
   and Krawinkel 1979).

   Our approach has been the isolation and subsequent serological and immunochemical characterization of T cell receptor
material, some properties of which we shall summarize and discuss in this paper. In contrast to the indirect functional analyses of T cell responses this system offers the opportunity
to study the T cell receptor molecule directly and in solution.
We shall end our discussion by listing up our preliminary
arguments in favour of the notion that we actually deal with
molecules isolated from the T cell surface.

ISOLATION AND SEROLOGICAL ANALYSIS OF B- AND T-CELL RECEPTOR
MATERIAL

   A method originally devised by H. Kiefer for the enrichment of hapten-specific B cells (Kiefer 1973) is used to obtain receptor material from B and T cells. As described in
detail in earlier publications (Krawinkel and Rajewsky 1976,
Krawinkel et al. 1977b, Cramer and Krawinkel 1979), sensitized
spleen cells are incubated with hapten-coupled nylon discs at
4°C. Binding of B and T cells to the discs is observed. A temperature shift to 25°C or 37°C releases the cells from the
hapten-coupled nylon. Hapten-specific material can subsequently be eluted from the nylon discs (Krawinkel and Rajewkky 1976,
Krawinkel et al. 1977b) and be titrated in a sensitive haptenated bacteriophage inactivation (HPI) assay (Becker and Mäkelä
1975, Krawinkel and Rajewsky 1976).

   By the use of insolubilized polyspecific anti-mouse immunoglobulin antiserum (a-MIg) the B cell receptor material,
i.e. the fraction which is bound to a-MIg and therefore called
the anti-Ig^{+} fraction, can be separated from the T-cell mate-

rial which does not bind to a-MIg and is therefore called the anti-Ig⁻ fraction (Krawinkel and Rajewsky 1976, Krawinkel et al. 1977a, b, Cramer and Krawinkel 1979).

Detailed immunoabsorption studies demonstrated the absence of serological determinants of immunoglobulin (Ig) heavy (H) and light (L) chain constant domains on our T cell receptor material (Krawinkel and Rajewsky 1976, Krawinkel et al. 1977b, Cramer et al. 1978, Cramer and Krawinkel 1979).

Similarly, structures encoded by genes in the H-2 locus (including the I region) (Cramer et al. 1978, Cramer and Krawinkel 1979), the Qat antigen (Cramer and Krawinkel 1979) and more recently the Lyt-1, Lyt-2 and Lyt-3 antigens (data not shown) were not found to be part of the isolated T cell receptor molecule. It should be mentioned, however, that the quality and the capacity of the immunosorbents used for the analysis of these alloantigens can not be properly controlled (for a detailed discussion of this problem see Cramer and Krawinkel 1979).

V_H EXPRESSION ON ISOLATED T CELL RECEPTORS

The available data demonstrating the presence of variable regions of immunoglobulin heavy chains (V_H) on functional and isolated T cell receptors have recently been reviewed (Lindahl and Rajewsky 1979, Cramer and Krawinkel 1979). The information obtained from studies with isolated hapten-specific T cell receptor material is summarized in Table 1.

Four points deserve special attention. (1) As it is obvious from Table 1 two types of V_H-markers were tested on our anti-Ig⁻ receptor material: Binding-site related markers like the NP^b-idiotype as detected by rabbit anti-idiotypic antibodies (Krawinkel et al. 1978, Imanishi-Kari et al. 1979) and the heteroclitic fine specificity marker (Imanishi and Mäkelä 1974) on the one side and V_H-framework markers like the NP^b-idiotype as detected by guinea pig anti-idiotypic antibodies (Jack et al. 1977), the rabbit a locus allotypes (Kindt 1975) and a rabbit antiserum raised against mouse V_H (Ben-Neriah et al. 1978) on the other side. Since all these markers are found on our T cell receptor material the conclusion seems inevitable that the entire V_H region is shared between B and T cell molecules. (2) Except for the rabbit anti-mouse V_H antiserum all our serological evidence on this point can be and in fact is genetically controlled and verified (Krawinkel et al. 1977a, b, c,1978). (3) It was found that the expression of V_H in the

Table 1. Expression of entire V_H regions on isolated T cell receptor molecules

| Anti-Ig receptor material | | Designation | V_H-markers | | References |
Origin	Hapten specificity [x]		Binding-site related	Framework related	
C57BL/6	NP	NP[b] idiotype	+	+	Krawinkel et al. 1977b, 1978
C57BL/6	NP	heteroclicity	+		Krawinkel et al. 1977b
BALB/c, SJL (C57BL/6xCBA)F_2	NP	rabbit anti- [xx] mouse V_H		+	Cramer et al. 1979
rabbit	NIP, DNP, NAP	a locus-allotypes		+	Krawinkel et al. 1977a, c

x) NP: 4-hydroxy-3-nitro-phenylacetyl, NIP: 4-hydroxy-5-iodo-3-nitro-phenylacetyl
DNP: 2,4-dinitro-phenyl. NAP: 4-azido-2-nitro-phenyl

xx) In contrast to the other systems: no genetic studies performed.

response to the hapten 4-hydroxy-3-nitrophenylacetyl (NP) follows different rules in the T and B cell compartments of SJL and C57BL/6 mice. SJL mice express the NP^b idiotype at the level of isolated NP-specific T cell receptor material but lack NP^b in their B cell receptors and antibodies (Cramer et al. 1979). Furthermore, NP-specific T cell receptor material obtained from C57BL/6 lymphocytes is restricted to the expression of "early" idiotypic determinants while the B cell receptors from the same mice are representative for a "late" idiotypic spectrum (Krawinkel et al. 1978). (4) Our data do <u>not</u> yield any information about the <u>extent</u> of overlap between the B-cell V_H- and the T-cell V_H-repertoires but this question is under study.

T-CELL ORIGIN OF THE HAPTEN-SPECIFIC RECEPTOR MATERIAL

Earlier work suggested that the receptor material in the anti-Ig$^-$ fraction is isolated from T lymphocytes, because the yield of HPI activity in this fraction correlates with the T cell content of the cell preparation from which the receptor material is obtained (Krawinkel and Rajewsky 1976, Krawinkel et al. 1977a, b, c). More recently, we have shown that the isolated receptor material is an endogenous T-cell product (Krawinkel et al. 1979). The design and results of these experiments are summarized in Table 2.

Thymusless nude mice were reconstituted with histocompatible thymocytes in such a way that in the very same animal the B-cell and the T-cell compartments differed genetically with respect to Igh allotype and therefore NP^b idiotype expression (compare Table 2, for details see Krawinkel et al. 1979). After sensitization of the reconstituted nude mice their serum antibodies, the anti-Ig$^+$ receptors, and the anti-Ig$^-$ receptors were assayed for the expression of NP^b idiotype (Table 2) and heteroclicity (Krawinkel et al. 1979). NP^b idiotype was expressed exclusively in the anti-Ig$^-$ receptor material, if the T cells originated from Igh^b mice but the B cells (and therefore the serum antibodies as well) were Igh^a while the reverse is true if the T cell input is Igh^a and the B cells express Igh^b (Table 2).

Taken together with the cellular enrichment studies mentioned above these data demonstrate that the anti-Ig$^+$ receptors are a B-cell product and the anti-Ig$^-$ receptors are an endogenous T-cell product (Krawinkel et al. 1979).

Table 2. T-cell origin of anti-Ig$^-$ receptor material

Cellular constitution of reconstituted nu/nu mice	Experimental group A	Experimental group B
B cells	Igh^a, NP^b −	Igh^b, NP^b +
T cells	Igh^b, NP^b +	Igh^a, NP^b −
Anti-NP response		
serum antibody	NP^b − x)	NP^b + xx)
anti-Ig$^+$ receptor fraction	NP^b −	NP^b +
anti-Ig$^-$ receptor fraction	NP^b +	NP^b −

x) NP^b−: less than 10% of NP-specific molecules carry the NP^b idiotype

xx) NP^b+: more than 45% of NP-specific molecules carry the NP^b idiotype.

BIOCHEMICAL STUDIES

Straightforward biochemical analyses of the isolated T cell material are hampered by both the very limited amount of material available and by the impurity of the receptor preparations which contain a considerable amount of non-antigen binding protein.

Nevertheless, some biochemical properties of the T cell receptor molecule could be determined: (1) Detailed studies of the haptenated phage inactivation assay (HPI) (Becker and Mäkelä 1975) led us to conclude that the molecule should carry more than one, probably two, hapten-specific binding sites (Cramer and Krawinkel 1979). (2) Molecular weight determinations using various denaturing and non-denaturing techniques suggest a molecular weight of the complete molecule close to that of 7S IgG (Cramer, Krawinkel and Rajewsky, manuscript in preparation) and (3) in contrast to the results obtained in other systems (Binz and Wigzell 1975, Binz et al. 1978, Lea et al. 1979 and Wigzell, this volume) isolated NP-specific T cell receptor molecules are built from two types of polypeptide chains with molecular weights of 50 000 Daltons and 25 000 Daltons, respectively (M. Cramer, manuscript in preparation).

SURFACE RECEPTORS ?

Three sets of arguments suggest that our isolated T cell material may represent surface receptor molecules. Firstly, the data of V_H expression on isolated hapten-specific T cell receptor material correlate well with the findings of V_H-carrying molecules on the surface of functional T cells described in other systems (Rajewsky and Eichmann 1977, Binz and Wigzell 1977, Krammer and Eichmann 1978, Lindahl and Rajewsky 1979). It is therefore tempting to speculate that both types of molecules actually represent one and the same entity, namely the surface receptor for antigen.

The second argument comes from the technique used for receptor preparation (compare 2nd section and Kiefer 1973). Kiefer demonstrated for the case of a hapten-specific B cell that the surface Ig receptors of this cell - probably induced by antigen binding - are collected in a "cap" adjacent to the hapten-coupled nylon disc (Kiefer 1973). We think that instead of endocytosis these cells leave their surface receptor molecules

Table 3. Influence of protease inhibitor and cell viability on the preparation
of NP-specific receptor material

Lymphocytes obtained from		Normalized HPI titer[x]	
		Total receptor	anti-Ig⁻ fraction
A)			
C57BL/6 spleen cells[xx]	no Trasylol(R) o)	135	29
	Trasylol(R) added§)	9	4
B)			
(C57BL/6 x DBA/2)F₁[xx] spleen cells	67% viable	4	1.5
	96% viable	3	0.7

x) As described by Krawinkel et al. 1977b the receptor material is titrated with NIP$_8$cap T4 bacteriophages and the 50% HPI titer thus obtained is normalized for 1 ml volume and 10^8 viable lymphocytes. xx) The receptor materials described in Table 3A and Table 3B were prepared under very different sets of circumstances apart from those stated in this table. Therefore, HPI titers from Table 3A can not be compared to HPI titers from Table 3B. o) Trasylol(R) is a trade mark of Bayer AG, Leverkusen, F.R.G. and was kindly donated by the manufacturer. §) Trasylol(R) was used at a final concentration of 1 mg/ml (6600 KIU/ml) during all the procedure of receptor preparation but was omitted at the step of receptor elution from the nylon discs via free hapten. Cell viability - as judged by trypan blue exclusion - was not detectably affected by the Trasylol(R) treatment.

behind on the hapten once the cell falls off the disc (Krawinkel and Rajewsky 1976). Speculative as it may be, a very similar process could exist for T cells as well.

Thirdly, it seems unlikely that anti-Ig⁻ receptor material is somehow secreted by T cells and then absorbed by the hapten-coupled nylon discs because even the products of splenic plasma cells, the serum antibodies, are not picked up by our discs, as we have shown earlier (Krawinkel et al. 1978).

The possibility remains that the antigen-specific T cell material leaks out of ruptured or dead cells. The data shown in Table 3 seem to rule this out. When protease inhibitor is added to an aliquot of sensitized lymphocytes under conditions which do not affect cell viability, the amount of receptor material obtained is dramatically decreased as compared to an untreated aliquot (Table 3A). It seems therefore that the processes involved in the release of the receptor material from the cells are active ones rather than passive leakage of hapten-specific material from dead cells. Further evidence comes from receptor preparations obtained from aliquots of sensitized cells of different viability, i.e. different ratios of living and dead cells (Table 3B). The HPI titers of the two receptor preparations normalized for 10^8 viable lymphocytes are very similar suggesting again that the receptor material originates from living and not from dead lymphocytes (Table 3B).

Future work will have to analyse the location of the T-cell receptor molecule on the cell surface by more direct methods and in more detail.

Acknowledgements. The authors wish to thank Drs. E.A. Boyse and F.W. Shen for the gift of anti-Lyt-antisera, the Bayer AG for the generous supply of Trasylol$^{(R)}$ and Ms. C. Schenkel for expert technical help. In addition, we are grateful to Dr. K. Rajewsky for many fruitful discussions and continuing support.

REFERENCES

Becker M, Mäkelä O (1975). Modification of bacteriophage with hapten ε-aminocaproyl-N-succinimide esters, increased sensitivity for immunoassay. Immunochem 7:329.

Ben-Neriah Y, Wuilmart C, Lonai P, Givol D (1978). Preparation and characterization of anti-framework antibodies to heavy chain variable region (V_H) of mouse immunoglobulins. Eur J Immunol 8:797.

Binz H, Frischknecht H, Mercolli C, Wigzell H (1978). Partial characterization of cell surface idiotypes on alloantigen-activated T lymphoblasts. Scand J Immunol 7:481.

Binz H, Wigzell H (1976). Shared idiotypic determinants on B and T lymphocytes reactive against the same antigenic determinant. V. Biochemical and serological characteristics of naturally occuring, soluble antigen-binding T-lymphocyte derived molecules. Scand J Immunol 5:559.

Binz H, Wigzell H (1977). Antigen-binding idiotypic T-lymphocyte receptors. Contemp Top Immunobiol 7:113.

Cazenave P-A, Cavaillon JM, Bona C (1977). Idiotypic determinants on rabbit B- and T-derived lymphocytes. Immunol Rev 34:34.

Cramer M, Krawinkel U (1979) Immunochemical properties of isolated hapten-specific T cell receptor molecules. In Pernis B, Vogel HJ (eds): "Regulatory T Lymphocytes", New York: Academic Press, in press.

Cramer M, Krawinkel U, Hämmerling GJ, Black SJ, Berek C, Eichmann K, Rajewsky K (1978). Antigen receptors on mouse T lymphocytes. In McDevitt HO (ed): "Ir Genes and Ia Antigens", New York: Academic Press, p 583.

Cramer M, Krawinkel U, Melchers I, Imanishi-Kari T, Ben-Neriah Y, Givol D, Rajewsky K (1979). Isolated hapten-binding receptors of sensitized lymphocytes. IV. Expression of immunoglobulin variable regions in (4-hydroxy-3-nitrophenyl)acetyl (NP)-specific receptors isolated from murine B and T lymphocytes. Eur J Immunol 9:332.

Finn OJ, Boniver J, Kaplan HS (1979). Induction, establishment in vitro, and characterization of functional, antigen-specific, carrier-primed murine T-cell lymphomas. Proc Nat Acad Sci USA 76:4033.

Haas W, von Boehmer H (1978), Techniques for separation and selection of antigen specific lymphocytes. Curr Top Microbiol Immunobiol 84:1.

Imanishi T, Mäkelä O (1974). Inheritance of antibody specificity. I. Anti-(4-hydroxy-3-nitrophenyl)acetyl of the mouse primary response. J Exp Med 140:1498.

Imanishi-Kari T, Rajnavölgyi E, Takemori T, Jack RS, Rajesky K (1979). The effect of light chain gene expression on the inheritance of an idiotype associated with primary anti-(4-hydroxy-3-nitrophenyl)acetyl (NP) antibodies. Eur J Immunol 9:324.

Jack RS, Imanishi-Kari T, Rajewsky K (1977). Idiotypic analysis of the response of C57BL/6 mice to the 4-hydroxy-3-nitrophenylacetyl group. Eur J Immunol 7:559.

Kiefer H (1973). Binding and release of lymphocytes by hapten-derivatized nylon fibers. Eur J Immunol 3:181.

Kindt TJ (1975). Rabbit immunoglobulin allotypes: structure, immunology and genetics. Advan Immunol 21:35.

Krammer P, Eichmann K (1978). Genetic control of idiotypes of T cell receptors for antigen. Behring Inst Res Commun 62:9.

Krawinkel U, Cramer M, Berek C, Hämmerling GJ, Black SJ, Rajewsky K, Eichmann K (1977a). On the structure of the T-cell receptor for antigen. Cold Spring Harb Symp Quant Biol 41:285.

Krawinkel U, Cramer M, Imanishi-Kari T, Jack RS, Rajewsky K, Mäkelä O (1977b). Isolated hapten-binding receptors of sensitized lymphocytes. I. Receptors from nylon-wool enriched mouse T lymphocytes lack serological markers of immunoglobulin constant domains but express heavy chain variable portions. Eur J Immunol 7:566.

Krawinkel U, Cramer M, Kindred B, Rajewsky K (1979). Isolated hapten-binding receptors of sensitized lymphocytes. V. Cellular origin of receptor molecules. Eur J Immunol 9: in press.

Krawinkel U, Cramer M, Mage RG, Kelus AS, Rajewsky K (1977c). Isolated hapten-binding receptors of sensitized lymphocytes. II. Receptors from nylon wool-enriched rabbit T lymphocytes lack serological determinants of immunoglobulin constant domains but carry the a locus allotypic markers. J Exp Med 146:792.

Krawinkel U, Cramer M, Melchers I, Imanishi-Kari T, Rajewsky K (1978). Isolated hapten-binding receptors of sensitized lymphocytes. III. Evidence for idiotypic restriction of T-cell receptors. J Exp Med 147:1341.

Krawinkel U, Rajewsky K (1976). Specific enrichment of antigen-binding receptors from sensitized murine lymphocytes Eur J Immunol 6:529.

Lea T, Förre ÖT, Michaelsen TE, Natwig JB (1979). Shared idiotypes on human peripheral blood B and T lymphocytes. J Immunol 122:2413.

Lindahl KF, Rajewsky K (1979). T cell recognition: genes, molecules, and functions. In Lennox ES (ed): "International Review of Biochemistry, Defense and Recognition, IIA, Cellular Aspects", Baltimore: University Park Press, 22:97.

Moseley JM, Beatty EA, Marchalonis JJ (1979). Molecular properties of T-lymphoma immunoglobulin. II. Peptide composition of the light chain. J Immunogen 6:19.

Rajewsky K, Eichmann K (1977). Antigen receptors of T helper cells. Contemp Top Immunobiol 7:69.

Taniguchi T, Saito T, Tada T (1979). Antigen-specific suppressive factor produced by a transplantable I-J bearing T-cell hybridoma. Nature 278:555.

Cosenza: We used Claflin and Davies' PC-binding site-specific antibody to label T cells. It was a rabbit antibody and we used fluorescent goat anti-rabbit to detect T cells with the idiotype, but we saw no fluorescence. However, we could enrich the T cells for 95% PC-specific Th using the fluorescence activated cell sorter. The receptor most likely has heavy chain and light chain equivalent variable regions because the PC-binding site requires heavy and light chains. If the smaller chain you describe is not a light chain, what is it?

Cramer: The L chain of the T cell,receptor definitely is not Ig, since there are no kappa or lambda determinants. The combining site is questionable. The size of the T cell receptor light chain is similar but not identical to the L chain of Ig.

Hood: Does not the receptor have to have V-lambda variable region?

Cramer: Yes. The combining site of the T cell receptor carries a variable region. Determinants seen by anti-idiotype sera are made up of both V-lambda and V_H chain in the NP system, but I don't know to what extent. It is possible that 98% of the idiotype determinants are not on the L chain, and only see 2% in this case.

Nisonoff: Green found that anti-idiotype sera suppressed delayed hypersensitivity to arsenate. The arsenate T_S activity is absorbed by anti-idiotype.

Hood: Can't you do peptide maps of T cell light chains and B cell light chains and look for differences?

Cramer: We tried to do this without success because the amounts of material we have to work with are too small. What we did try was to see if two chains are needed to make the binding site.

Sarmiento: Have you done either of the following experiments:
(1) Determine if the T cell receptor can compete in CTL?

(2) Determine if antibody to the T cell
receptor can block CTL?

Cramer: We have no information yet on your first
question. In response to your second question,
we tried to get antisera to T cell receptors,
but the rabbits gave weak Ab, and we could not
determine its effect.

Sehon: Can you stain T cells by anti-idiotype
antibodies?

Cramer: The antisera used stained about 1% of all
spleen cells. We felt this was too high and
not specific enough to do those studies.

Gearhart: How do you get Id^+ T cell receptors from SJL
mice who do not express the idiotype?

Cramer: The antibodies in SJL mice do not form the
idiotype because of a lack of lambda light
chain production in these mice. The T cells do
contain the idiotype. This is further evidence
that L chain from Ig and light chain of T cell
receptors are not identical.

Pages 359–370, Membranes, Receptors, and the Immune Response
© 1980 Alan R. Liss, Inc., 150 Fifth Avenue, New York, NY 10011

IDIOTYPIC NETWORK : THE MOPC 460 SYSTEM

P.-A. Cazenave[°], C. Le Guern[°], C. Bona[°] and
G. Buttin[°°]
[°]Unité d'Immunochimie Analytique, Institut Pasteur, 28 rue du Dr. Roux, 75724 Paris Cédex 15, and
[°°]IRBM, 4 Place Jussieu, 75230 Paris Cédex 05.
FRANCE.

During a long time the immune system was viewed as a procaryotic world of independent clones waiting for non self antigens.

A number of important findings (interactions between T and B lymphocytes, functional specialization of subsets of lymphocytes, H2 restriction phenomenom, involvement of idiotopes in clonal interactions) have shown that the immune system is an encaryotic world in which each clone speaks to each other and that self antigens are involved in its regulation.

Five years ago, Niels Jerne (1974a, b) proposed that, the number of idiotopes (idiotypic determinants) being of the same order of magnitude as the number of paratopes (combining sites), every immunoglobulin is in fact an antiidiotypic antibody recognizing a given idiotope present in the same immunological repertoire.

A number of observations suggest that this formal network could lead to a functional network:
- Auto-antibody against a given idiotype ca be induced (Rodkey, 1974; Eichmann, 1974; Urbain, 1977; Aguet *et al.*, (1978) or can occur spontaneously (Kluskens and Köhler, 1974; McKearn *et al.*, 1974; Cosenza, 1976; Bona *et al.*, 1978; Tasiaux *et al.*, 1978; Brown and Rodkey, 1979) during the immune response.
- T lymphocytes bearing idiotypic determinants or antiidiotypic receptors have been detected both in the helper and in the suppressor compartments (Binz *et al.*, 1979; Hetzelberger and Eichmann, 1979; Bona and Paul, 1979).
- Antibodies against idiotypes can mimic antigens (Eichmann

and Rajewsky, 1975; Binz *et al.*, 1979).

Two rabbits, A and B, synthezis different idiotypic IdA and IdB against the same antigen X (Oudin and Michel, 1963). If rabbit B possesses in its immune repertoire silent lymphocytes precommited for the synthesis of IdA or idiotypes cross-reacting with anti-IdA, it is reasonable to assume that their non expression is due to specific suppressors bearing auto anti-IdA receptors. If the suppressors of IdA are suppressed in rabbit B we would expect to favor the synthezis of IdA in rabbit B against the antigen X. This hypothesis can be tested by inducing in rabbit B an immune response against the anti-IdA suppressor if, as additionnal hypothesis, we suppose that anti-idiotypic antibodies produced by different animals of the same species against the same idiotype possesses some idiotypic similarity.

In the rabbit antibodies against ribonuclease (Ab 1) were injected in a second animal which produced anti-idiotypic antibodies (Ab2). Ab2 was used to preimmunize a third animal which produced anti-(anti-idiotypic) antibodies (Ab3). Under these conditions, the idiotypic specificities expressed by anti-ribonuclease antibodies (Ab1') induced in the third animal against this antigen are similar to the idiotypic specificities of the Ab1 antibodies (Cazenave, 1977) (fig.1). An identical result was

AgX

↓

ANIMAL 1 : Ab 1

↓

    ANIMAL 2 : Ab2

       ↓

       ANIMAL 3   : Ab_3

       ANIMAL 3 (Ab3) : Ab1'

       ↑

       AgX

Figure 1: Summary of the different immunizations

obtained when the antigen was *Micrococcus lysodeikticus* carbohydrate (Urbain *et al.*, 1977). These results showed that a large proportion of rabbits possess closely related idiotypic repertoire.

In the mouse, we have studied the molecular and cellular basis of regulation of expression of the MOPC460 idiotype. The results that we have obtained are summarized in the present communication.

Genetics of M460 idiotype

DNP binding MOPC460 myeloma protein expresses an idiotype which does not cross-react with other DNP binding myeloma proteins such as MOPC 315 and XRPC 25 (Table 1).

Table 1.- Inhibition by several reagents of the binding of ^{125}I-M460 Fab to isogeneic BALB/c anti-M460 Id.

Inhibitor	% Inhibition
M460 7s, 20ng	100
M315 7s, 2000ng	3
X25 7s, 2000ng	2
Normal BALB/c serum, 3µl	3
DNP-glycine 16mM	95

Nevertheless it was found that idiotypic determinants of MOPC 460 myeloma protein (460 Id) are shared with BALB/c anti-TNP antibodies elicited following immunizations with various thymus independent (TI) and thymus dependent (TD) antigens. Therefore, we studied the distribution of 460Id in various strains in the response to immunizations with TI and TD antigens such as TNP-Ficoll and DNP-ovalbumin (DNP-OVA). The expression of the 460Id was studied by inhibition of radioimmunoassay using BALB/c anti-460Id antibodies and iodine labelled Fab fragment of M460 myeloma protein. The specificity of anti-460 Id serum and its interaction with combining-site associated idiotypic determinants of M460 myeloma protein is illustrated on Table 1. As can be seen in Table 2 anti-TNP antibodies bearing 460-Id were only detected in BALB/c, B.C8, 129, CXBJ and CXBG-strains of mice. By contrast, CAL.20, C.B 20, DBA/2, NZB and CXBI strains of mice failed to express 460Id in the sera. This result assessed for a linkage of 460IdV region genes to $IghC^{\alpha}$ haplotype. It should be mentioned that

Table 2.- 460 Id expression is controlled by gene(s) linked
to the CH allotype locus of the mouse

Strains	IghC	H2	460 Id
BALB/c	a	d	+
C.AL 20	d	d	0
C.B 20	b	d	0
B.C 8	a	b	+
DBA/2	c	d	0
NZB	e	d	0
129/SV	a	b	+
(CXB)G	a	b	+
(CXB)J	a	b	+
(CXB)I	b	b	0

similar results were obtained using a rabbit anti-460 Id
serum (Zeldis *et al.*, 1979). A linkage of VH idiotypic
markers to *IghC* haplotypes was also observed in inulin
(Lieberman *et al.*, 1976), streptococcal A-S117 Id, and
A5A Id (Eichman and Berek 1973, Berek *et al.*, 1976),
arsonate (Pawlak *et al.*, 1973), NP (Mäkelä and Karjalainen,
1977) an dextran (Blomberg *et al.*, 1972) antigenic
systems.

Induction of 460 Id in BALB/c and DBA/2 mice with immunity
to heterogeneous anti-460 Id antibodies.
 As we mentioned above while BALB/c mice develop a
460 Id positive anti-TNP antibodies, the DBA/2 mice after
immunization with TI and TD antigens failed to produce
460 Id positive molecules. By contrast, both strains were
able to produce anti-460 Id antibodies after immunization
with M460 myeloma protein. DBA/2 and BALB/c chromatography
affinity purified anti-460 Id antibodies were used to
induce an anti-(anti-460 Id) antibody response in both DBA/2
and BALB/c mice. After such immunization both strains
developped an Ab3 type of response. Therefore, when these
mice (Ab3) were immunized with TNP-Ficoll or DNP-OVA we
observed the appearance of anti-TNP antibodies expressing
460 Id. In BALB/c mice the titer of 460 Id positive anti-
TNP antibodies as well as the number of plaques expressing
this idiotype were substantially increased as compared to
normal BALB/c mice immunized with the same TNP-conjugates.
Parallel increase of anti-TNP antibody titer and of plaques
specific for TNP clearly indicate that in Ab3 mice we

observed a real enhancement of 460 Id positive component of the anti-TNP response. Interestingly, DBA/2 mice which failed to produce 460 Id positive molecules after immunization with TI and TD antigens synthezised 460 Id positive anti-TNP antibodies when they previsouly develop an immunity to DBA/2 anti-M460 Id antibodies (Le Guern *et al.*, 1979).

These results clearly indicate that the 460 Id positive anti-TNP antibody response was enhanced in BALB/c mice which have 460 Id in their available repertoire. It appears that DBA/2 also have the potency to express 460 Id but only in particular situation i.e. when an immunity against anti-460 Id was provoked.

Induction of 460 Id in DBA/2 mice with immunity to homogeneous BALB/c anti-460 Id antibody.

A BALB/c homogeneous anti-460 Id antibody (Buttin *et al.*, 1978) was used to induce an Ab3 type response in DBA/2 mice. Similarly, an 460 Id positive anti-TNP response was obtained in DBA/2 (Ab3) mice immunized with anti-460 Id hybridoma and challenge with TNP-Ficoll. As can be seen in fig.2, the sera from these mice competed as well as M460 myeloma protein in the inhibition of radioimmunoassay indicating that main idiotopes borne by M460 myeloma protein were shared by DBA/2 anti-DNP antibodies. From these DBA/2 (Ab3) mice, by cell fusion, we prepared several hybridomas from which three were specific for TNP. By radioimmunoassay we were able to determine that two of them expressed 460Id (Buttin *et al.*, 1979). These results represent an additional prove that 460 Id anti-TNP clone(s) could emerge as result of anti-(anti-460 Id) antibody response in a strain of mice which lacks *a* allelic form of allotypes. The possible cellular mechanism of enhancement of 460 Id positive component of anti-TNP response in BALB/c mice and of stimulation of silent 460 Id positive clone(s) in DBA/2 mice will be discussed in the next section.

Regulation of 460 Id bearing anti-TNP antibodies by T cells.

In vitro experiments indicated that the 460 Id component of the anti-TNP response was substantially greater in anti-Thy 1.2 and complement pretreated spleen cells that in unseparated spleen cells. Addition of nylon wool enriched T cells to positively selected B cells strongly inhibited 460 Id component of anti-TNP response (Bona and Paul, 1979). This result clearly indicated that T cells population contained a discrete subset which regulates the clone(s) able to make anti-TNP antibody bearing 460 Id.

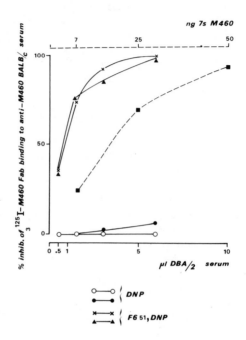

Figure 2: Inhibition of the binding of ^{125}I-Fab M460 to
BALB/c anti-M460 idiotype antibodies: 7S M460 protein
(●--●--●); sera from two normal DBA/2 mice immunized
against DNP-ovalbumin (o———o , ●———●): sera from two
DBA/2 mice preimmunized against homogeneous anti-M460
antibody F6(51) and subsequently immunized against DNP-
ovalbumin (▲———▲, X – X): this inhibition is no longer
observed if anti-DNP antibodies are removed on DNP-lysine-
Sepharose.

The properties of these regulatory cells were characterized as follows:

a - These regulatory cells are specific for 460 Id. Indeed they were removed after incubation on Petri dishes coated with M460 myeloma protein and not with other IgA κ BALB/c myeloma proteins which express an unrelated idiotype(Bona and Paul, 1979).

b - The suppressor activity of these 460 Id specific suppressor T cells was ablated by pretreatment with anti-Lyt 2.2 and Qal sera and complement (Bona and Paul in press).

c - It seems that these suppressor T cells occur only in the strains of mice having a allelic form of allotypes (Bona and Paul, in press).

The properties of these suppressor T cells are illustrated in Table 3.

Table 3. Properties of 460 Id specific suppressor T cells

B cells incubated with:	460Id + anti TNP response
—	+++
unseparated T cells	+
T cells adsorbed on MOPC 460 plates	+++
T cells recovered from MOPC 460 plates	—
T cells adsorbed on E109 plates	+
T cells recovered from E109 plates	+++
T cells adsorbed on anti-460 Id plates	—
T cells recovered from anti-460 Id plates	+++
T cells incubated with C	+
T cells incubated with anti Lyt 1-2 + C	++
T cells incubated with anti Lyt 2.2 + C	+++
T cells incubated with anti Qal + C	+++

The degree of response designated in a - to +++ scale was determined from 3-5 individual experiments. Cells were cultured with TNP-NWSM (3μg/ml). Total number of anti-TNP-PFC and the number of PFC secreting 460 Id bearing molecules were measured 4 days latter.

Cellular basis of enhancement of 460 Id positive component
of anti-TNP response by anti-(anti-460 Id) antibodies
As we mentioned above a significant increase of 460Id
positive component of the anti-TNP antibody titer and plaque
forming cells response was observed in BALB/c mice which
develop an Ab3 type of response and were challenged with
TNP conjugates. This increased 460 Id positive response was
also obtained after pretreatment of BALB/c mice with 100μg
of ammonium sulfate fraction of Ab3 serum. It should be
mentioned that these antibodies (i.a. Ab3) lack specificity
for TNP ligands (Le Guern et al., 1979).
    The increase in the 460 Id positive response in Ab3
mice was correlated with an absence of 460 Id specific
suppressor T cells (Bona et al., 1979). The simplest explanation for the absence of these suppressor cells in the
BALB/c mice which actively produced anti-(anti-460 Id) antibodies (Ab3) is that these antibodies react with and eliminate suppressor cells. This of course implies that the
receptor of 460 Id specific suppressor T cells share idiotypic determinants of anti-460 Id antibodies used as immunogen. to raise an Ab3 type response.

Conclusions
    The results presented in this communication show very
clearly that the mice with $IghC^{\alpha}$ haplotype can produce anti-
TNP antibodies from which a fraction share the idiotypic
determinants expressed on M460 myeloma protein. Nevertheless
the gene(s) which encode(s) this specificity, is present in
the repertoire of strains of mice which have not this haplotype. As in DBA/2 mice this silent clone(s) can be stimulated by an appropriate immunological manipulation and
their progeny even can be frozen in hybridomas.
    The expression of 460 Id positive anti-TNP antibody
forming cells is regulated by T cells in BALB/c mice. These
T cells are specific for 460 Id and share the idiotypic
determinants of anti-460 Id antibodies since they were not
found in BALB/c mice with an Ab3 type of response.

Berek C., Taylor B.A. and Eichmann K. (1976). Genetics
    of the idiotype of BALB/c myeloma S117: multiple chro-
    mosomal loci for V_H genes encouding specificity for
    group A streptococcal carbohydrate. J. Exp. Med.,
    144: 1164.

Binz H., Frischknecht H. and Wigzell H. (1979). Some studies on idiotypes and anti-idiotypic reactions and receptors in anti-allo-MHC T-cell immunity. Ann. Immunol.(Inst. Pasteur) 130C: 273.

Blomberg B., Geckeler W. and Weigert M. (1972). Genetics of the antibody response to dextran in mice. Science (Wash. D.C.) 177: 178.

Bona, C., Lieberman R., Chien C.C., Mond J. House S., Green I., and Paul W.E. (1978). Immune response to levan I.kinetics and ontogeny of antilevan and anti-inulin antibody response and of expression of cross-reactive idiotype. J. Immunol. 120: 1976.

Bona C. and Paul W.E., (1979). Cellular basis of regulation of expression of idiotype.I. T-suppressor cells specific for MOPC 460 idiotype regulate the expression of cells secreting anti-TNP antibodies bearing 460 idiotype. J. Exp. Med., 149, 992.

Bona, C., Hooghe R., Cazenave P.-A., Le Guern C. and W.E. Paul (1979). Cellular basis of regulation of expression of idiotype II. Immunity to anti-MOPC 460 idiotype antibodies increases the level of anti-trinitrophenyl antibodies bearing 460 idiotypes. J. Exp. Med., 149,815.

Bona C. and Paul W.E.(1979). Cellular basis of the regulation of anti-TNP antibodies carrying MOPC 460 idiotype, in ICN-UCLA Symposium on T and B lymphocytes:Recognition and function F. Bach, B.Bonavida and E. Vitetta eds. Acad. Press Inc. New York in press.

Brown J.C. and Rodkey L.S. (1979). Autoregulation of an antibody response via network-induced auto-anti-idiotype J. Exp. Med., 150,67.

Buttin G., Le Guern, C., Phalente L., Lin E.C.C., Medrano L., and Cazenave P.-A. (1978).Production of hybrid lines secreting monoclonal anti-idiotypic antibodies by cell fusion on membrane filters in "Lymphocyte hybridomas" Ed. by F. Melchors, M. Potter, N. Warner, Cur.Top. Microbiol. Immunol., 81, 27.

Buttin G., Juy D., Medrano L., Legrain P., Le Guern C. and Cazenave P.-A. (1979). Hybridomas as tool for the analysis of antibody diversity in "Cellular and Molecular basis of lymphocyte function". Proc. 13th leucocyte culture conference. Elsevier-North Holland (in press).

Cazenave P.-A. (1977).Idiotypic anti-idiotypic regulation of antibody synthesis in rabbits, Proc.Nat.Acad.,Sci. U.S.A., 74, 5122.

Cosenza H. (1976). Detection of anti-idiotype reactive cells in the response to phosphorylcholine, Eur.J. Immunol., 6, 114.

Eichmann K. and Rajewsky K. (1975) Induction of T and B cell immunity by antiidiotypic antibody. Eur. J. Immunol., 5, 661.

Eichmann K. and Berek C. (1973). Mendelian segregation of a mouse antibody idiotype. Eur. J. Immunol. 3, 599.

Hetzelberg D. and Eichmann K. (1978). Recognition of idiotypes in lymphocyte interactions I. Idiotypic selectivity in the cooperation between T and B lymphocytes. Eur. J. Immunol. 8, 846.

Jerne N.K. (1974a). Towards a network theory of the immune system. Ann. Immunol. (Inst. Pasteur), 125C: 373.

Jerne N.K. (1974b). The immune system: a web of V domains, Harvey Lect., 70, 93.

Kluskens L. and Köhler H. (1974). Regulation of immune response by autogeneous antibody against receptor. Proc. Nat. Acad. Sci. USA, 71, 5083.

Le Guern C., Ben Aïssa F., Juy D., Mariamé B., Buttin G. and Cazenave P.-A. (1979). Expression and induction of MOPC 460 idiotopes in different strains of mice. Ann. Immunol. (Inst. Pasteur), 130C, 293.

Lieberman R., Potter M., Humphrey W. and Chien C.C. (1976). Idiotypes of inulin binding antibodies and myeloma proteins controlled by genes linked to the allotype locus of the mouse. J. Immunol., 117, 2105.

Mäkelä O., and Karjelainen K. (1977). Inherited immunoglobulin idiotypes of the mouse. Immunol. Rev.34, 119.

McKearn T.J., Stuart F.P. and Fitch F.W. (1974). Anti-idiotypic antibody in rat transplantation immunity. I. Production of anti-idiotypic antibody in animals repeatedly immunized with alloantigens. J. Immunol. 113, 1876.

Oudin J.and Michel M. (1963). Une nouvelle forme d'allotypie des globulines du sérum de lapin, apparemment liée à la fonction et à la spécificité anticorps. C.R. Acad. Sci (Paris), 257, 805.

PawlakL.L., Mushinsky E.B., Nisonoff A. and Potter M.(1973). Evidence for the linkage of the IgC$_H$ locus to a gene controlling the idiotype specificity of anti-p-220 phenylarsonate antibodies in strain A mice. J. Exp. Med. 137, 22.

Rodkey L.S. (1974). Studies of idiotypic antibodies. Production and characterization of autoantiidiotypic antisera. J. Exp. Med., 139, 712.

Tasiaux N.,Leuwenkroon R., Bruyns C. and Urbain J. (1978). Possible occurrence and meaning of lymphocytes bearing autoanti-idiotypic receptors during the immune response Eur. J. Immunol., 8, 464.

Urbain J. (1977). L'idiotypie et la regulation dans le système immunitaire. Ann. Immunol. (Inst. Pasteur),128C, 445.

Urbain J., Wickler M., Franssen J.D. and Collignon C. (1977) Idiotypic regulation of the immune system by the induction of antibodies against anti-idiotypic antibodies, Proc.Nat. Acad. Sci. USA, 74, 5126.

Zeldis J.B., Riblet R., Konigsberg W.H., Richards F.F. and Rosenstein R.W. (1979). The location and expression of idiotypic determinants in the immunoglobulin variable region III. Expression of the protein 315 and 460 idiotypic determinants in mouse anti-DNP antibodies. Mol. Immunol., 16, 657.

Sehon: Is the response to TNP-levan T-independent?
Cazenave: Yes.

Sehon: Have you ever used a T-dependent TNP antigen?
Cazenave: In vitro, no.

Cramer: The network theory has been criticized
because it doesn't include T and B cell
interaction. Are you theorizing that this is
a way T and B cells interact?
Cazenave: Yes.

Pages 371–380, Membranes, Receptors, and the Immune Response

REARRANGEMENTS OF AN ALPHA IMMUNOGLOBULIN HEAVY CHAIN GENE *

L. Hood and J. Schilling

Division of Biology
California Institute of Technology
Pasadena, California 91125

INTRODUCTION

Our understanding of molecular immunology has gone
through an explosive expansion in the last few years due
mostly to the introduction of recombinant DNA techniques
(Brack et al., 1978; Seidman et al., 1978; Early et al.,
1979). Protein and nucleic acid chemistry have demonstrated
unequivocally several startling features of antibody genes
and molecules. First, the antibody molecule is composed of
distinct molecular domains--the variable (V) domains are
responsible for the antigen-binding function and the constant
(C) domains perform the effector functions of the antibody
molecule (Amzel et al., 1974). Second, the V regions of
light chains are encoded by two distinct gene segments--the
variable (V_L) gene segment and the joining (J_L) gene segment
(Fig. 1) (Brack et al., 1978). Third, a DNA rearrangement
of light chain gene segments occurs during the differentiation
of the antibody-producing or B cell (Fig. 1). This DNA rearrangement joins together the V_L and J_L gene segments,
presumably deleting the intervening DNA between these gene
segments. Accordingly, a DNA rearrangement appears to be at
least one of the molecular events which commits the B cell
to the expression of a single type of antibody light chain.
Finally, a high molecular weight nuclear transcript is
produced from the rearranged $V_L J_L C_L$ gene in which intervening
DNA sequences between the leader (L) and V_L gene segments
and between the J_L and C_L gene segments are removed by RNA
splicing (Fig. 1) (Gilmore-Hebert and Wall, 1978). A general
consideration of the events in B-cell differentiation suggests
that additional types of DNA rearrangements must occur in
heavy chain genes.

*In the Table of Contents, this article is part of Session III.

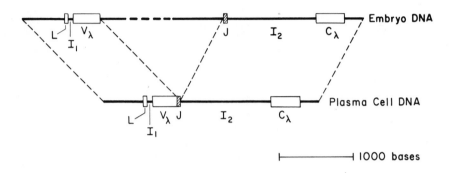

Fig. 1. Model of the mouse λ gene in undifferentiated (embryo) and differentiated (plasma cell) DNAs. L denotes the leader gene segment, I the various intervening DNA sequences, V_λ the variable gene segment, J the joining gene segment, and C_λ the lambda constant gene segment. Dotted lines indicate equivalent regions in the undifferentiated and differentiated clones. The intervening DNA sequence between the V_λ and J gene segments in the embryo DNA is apparently deleted in the plasma cell DNA. From Brack et al. (1978).

A Differentiating B Cell Exhibits Immunoglobulin Class Switching and the Commitment to a Single V Domain

   The bone-marrow stem cell for B-cell development initially becomes committed to the expression of cytoplasmic μ chains as it differentiates into a pre B cell (Fig. 2) (Burrows, LeJeune and Kearney, 1979). Subsequently, the pre B cell expresses light chains and the $(\mu L)_2$ or IgM molecule is placed on the plasma membrane, presumably to serve as an antigen receptor which can trigger further differentiation and proliferation (Warner, Leary and McLaughlin, 1979). The B cell with receptor IgM molecules can then differentiate along one of several different pathways to eventually produce terminally differentiated plasma cells capable of synthesizing any one of the different classes of immunoglobulin--IgG (γ), IgA (α), IgE (ε) or IgD (δ) (Fig. 2).

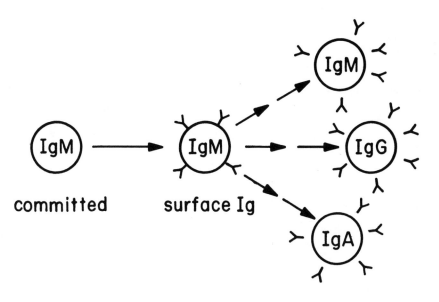

committed   surface Ig

secreting Ig

Fig. 2. A model of the differentiation of an antibody-
producing or B cell (see text).

In each case, it is the heavy chain constant (C_H) region
which determines the immunoglobulin class (i.e., C_μ-IgM,
C_α-IgA, C_γ-IgG, etc.). During the differentiation of an
individual B cell, two phenotypic events stand out--1) the
V domain remains invariant throughout and 2) the B cell can
switch from the expression of one immunoglobulin class to
another (C_H switch). We will now demonstrate that the
invariance of the V domain and C_H switching are mediated by
two distinct types of DNA rearrangement events.
    The heavy chain is encoded by L, V_H, J_H and C_H gene
segments. cDNA probes have been prepared for α and μ genes

(Early et al., 1979; Calame et al., 1980). We have used
these probes to screen two types of genomic libraries--a
sperm library of genomic clones that are undifferentiated
(unrearranged) with regard to antibody gene segments and
a library from an IgA myeloma cell committed to the expression
of an α heavy chain gene (Davis et al., 1980). This IgA
molecule binds phosphorylcholine (PC) and has V_H and J_H
regions that we will denote as V_{PC} and J_{PC}, respectively.
Our α cDNA probe has been used to isolate V_{PC} and J_{PC} gene
segments from the sperm or germline library (Davis et al.,
1980). DNA sequence analysis of these gene segments demonstrate that the heavy chain gene, like its light chain
counterpart, has L, V_H, J_H and C_H gene segments (Fig. 3)
(Early et al., 1980).

	96	97	98	99					100	101	102	103	104	105
Germline V_{PC}	TGT	GCA	AGA	GAT	GCA	CAC	AGT	GAG	AGG	ACG	TCA	TTG	TGA	GCC	CAG

Germline J_{PC}	ACA	GAG	GCA	GAA	CAG	AGA	CTG	TGC	TAC	TGG	TAC	TTC	GAT	GTC	TGG

————V_{PC}————   ————————J_{PC}————————

Fig. 3. DNA sequences of germline V_{PC} and J_{PC} gene segments.
The V gene segment ends at position 99. The J gene segment
starts at codon 100. * denotes a termination codon. The
boxes indicate palindromes or inverted repeats that are
believed to be involved in V-J joining (see Early et al.,
1980; Sakano et al., 1979, Max, Seidman and Leder, 1979).
Adapted from Early et al. (1980).

The rearranged $V_{PC}J_{PC}C_\alpha$ clone also has been isolated
from the IgA genomic library (Early et al., 1979) and DNA
sequence analyses and restriction mapping analyses show that
the V_{PC} and J_{PC} gene segments have been joined together by a
DNA rearrangement event (Fig. 4) (Davis et al., 1980; Early
et al., 1980). Moreover, the V_{PC} coding region is separated

from the C_α coding region by an intervening sequence of 6800 nucleotides (Fig. 4) (Early et al., 1979). Thus, heavy chain genes resemble their light chain counterparts in several features--they exhibit similar gene segments (L, V_H, J_H and C_H) and a V-J joining that occurs by a DNA rearrangement. However, heavy and light chain genes differ in at least one significant feature.

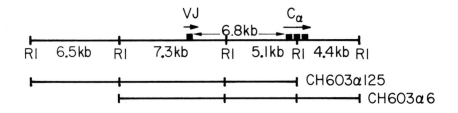

Fig. 4. Alpha genomic clones from the DNA of the IgA-producing myeloma M603. kb denotes kilobases. RI designates sites of cleavage by the restriction enzyme EcoRI. Two distinct types of rearranged α clones have been isolated (α6 and α125).

An α heavy chain gene is made up of three distinct germline gene segments. The intervening DNA sequence between the J_λ and C_λ gene segments comes entirely from DNA 5' to the C_λ gene segment (Fig. 1). In contrast, we were readily able to demonstrate by restriction mapping analysis that only a portion of the intervening DNA sequence between the V_{PC} (J_{PC}) and C_α gene segments is derived from DNA 5' to the germline C_α gene segment. What was the origin of the remainder of the intervening DNA? Our earlier analysis of B-cell differentiation noted that all B cells go through an initial differentiation stage in which IgM molecules are expressed (i.e., a C_μ gene segment). Accordingly, it was logical to suggest that perhaps a portion of the intervening DNA sequence in the α gene arose from a DNA segment that was 5' to the C_μ gene. Hence, we employed our μ cDNA probe to isolate a C_μ genomic clone from the sperm (undifferentiated) library (Davis et al., 1980). Then we compared the sperm V_{PC}, C_μ, and C_α clones to the rearranged myeloma α clone by

the technique of heteroduplex analysis. This analysis
allows one to determine which portions of two genomic clones
are identical. These heteroduplex analyses revealed a
striking relationship between the rearranged myeloma α gene
and the germline V_{PC}, C_μ and C_α clones. The myeloma α gene
is a tripartite structure composed of a germline V_{PC} gene
segment, a germline J_{PC} gene segment associated with approximately 5000 nucleotides 5' to the C_μ gene, and a C_α gene
segment with its attendent 5' and 3' flanking sequences
(Fig. 5). Clearly this tripartite rearranged α gene must
arise from DNA rearrangements at two separate and distinct
sites (Davis et al., 1980).

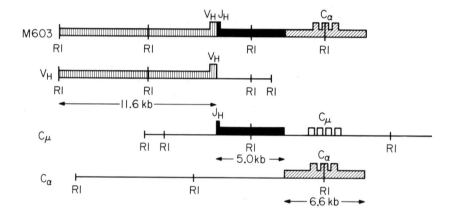

Fig. 5. Origins of the three germline components of the
M603 myeloma α heavy chain gene. Various types of shading
indicate homology by heteroduplex analyses and by restriction
enzyme analyses. From Davis et al. (1980).

The α heavy chain gene is created by two distinct DNA
rearrangements--a V-J joining and a C_H switch. The two DNA
rearrangements that are necessary to create a tripartite
α gene explain two fundamental features of B-cell differentiation (Fig. 6). The first DNA rearrangement joins together
the V_H and J_H gene segments. This V-J joining creates a V_H

gene and commits the B cell to the expression of a particular
V domain (Fig. 6). Since the J_H gene segment is associated

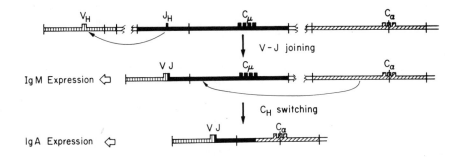

Fig. 6. Two types of DNA rearrangements leading to the
creation of the M603 myeloma α heavy chain gene--V-J joining
and C_H switching. V-J joining indicates a DNA rearrangement
that joins the V_H and J_H gene segments. Because the J_H gene
segments appear to be associated with the germline C_μ gene
segment (Early et al., 1980), V-J joining permits a μ chain
and IgM molecules to be expressed by the differentiating
B cell. C_H switching denotes a second DNA rearrangement
that replaces the C_μ gene segment with a C_α gene segment.
This DNA rearrangement presumably permits an α chain and
IgA molecules to be expressed by the now fully differentiated
lymphocyte. From Davis et al. (1980).

in the germline with a C_μ gene segment, V-J joining allows
the B cell to initially express the C_μ gene segment or an
IgM molecule. Thus, the first DNA rearrangement, V-J
joining, explains why a B cell is always initially committed
to express IgM molecules. The second DNA rearrangement,
the C_H switch, replaces the C_μ gene segment with a C_α gene
segment (Fig. 6). Thus, the B cell can now express the
C_α gene segment or the IgA molecule. Accordingly, these
two types of DNA rearrangements occur at two different sites
and explain two dominant features of B-cell differentiation--
the invariance of the V domain (V-J joining) and the switching
of immunoglobulin classes (C_H switching). It is striking to
note that one can study the organization of antibody heavy
chain genes to deduce pathways of DNA rearrangements that

correlate with B-cell differentiation. It will be interesting
to analyze additional heavy chain genes of the α class and
of other classes to determine the number of different switch
sites and the various pathways by which class switching may
occur in B-cell differentiation. Thus, DNA rearrangements
of several different types appear to play an integral role
in B-cell differentiation.

How general are DNA rearrangements in eukaryotic
differentiation? The antibody genes provide one of the few
examples of the strategy whereby information is amplified
by virtue of the rearrangements of gene segments. It is
our feeling that the evolution of the split gene and DNA
rearrangement strategies evolved long before the emergence
of the vertebrate immune system (Hood, Huang and Dreyer,
1977). Indeed, it is attractive to postulate that these
strategies evolved with the emergence of the first multi-
gene families--possibly at the time when metazoa evolved
with their enormously increased informational requirements
for cell-surface recognition molecules (Fig. 7). If this
assumption is correct, many other contemporary eukaryotic
gene families with complex informational requirements also
may employ the split gene and DNA rearrangement strategies.
The question for future studies is where can we go to find
these intriguing informational gene families?

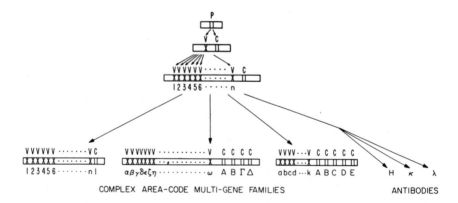

COMPLEX AREA-CODE MULTI-GENE FAMILIES   ANTIBODIES

Fig. 7. A hypothetical model for the evolution of complex
multigene families or area-code gene families. The hypothesis
is that the evolution of split gene, multigene, and DNA
rearrangement steategies antedated the evolution of the
vertebrate immune system. From Hood, Huang and Dreyer (1977).

ACKNOWLEDGEMENTS

These studies were made possible by grants from NSF and NIH.

REFERENCES

Amzel L, Poljak R, Saul F, Varga J, Richard F (1974). The three dimensional structure of a combining region-ligand complex of immunoglobulin NEW at 3.5-Å resolution. Proc Natl Acad Sci USA 71:1427.

Brack C, Hirama M, Lenhard-Schuller R, Tonegawa S (1978). A complete immunoglobulin gene is created by somatic recombination. Cell 15:1.

Burrows P, LeJeune M, Kearney JF (1979). Evidence that murine pre-B cells synthesize µ heavy chains but no light chains. Nature 280:838.

Calame K, Rogers J, Early PW, Davis MM, Livant DL, Wall R, Hood L (1980). The mouse C_μ heavy chain immunoglobulin gene segment contains three intervening sequences which separate domains. Nature in press.

Davis MM, Calame K, Early PW, Livant DL, Joho R, Weissman IL, Hood L (1980). An immunoglobulin heavy chain gene is formed by at least two recombinational events. Nature in press.

Early PW, Davis MM, Kaback DB, Davidson N, Hood L (1979). Immunoglobulin heavy chain gene organization in mice: Analysis of a myeloma genomic clone containing variable and α constant regions. Proc Natl Acad Sci USA 76:857.

Early PW, Huang H, Davis M, Calame K, Hood L (1980). An immunoglobulin heavy chain variable region gene is generated from three segments of DNA: V_H, D, and J_H. Cell in press.

Gilmore-Hebert M, Wall R (1978). Immunoglobulin light chain mRNA is processed from large nuclear RNA. Proc Natl Acad Sci USA 75:342.

Hood L, Huang H, Dreyer WJ (1977). The area-code hypothesis: The immune system provides clues to understanding the genetic and molecular basis of cell recognition during development. J Supramolec Struct 7:531.

Max EE, Seidman JG, Leder P (1979). Sequences of five potential recombination sites encoded close to an immunoglobulin κ constant region gene. Proc Natl Acad Sci USA 76:3450.

Sakano H, Höppi K, Heinrich G, Tonegawa S (1979). Sequences at the somatic recombination sites of immunoglobulin light-chain genes. Nature 280:288.
Seidman JG, Leder A, Nau M, Norman B, Leder P (1978). Antibody diversity. Science 202:11.
Warner NL, Leary JF, McLaughlin S (1979). Analysis of murine B cell lymphomas as models of B cell differentiation arrest. In Cooper M, Mosier DE, Scher I, Vitetta ES (eds): "B Lymphocytes in the Immune Response," New York: Elsevier/North Holland, p 371.

Index

Author Index

DATE DUE